**Evidence-based Clinical Chinese Medicine**

Co Editors-in-Chief

## Charlie Changli Xue
RMIT University, Australia

## Chuanjian Lu
Guangdong Provincial Hospital of Chinese Medicine, China

# Volume 19
# Irritable Bowel Syndrome

Lead Authors

## Shefton Parker
RMIT University, Australia

## Yingting Li
Guangdong Provincial Hospital of Chinese Medicine, China

**World Scientific**

NEW JERSEY · LONDON · SINGAPORE · BEIJING · SHANGHAI · HONG KONG · TAIPEI · CHENNAI · TOKYO

*Published by*

World Scientific Publishing Co. Pte. Ltd.

5 Toh Tuck Link, Singapore 596224

*USA office:* 27 Warren Street, Suite 401-402, Hackensack, NJ 07601

*UK office:* 57 Shelton Street, Covent Garden, London WC2H 9HE

**Library of Congress Cataloging-in-Publication Data**

Names: Xue, Charlie Changli, author. | Lu, Chuan-jian, 1964–    author.
Title: Evidence-based clinical Chinese medicine / Charlie Changli Xue, Chuanjian Lu.
Description: New Jersey : World Scientific, 2016. | Includes bibliographical references and index.
Identifiers: LCCN 2015030389| ISBN 9789814723084 (v. 1 : hardcover : alk. paper) |
    ISBN 9789814723091 (v. 1 : paperback : alk. paper) |
    ISBN 9789814723121 (v. 2 : hardcover : alk. paper) |
    ISBN 9789814723138 (v. 2 : paperback : alk. paper) |
    ISBN 9789814759045 (v. 3 : hardcover : alk. paper) |
    ISBN 9789814759052 (v. 3 : paperback : alk. paper)
Subjects: | MESH: Medicine, Chinese Traditional--methods. | Clinical Medicine--methods. |
    Evidence-Based Medicine--methods. | Psoriasis. | Pulmonary Disease, Chronic Obstructive.
Classification: LCC RC81 | NLM WB 55.C4 | DDC 616--dc23
LC record available at http://lccn.loc.gov/2015030389

**Volume 19: Irritable Bowel Syndrome**
ISBN  978-981-126-150-3 (hardcover)
ISBN  978-981-126-151-0 (ebook for institutions)
ISBN  978-981-126-152-7 (ebook for individuals)

**British Library Cataloguing-in-Publication Data**
A catalogue record for this book is available from the British Library.

For any available supplementary material, please visit
https://www.worldscientific.com/worldscibooks/10.1142/13000#t=suppl

# Disclaimer

The information in this monograph is based on systematic analyses of the best available evidence for Chinese medicine interventions, both historical and contemporary. Every effort has been made to ensure the accuracy and completeness of the data in this publication. This book is intended for clinicians, researchers and educators. The practice of evidence-based medicine considers the best available evidence, practitioners' clinical experience and judgement, and patients' preference. Not all interventions are acceptable in all countries. It is important to note that some of the substances mentioned in this book may no longer be in use, toxic, prohibited, or restricted under the provisions of the Convention on International Trade in Endangered Species of Wild Fauna and Flora (CITES). Practitioners, researchers and educators are advised to comply with the relevant regulations in their country and with the restrictions on the trade of the species included in CITES appendices I, II and III. This book is not intended as a guide for self-medication. Patients should seek professional advice from qualified Chinese medicine practitioners.

# Foreword

Since the late 20<sup>th</sup> century, Chinese medicine, including acupuncture and herbal medicine, has been increasingly used throughout the world. The parallel development and spread of evidence-based medicine have provided challenges and opportunities for Chinese medicine. The opportunities have been evidence-based medicine's emphasis on the effective use of the best available clinical evidence, incorporating the clinicians' clinical experience, subject to patients' preference. Such practices have a patient focus that reflects the historical nature of Chinese medicine practice. However, the challenges are also significant due to the fact that, despite the long-term development and very rich literature accumulated over 2,000 years, there is an overall lack of high-level clinical evidence for many of the interventions used in Chinese medicine.

To address this knowledge gap, we need to generate clinical evidence through high-quality clinical studies and evaluate evidence to enable the effective use of such available evidence to promote evidence-based Chinese medicine practice.

Modern Chinese medicine is rooted in its classical literature and the legacies of ancient doctors, grounded in the practice of expert clinicians and increasingly informed by clinical and experimental research efforts. In recognition of the unique features of Chinese medicine, for each of the conditions in this series, a "whole-evidence" approach is used to provide a synthesis of different types and levels of evidence to enable practitioners to make clinical decisions informed by the current best evidence.

There are four main components of this "whole-evidence" approach. Firstly, we present the current approaches to the diagnosis, differentiation and treatment of each condition based on expert consensus in published textbooks and clinical guidelines. This provides an overview of how the condition is currently managed. The second section provides an analysis of the condition in historical context based on systematic searches of the *Zhong Hua Yi Dian*, which includes the full texts of more than 1,000 classical medical books. These analyses provide objective views on how the condition has been treated over two millennia, reveal continuities and discontinuities between traditional and modern practice, and suggest avenues for future research.

The third component is the assessment of evidence derived from modern clinical studies of Chinese medicine interventions. The methods established by the *Cochrane Collaboration* are used as the basis for conducting systematic reviews and undertaking meta-analyses of outcome data for randomised controlled trials (RCTs). In addition, the clinical relevance of meta-analysis data is enhanced by examining the herbal formulae, individual herbs, and acupuncture treatments that were assessed in the RCTs, and the evidence base is broadened by the inclusion of data from controlled clinical trials and non-controlled studies. The fourth component is to determine how the herbal medicine interventions may achieve the effects indicated by the clinical trials. Thus for each of the most frequently used herbs, we provide reviews of their effects in pre-clinical models and their likely mechanisms of action.

For each condition, this "whole-evidence" approach links clinical expertise, historical precedent, clinical research data, and experimental research to provide the reader with assessments of the current state of the evidence of efficacy and safety for Chinese medicine interventions using herbal medicines, acupuncture and moxibustion, and other health care practices such as *tai chi*.

Since these books are available in Chinese and English, they can benefit patients, practitioners and educators internationally and enable practitioners to make clinical decisions informed by the current best evidence.

These publications represent a major milestone in Chinese medicine development and make a significant contribution to the evidence-based Chinese medicine development globally.

**Co-Editors-in-Chief**
Distinguished Professor Charlie Changli Xue,
RMIT University, Australia
Professor Chuanjian Lu, Guangdong Provincial Hospital of
Chinese Medicine, China

# Purpose of the Monograph

This book is intended for clinicians, researchers and educators. It can be used to inform tertiary education and clinical practice by providing systematic, multi-dimensional assessments of the best available evidence for using Chinese medicine to manage each common clinical condition.

## How to Use This Monograph

### Some Definitions

A glossary is included, containing terms and definitions that frequently appear in the book. It also describes the definitions of statistical tests, methodological terms, evaluation tools, and interventions. For example, in this book, Integrative Medicine refers to the combined use of a Chinese medicine treatment with conventional medical management, and Combination Therapies refer to two or more Chinese medicines from different therapy groups (Chinese herbal medicine, acupuncture or other Chinese medicine therapies) administered together. The terminology used throughout the monograph is based on the World Health Organization's *Standard Terminologies on Traditional Medicine in the Western Pacific Region* (2007) where possible or from the cited reference.

### Data Analysis and Interpretation of Results

In order to synthesise the clinical evidence, a range of statistical analysis approaches are used. In general, the effect size for dichotomous data is reported as a risk ratio (RR) with a 95% confidence interval (CI), and for continuous data, they are reported as mean difference (MD) with a 95% CI. Statistically significant effects are indicated with an asterisk. Readers should note that being statistically significant does not necessarily correspond with a clinically important effect. Interpretation of results should take into consideration of the clinical significance, quality of studies (expressed as "high", "low" or "unclear" risk of bias in this book), and heterogeneity amongst the studies. Tests for heterogeneity are conducted using the $I^2$ statistic. An $I^2$ score greater than 50% may indicate substantial heterogeneity.

## Use of Evidence in Practice

The Grading of Recommendations Assessment, Development and Evaluation (GRADE) approach was used to summarise the quality of evidence and results of the strength of evidence for critical and important comparisons and outcomes. Due to the diverse nature of Chinese medicine practice, treatment recommendations are not included with the summary of findings tables. Therefore readers will need to interpret the evidence with reference to the local practice environment.

## Limitations

Readers should note some of the methodological limitations on classical literature and clinical evidence.

- Search terms used to search the *Zhong Hua Yi Dian* database may not include all terms that have been used for the condition, which may alter the findings.
- The Chinese language has changed over time. Citations have been interpreted for analysis, and such interpretations may be subject to disagreement.
- The Chinese medicine theory has evolved over time. As such, concepts described in classical Chinese medical literature may no longer be found in contemporary works.

- Symptoms described in citations may be common to many conditions, and a judgement was required to determine the likelihood of the citation being related to the condition. This may have introduced some bias due to the subjective nature of the judgement.
- The vast majority of the clinical evidence for Chinese medicine treatments has come from China. The applicability of the findings to other populations and countries requires further assessment.
- Many studies included participants with varying disease severity. Where possible, subgroup analyses were undertaken to examine the effects in different sub-populations. As this was not always possible, the findings may be limited to the population included and not to sub-populations.
- The potential risk of bias found in many included studies suggested methodological limitations. The findings for GRADE assessments based on studies of very low to moderate quality evidence should be interpreted accordingly.
- Nine major English and Chinese language databases were searched to identify clinical studies, in addition to clinical trial registers. Other studies may exist that were not identified through searches and which may alter the findings.
- The calculation of the frequency of herbal formula use was based on formula names only. It is possible that studies evaluated herbal treatments with the same or similar herb ingredients but were given different formula names. Due to the complexity of herbal formulas, it was considered not appropriate to make a judgement as to the similarity of the formulas for analysis. As such, the frequency of the formulas reported in Chap. 5 may be underestimated.
- The most frequently utilised herbs that may have contributed to the treatment effect have been described in Chap. 5. These herbs may provide leads for further exploration. Calculation of the herbs with potential effect is based on the frequency of formulae reported in the studies and does not take into consideration the clinical implications and functions of every herb in a formula.

# Authors and Contributors

**Co-Editors-in-Chief**
Distinguished Prof. Charlie Changli Xue (*RMIT University, Australia*)
Prof. Chuanjian Lu (*Guangdong Provincial Hospital of Chinese Medicine, China*)

**Co-Deputy Editors-in-Chief**
Prof. Anthony Lin Zhang (*RMIT University, Australia*)
Dr. Brian H May (*RMIT University, Australia*)
Prof. Xinfeng Guo (*Guangdong Provincial Hospital of Chinese Medicine, China*)
Prof. Zehuai Wen (*Guangdong Provincial Hospital of Chinese Medicine, China*)

**Lead Authors**
Dr. Shefton Parker (*RMIT University, Australia*)
Dr. Yingting Li (*Guangdong Provincial Hospital of Chinese Medicine, China*)

**Co-Authors:**
*RMIT University (Australia)*:
Dr. Yuan Ming Di
Dr. Mary Xinmei Zhang
Prof. Anthony Lin Zhang
Distinguished Prof. Charlie Changli Xue
*Guangdong Provincial Hospital of Chinese Medicine (China)*:
Prof. Shaogang Huang
Prof. Xinfeng Guo
Prof. Xianyu Tang

# Member of Advisory Committee and Panel

CO-CHAIRS OF PROJECT PLANNING COMMITTEE
Prof. Peter J Coloe (*RMIT University, Australia*)
Prof. Yubo Lyu (*Guangdong Provincial Hospital of Chinese Medicine, China*)
Prof. Dacan Chen (*Guangdong Provincial Hospital of Chinese Medicine, China*)

CENTRE ADVISORY COMMITTEE (ALPHABETICAL ORDER)
Prof. Keji Chen (*The Chinese Academy of Sciences, China*)
Prof. Aiping Lu (*Hong Kong Baptist University, China*)
Prof. Caroline Smith (*Western Sydney University, Australia*)
Prof. David F Story (*RMIT University, Australia*)

METHODOLOGY EXPERT ADVISORY PANEL (ALPHABETICAL ORDER)
Prof. Zhaoxiang Bian (*Hong Kong Baptist University, China*)
Prof. Lixing Lao (*The University of Hong Kong, China*)
The Late Prof. George Lewith (*University of Southampton, United Kingdom*)
Prof. Jianping Liu (*Beijing University of Chinese Medicine, China*)
Prof. Frank Thien (*Monash University, Australia*)
Prof. Jialiang Wang (*Sichuan University, China*)

CONTENT EXPERT ADVISORY PANEL (ALPHABETICAL ORDER)
Prof. Xudong Tang (*China Academy of Chinese Medical Sciences, China*)
Prof. Shengsheng Zhang (*Beijing Hospital of Traditional Chinese Medicine, China*)

# Distinguished Professor
# Charlie Changli Xue, PhD

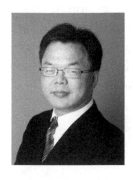 Distinguished Professor Charlie Changli Xue holds a Bachelor of Medicine (majoring in Chinese Medicine) from Guangzhou University of Chinese Medicine, China (1987), and a PhD from RMIT University, Australia (2000). He has been an academic, researcher, regulator, and practitioner for over three decades. Distinguished Professor Xue has made significant contributions to evidence-based educational development, clinical research, regulatory framework and policy development, and provision of high-quality clinical care to the community. Distinguished Professor Xue is recognised internationally as an expert in evidence-based traditional medicine and integrative healthcare.

Distinguished Professor Xue was appointed by the Australian Health Workforce Ministerial Council in 2011 as the Inaugural National Chair of the Chinese Medicine Board of Australia, and he was reappointed in 2014 and 2017 for second and third terms. Since 2007, he has been a Member of the World Health Organization's (WHO) Expert Advisory Panel for Traditional and Complementary Medicine, Geneva. Distinguished Professor Xue is also an Honorary Senior Principal Research Fellow at the Guangdong Provincial Academy of Chinese Medical Sciences, China.

At RMIT, Distinguished Professor Xue is an Associate Deputy Vice-Chancellor (International). He is also the Director of WHO's Collaborating Centre for Traditional Medicine.

Between 1995 and 2010, Distinguished Professor Xue was Discipline Head of Chinese Medicine at RMIT University. He leads the development of five successful undergraduate and postgraduate degree programs in Chinese Medicine at RMIT University, which is now a global leader in Chinese medicine education and research.

Distinguished Professor Xue's research has been supported by over AU$15 million in research grants, including six project grants from the Australian Government's National Health and Medical Research Council (NHMRC) and two Australian Research Council (ARC) grants. He has contributed over 200 publications and has been frequently invited as keynote speaker for numerous national and international conferences. Distinguished Professor Xue has contributed to over 300 media interviews on issues related to complementary medicine education, research, regulation, and practice.

# Professor Chuanjian Lu, MD

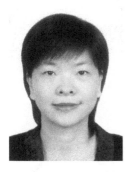 Professor Chuanjian Lu, Doctor of Medicine, is the Vice President of Guangdong Provincial Hospital of Chinese Medicine (Guangdong Provincial Academy of Chinese Medical Sciences, Second Clinical Medical College of Guangzhou University of Chinese Medicine). She also is the chair of the Guangdong Traditional Chinese Medicine (TCM) Standardization Technical Committee and the vice-chair of the Immunity Specialty Committee of the World Federation of Chinese Medicine Societies (WFCMS).

Professor Lu has engaged in scientific research into TCM, clinical practice, and teaching for some 25 years. Her research has been devoted to integrated traditional and western medicine. She has edited and published 12 monographs and 120 academic research articles as the first author and corresponding author, with over 30 articles being included in SCI journals.

She has received widespread recognition for her achievements with awards for "Excellent Teacher of South China", "National Outstanding Women TCM Doctor", and "National Outstanding Young Doctor of TCM". She also received "The Science and Technology Star of the Association of Chinese Medicine", the "National Excellent Science and Technology Workers of China Award", and the "Five-Continent Women's Scientific Awards of China Medical Women's Association".

Professor Lu has won the "Award of Science and Technology Progress" over 10 times from the Guangdong Provincial Government, China Association of Chinese Medicine, and Chinese Hospital Association.

# Acknowledgements

The authors and contributors would like to acknowledge the valuable contributions of the following people who assisted with database searches, data extraction, data screening, data assessment, translation of documents, editing, and/or administrative tasks: Ms Mary-Jo O'Rourke AE, Ms Anje Scarfe, and Huan Zheng.

# Contents

Contents

Contents

# List of Figures

# List of Tables

# 1

# Introduction to Irritable Bowel Syndrome

## OVERVIEW

This chapter provides an overview of the diagnosis and pathophysiology of irritable bowel syndrome (IBS). The subtypes of IBS are differentiated, and clinical guidelines are summarised to provide a brief overview of the various treatments that are commonly recommended for IBS. Measures for the clinical severity of IBS and its management and treatment are also discussed.

## Definition of Irritable Bowel Syndrome

Irritable bowel syndrome (IBS) is a type of functional bowel disorder causing symptoms of abdominal pain and altered bowel habits such as diarrhoea or constipation.[1,2]

## Clinical Presentation

Generally people with IBS clinically present with at least 6 months of abdominal pain that is associated with a change in bowel habits.[3] A patient's defecation urgency, stool form and/or frequency may be abnormal, with symptoms such as straining during defecation and a feeling of incomplete evacuation.[4] Diarrhoea and/or constipation may be accompanied by symptoms of bloating or distension, or mucous in the stools.[5] These features are typical of IBS, but they are not unique only to IBS. Further differential diagnosis by the clinician is needed for a definitive diagnosis of IBS.[4]

## Subtypes of Irritable Bowel Syndrome

IBS has been classified into several subtypes based on the sufferer's predominant clinical bowel habits.[3] Currently, four subtypes are recognised clinically:

 i) IBS with predominant constipation (IBS-C);
 ii) IBS with predominant diarrhoea (IBS-D);
 iii) IBS with mixed bowel habits (IBS-M) consisting of both constipation and diarrhoea; and
 iv) IBS unclassified (IBS-U), when a sufferer's condition does not fall under one of the above three subtypes.

People can be classified as a specific subtype; however, it is common for sufferers to transition between subtypes, more so in those diagnosed as subtypes IBS-M or IBS-C.[6]

## Epidemiology

Historically, global variation in the utilisation of IBS criteria impacted the reporting of IBS diagnosis prevalence rates.[7] For instance, when using the Manning criteria, prevalence has been estimated to be up to 20.4% compared to 8.5% prevalence when using the Rome criteria.[7] The average international IBS prevalence is estimated to be around 11.2%,[8] with prevalence estimates as high as 31.6% in Nigeria[9] and as low as 4.7% in France.[10] The pooled prevalence for Asia has been calculated to be 9.6%, with North America, Europe, Australia and New Zealand estimated to have a pooled prevalence of 8.1%.[11]

Global variations in prevalence may also be explained in part by inconsistencies in assessment methods. In an attempt to reduce variation in assessment, the most recent Rome IV criteria use simplified language when describing symptoms.[12]

A Japanese study reported higher IBS-D prevalence in males than females and higher IBS-C prevalence in females than males.[13] Overall, the prevalence has been reported to be 1.6 times higher in females than in males, with people over 50 years of age reported to have the lowest prevalence. These prevalence figures support research suggesting that, with increasing age, there is decreased incidence of IBS.[8]

## Burden

Generally, IBS sufferers seek healthcare more often, and there is an increased burden on their quality of life.[14] For people with IBS-C, quality of life deficits, decreased work productivity, and elevated care utilisation are evidenced to be significantly worse than those with chronic disease such as asthma, migraine and rheumatoid arthritis.[15]

In the United Kingdom (UK) and the United States (US), economic losses in work productivity due to IBS are estimated to be between 8.5 and 21.6 days per year.[16] Research suggests some IBS sufferers unnecessarily utilise primary and secondary care pathways, with an overuse of investigative procedures, such as endoscopy and practitioner prescribing, increasing unnecessary cost burdens to health care systems.[17] Studies in the US show that people with IBS have increased medical service usage, with a higher mean number of hospitalisations and greater costs of between US$2,200 and US$2,500 per patient per year.[18]

In China, similar health system costs have been reported in people with IBS, with annual costs estimated at US$2,933 per person, an annual national cost of approximately US$1.99 billion.[19] Similar costs have been estimated for IBS in Europe; in the Netherlands, costs are 2,328 Euros higher in people with IBS.[20]

## Risk Factors

A study of IBS family clusters has indicated that possible genetic and/or shared environmental exposures may increase a person's susceptibility to the development of IBS.[21] The strongest research indicating potential IBS genetic links has been in a study of monozygotic twins, with correlations shown between IBS aetiology and major depressive disorders.[22] Identification of the genetic components related to IBS is still unclear.[23]

Stress appears to be both an initiating factor and an aggravating factor in IBS symptoms.[24] Approximately, half of IBS patients can be diagnosed as depressed, anxious or hypochondriacal.[25]

In close to 90% of people with IBS, food such as cereals and spicy foods are reported by patients as triggering or aggravating their IBS-related symptoms.[26]

Research indicates that, for some chronic pain disorders such as fibromyalgia, there is an increased incidence of IBS and greater severity of symptoms in these populations.[27] Mucosal inflammatory disorders such as ulcerative colitis show a correlation with increased IBS incidence; however, a biological explanation for the link is yet to be found.[28] A substantial proportion of the IBS population report a history of infectious gastroenteritis or enterocolitis, with a post-infection incidence of IBS increased up to 6–7 times.[29] Coexisting functional dyspepsia and gastroesophageal reflux disease (GERD) have twice the likelihood in people with IBS compared to non-IBS populations.[30]

# Pathological Processes

Symptoms of stool irregularity such as constipation and diarrhoea have been attributed to disturbances in gut transit times due to abnormalities in gastrointestinal motility and visceral hypersensitivity related to gut permeability and/or abnormal neurological stimulation.[31] Further, abnormalities in neurological links between the gut and central nervous system are also implicated in IBS pathogenesis.[32] The brain-gut interactions understood to cause IBS symptoms are complex, with experimental models suggesting potential abnormal microbiome, intestinal permeability, and endocrine and immune system involvement.[33]

## Gastrointestinal Motility

Research has shown stool form and frequency abnormalities in people with IBS are related to disturbances in gastrointestinal transit time.[34] Transit time irregularities have been shown to be related to abnormal gastrointestinal motility.[35] People with IBS-C typically experience delayed transit times, while people with IBS-D experience accelerated transit times.[34] Due to its role as a signalling molecule to regulate intestines, serotonin bioavailability likely also plays a role in the disturbance of normal gastrointestinal motility.[36] Observation has shown that in IBS, there is increased serotonin release in the colonic mucosa.[37]

While gastrointestinal motility can contribute to stool form and frequency symptoms in IBS, this does not completely explain other symptoms commonly associated with IBS, such as bloating, flatulence and abdominal pain, which indicates that other mechanisms also contribute to the condition.[34]

## Visceral Hypersensitivity

Visceral hypersensitivity occurs when distensions and contractions of the gastrointestinal visceral organs cause pain or discomfort. Abnormal stimulation by the central and/or peripheral sensory nervous systems, intestinal infection from gut microbiota, and immunological inflammation from diet sensitivities can contribute to visceral hypersensitivities.[38] Some potential aggravators to mucosa permeability are known to include, among others, stress, some foods, bile and infection.[31]

In IBS, these visceral hypersensitivity symptoms are understood to be caused by interactions between gut contents, such as food and bacteria, and the permeability of mucosa, with hypersensitivity-related inflammation leading to and triggering neural sensations such as pain.[39] Visceral hypersensitivity has been attributed to abnormal activation of mast cells and the release of serotonin in gastrointestinal nerve regions.[40]

In IBS, there is a decreased threshold to stimuli from visceral inflammation and other causes of visceral nerve stimulation.[38]

## Brain-Gut Axis

The relationship between the physiological functions of the gut and those of the central nervous system is termed the brain-gut axis. The brain-gut axis is the basis of a popular theory explaining the patho-physiology of IBS, with emotional/psychological changes to the neurological brain function shown to impact the autonomic, enteric and central nervous systems.[41]

It is evidenced that emotional responses impacting central nerv-ous responses can result in peripheral nervous system changes, affecting gastrointestinal transit and causing disturbances to bowel habits.[42] Similarly, physiological responses such as changes in the bioavailability of serotonin can affect the central nervous system and regulation of the brain-gut axis.[43] Subsequent biological responses affect the quantity of various hormones released and eventually the quantities and types of microbiota present in the gut.[44]

Gastrointestinal tract dysfunction from inflammation or obstruction can further loop back on the nervous system and result in alterations to normal mental functions and can cause anxiety or depression.[45]

## Overview of Pathological Processes

The pathological causation of IBS development is complex, with a number of theories implicated, including gastrointestinal motility dysfunction, visceral hypersensitivity from inflammation, and sero-tonergic physiological dysfunction.[46] The physiological impairment of cells that modulate gastrointestinal motility and visceral hypersen-sitivity can cause impaired mucosal secretion, altered autonomic nervous system function, and/or abnormal activation of hormones.[47] When promoted by psychological stressors, physiological gastroin-testinal imbalances can affect gut physiology and cause or exacerbate IBS symptoms.[48]

# Diagnosis

There is no quick laboratory test for the diagnosis of IBS; instead, generally, a diagnosis is clinically established by comparing a per-son's recent medical history with defined IBS symptom criteria.[1] The symptom criteria defining IBS have varied over time, and a number of criteria have been used. Table 1.1 provides a chronological list of

**Table 1.1.   Development of Irritable Bowel Syndrome Diagnosis Criteria**

| Diagnosis Criteria |
| --- |
| Manning[50] |
| Kruis Criteria (1984)[51] |
| Rome Guidelines for IBS (1989) |
| Rome Classification System for FGIDs (1990) |
| Rome I Criteria for IBS and Rome I Criteria for FGIDs (1992–94)[52] |
| Rome II Criteria for IBS (2000)[53] |
| Rome III Criteria for FGIDs[54] |
| Rome IV Criteria for FGIDs[3] |

Abbreviations: IBS, irritable bowel syndrome; FGIDs, functional gastrointestinal disorders.

the most commonly recognised IBS criteria, with the most well-developed criteria to date being the latest version of the Rome criteria.[12] Variations between earlier and more recent criteria show that earlier criteria were not IBS specific and had considerable overlap between subtypes.[49]

Currently, the Rome criteria are the most widely utilised for the clinical diagnosis of IBS. The most recent version (Rome IV) stipulates that the criteria for the diagnosis of IBS consist of recurrent abdominal pain of at least one event per day per week in the last three months and associated with at least two of the following:

- Related to their defecation;
- Associated with change to the frequency of bowel movements;
- Associated with change to the form/appearance of stool.

The onset of these symptoms should have first occurred at least six months prior to diagnosis.[3]

Clinically, a diagnosis of IBS is assisted by the use of the Bristol stool form chart (Fig. 1.1) to identify whether a stool is abnormal and determine the sufferer's IBS subtype.[55] Rome IV criteria suggest subtype diagnosis can be categorised into the following four types.[3]

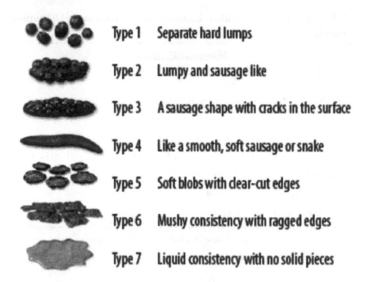

| | | |
|---|---|---|
| | Type 1 | Separate hard lumps |
| | Type 2 | Lumpy and sausage like |
| | Type 3 | A sausage shape with cracks in the surface |
| | Type 4 | Like a smooth, soft sausage or snake |
| | Type 5 | Soft blobs with clear-cut edges |
| | Type 6 | Mushy consistency with ragged edges |
| | Type 7 | Liquid consistency with no solid pieces |

**Fig. 1.1.**   Bristol Stool Chart[55] (image used under Creative Commons license https://creativecommons.org/licenses/by-sa/3.0)

## Irritable Bowel Syndrome with Predominant Diarrhoea

On the Bristol scale, stool types 6 (fluffy pieces with ragged edges, a mushy stool) and 7 (watery, no solid pieces, entirely liquid) are associated with IBS-D, and stools should make up more than 25% of bowel motions forms, while less than 25% of bowel motions are types 1 (separate hard lumps, like nuts [hard to pass]) or 2 (sausage-shaped but lumpy).[12]

## Irritable Bowel Syndrome with Predominant Constipation

On the Bristol scale, types 1 (separate hard lumps, like nuts [hard to pass]) and 2 (sausage-shaped but lumpy) are associated with IBS-C and stools should make up more than 25% of bowel motions, while less than 25% of bowel motions should be of types 6 (fluffy pieces with ragged edges, a mushy stool) or 7 (watery, no solid pieces, entirely liquid).[12]

## Irritable Bowel Syndrome with Mixed Bowel Habits

On the Bristol scale, more than 25% of bowel movements stool should be of type 1 (separate hard lumps, like nuts (hard to pass)) or 2 (sausage-shaped but lumpy) and more than 25% of bowel motions should be of types 6 (fluffy pieces with ragged edges, a mushy stool) and 7 (watery, no solid pieces, entirely liquid).[12] This subtype is IBS with mixed bowel habits (IBS-M).

## Irritable Bowel Syndrome Unclassified

A sufferer who meets the diagnostic criteria for IBS but their bowel habits are not sufficiently consistent in type to fit into one of the above subtypes is classified as IBS that is unclassified (IBS-U).[12]

# Differential Diagnosis

Clinically, a diagnosis of IBS is typically made based on patient's clinical history and their physical examination; however, as IBS symptoms are not unique, further laboratory tests and/or investigational procedures may be required in order to differentiate IBS from other disorders.

For people presenting with IBS-like symptoms without pain, their bowel dysfunction is typically labelled either "functional constipation" or "functional diarrhoea".[56] Those with IBS-like symptoms who experience continuous pain may be diagnosed with functional abdominal pain.[57] A clear separation between chronic idiopathic constipation (CIC) and IBS-C may be challenging and studies show there is considerable overlap, with patients sometimes shifting between these diagnoses over time.[58]

For people who clinically meet IBS criteria, clinicians should also consider additional testing of bloods and antibodies to rule out conditions with similar symptoms to IBS, such as coeliac disease.[2]

Other conditions from which clinicians might consider differentiating IBS include lactose intolerance, functional dyspepsia and

GERD. Many people who clinically report severe lactose intolerance do, in fact, absorb lactose normally and may actually have IBS.[59] For GERD and functional dyspepsia, there is some symptom overlap, with epigastric pain, nausea, vomiting and fullness being signs less likely to indicate IBS.[60]

A number of potential alarm symptoms are recognised clinically, which can indicate the presence of a different disease. Clinicians should pay particular attention to presentations with anaemia, unexplained/unintentional weight loss, unexplained fever, blood in stool, age of over 60 years (lower in some ethnicities), a family history of bowel cancer or ovarian cancer, abdominal masses, rectal masses, or inflammatory markers for inflammatory bowel disease.[61] Investigations may also include a sigmoidoscopy or colonoscopy to rule out inflammation, tumours or melanosis coli caused by regular laxative use.[2] Other investigations that may be useful in the differential diagnosis of IBS from other organic diseases include upper gastrointestinal endoscopy, abdominal ultrasonography, abdominal CT scan, abdominal magnetic resonance imaging (MRI), and X-ray of the abdomen.[62]

# Management

## Prevention

As IBS triggers are evidenced to be multifactorial, strategies for its prevention vary. The clinical purposes of prevention in IBS are typically to avert bowel hypersensitivity and gastrointestinal inflammation, maintaining normal bowel motility, and control emotions. Prevention may include a controlling diet to avoid foods causing mucosa sensitivity and inflammation,[63] taking probiotics to maintain intestinal flora and prevent inflammation, undertaking regular exercise[64] to promote normal bowel motility and manage one's psychological state, or behavioural aid techniques such as mindfulness to reduce the risk of the brain-gut axis being triggered psychologically.[65]

## Pharmacological Management

A lack of specificity in early-developed IBS criteria and subsequent changes to IBS criteria have made it difficult for clinicians to stand-ardise and optimise IBS treatment globally.[66] Historically, IBS was often referred to as a "spastic" or "irritable" colon, as it was primarily understood to be a disorder of gut motility. Thus pharmacological options routinely include antispasmodics or anticholinergics to relax smooth muscle and reduce IBS-related pain and bloating.[56] Clinically, national and regional treatment guidelines generally recommend that IBS pharmacotherapy should be selected based on the patient's IBS subtype.[2,56,67–69] Early interventions for IBS-C commonly consist of laxatives, while pharmacotherapy for IBS-D is generally intended to slow gut motility and may include anti-diarrhoeals (Table 1.2).

The instability of bowel habit subtypes suggests that relatively few patients should expect relief by taking the same motility-active drug regularly for long periods.[70] As the understanding of IBS pathogenesis has improved and clinicians have targeted therapies to address other IBS-causing mechanisms, the limitations of antispasmodic efficacy have been recognised. The relationships between IBS symptoms and mucosal hypersensitivity, gut inflammation, and the brian-gut axis now see a variety of pharmacological therapies utilised,[71] with therapies such as antidepressants, anti-allergics, and serotonin antagonists also routinely prescribed for the management of IBS.[72]

## Non-pharmacological Management

Various non-pharmacological therapies are recommended by guide-lines for benefit in IBS, including diet, exercise and behavioural therapies (Table 1.2).[1,2,56,67]

## Diet and Lifestyle

A key management method for IBS symptoms is through diet modifi-cation, as some foods with high carbohydrate content and fat such as

**Table 1.2.   Guideline-recommended Treatments for Irritable Bowel Syndrome**

| IBS Type | Symptom | First-line Therapies | Second-line Therapies |
|---|---|---|---|
| All types | Abdominal pain | — Antispasmodics (e.g., mebeverine)<br>— Anticholinergics (e.g., dicyclomine) | — Tricyclic antidepressives |
| | Gut hypersensitivity | — Anti-allergics (e.g., cromolyn, ketotifen) | N/A |
| | Bloating and distension | — Diet therapy | — Probiotics<br>— Tricyclic antidepressives |
| | Depressed mood | — Tricyclic antidepressants<br>— Selective serotonin reuptake inhibitors<br>— Relaxation therapy (e.g., mindfulness, hypnotherapy, cognitive behavioural therapy) | N/A |
| IBS-C | Constipation | — Dietary fibre supplementation (e.g., psyllium husk)<br>— Laxatives such as stool softeners and lubricants (e.g., methylcellulose, lactulose syrup, calcium polycarbophil) | — 5-HT4 agonist (e.g., tegaserod)<br>— Guanylate cyclase-C agonists (e.g., linaclotide)<br>— Other laxatives (e.g., lubiprostone, magnesium hydroxide)<br>— Enema |
| | Bloating and distension | Polyethylene glycols (osmotic laxative) | N/A |
| IBS-D | Diarrhoea | — Low fermentable oligosaccharides, disaccharides, monosaccharides and polyols (FODMAP) diet<br>— Anti-diarrheals (e.g., loperamide hydrochloride)<br>— Cholestyramine | — 5-HT3 antagonist (e.g., alosetron hydrochloride)<br>— Antibiotics (e.g., rifaximin) |

Abbreviations: IBS, irritable bowel syndrome; IBS-C, IBS with predominant constipation; IBS-D, IBS with predominant diarrhoea.

Adapted from guidelines from: Clinical Services Committee of British Society of Gastroenterology,[56] National Institute for Health and Care Excellence,[2] American Gastroenterological Association Institute,[68] Japanese Society of Gastroenterology,[69,79] and Gastroenterological Society of Australia.[67]

dairy products, beans and fried foods have been shown to trigger IBS symptoms.[73] Restricting high-fat and spicy foods, limiting alcohol and reducing the intake of caffeine can assist in managing IBS symptoms.[74]

For flatulence and bloating symptoms, it is recommended that gas-promoting foods such as legumes are reduced, and the dietary inclusion of oats or linseeds increased. Research indicates that, for IBS-C, whole grains, oats and vegetables that are high in fibre can assist in softening stools for ease of passing.[2] For IBS-D, restricting the dietary intake of fermentable oligosaccharides, disaccharides, monosaccharides and polyols (FODMAPs) can improve IBS symptoms.[75]

Exercising 3–5 times per week has shown to reduce the symptoms of IBS.[76]

## Probiotics and Prebiotics

The use of probiotics has been shown to be efficacious for IBS, and they are commonly recommended clinically; however, the magnitude of their effects varies between administered species. The role of prebiotics for IBS requires further evidence.[77]

## Herbal Medicine

Research on herbal medicine shows some positive effects in the control of IBS symptoms; however, to date, the majority of conventional guidelines indicate that evidence is insufficient for recommendation clinically. The UK's National Institute for Health and Care Excellence guidelines state there is a need for "a large randomised placebo-controlled trial comparing Chinese and non-Chinese herbal medicines (both single and multiple compounds available in the UK) as standard preparations".[2] A number of Chinese guidelines recommend various herbal formulations for IBS (see Chap. 2), as do guidelines from the Japanese Society of Gastroenterology, which recommend the use of peppermint oil and *kampo* therapy.[69] A systematic review of peppermint oil for IBS concluded it is safe and effective for short-term relief of IBS symptoms, including pain.[78]

## Other Non-pharmacological Therapies

Hypnotherapy has been recommended to be of some benefit for people with IBS but without accompanying major psychiatric disease.[56] Various relaxation therapies and psychotherapy methods such as cognitive behavioural therapy are also recommended to be useful for IBS.[2]

In summary, there is no cure for IBS, with current guidelines recommending therapies aimed to manage its symptoms by reducing the frequency and severity of constipation, diarrhoea and pain. As IBS symptoms vary and there is no one drug to treat all a sufferer's symptoms, practitioners are often required to prescribe multiple therapies to manage the condition.[80] As the condition is typically chronic, the ongoing associated drug treatment costs can be high; further, there can be increased risks to health, dependence concerns or reductions in a drug's effectiveness with its ongoing use.[81] Drugs such as antispasmodics used to manage abdominal pain and tricyclic antidepressants used for IBS-related depression can cause constipation, which can further aggravate the severity in IBS-C sufferers.[82] Other antidepressants such as selective serotonin reuptake inhibitors (SSRIs) can have side effects such as nausea, sweating, headaches and sexual dysfunction, so these are not appealing to all sufferers.[81] People with IBS receiving stimulant laxatives can experience cramping.[83]

Antispasmodics and anticholinergic drugs used to improve stool regularity have been evidenced to be most effective during acute IBS attacks, as they can lose their effectiveness when used chronically.[80]

Drugs acting as serotonin type 4 (5-HT4) receptor agonists have been shown in some trials to lead to carcinogenicity and cardiac toxicity in animal studies, so approved drugs targeting these pathways are clinically used cautiously.[81]

Diet and lifestyle modifications have been shown to improve symptoms in some sufferers with IBS; however, in others, there has been no symptom improvement.[84] In people with IBS symptoms of bloating, the bloating and distension symptoms can be exacerbated by fibre supplementation.[81]

# Prognosis

Patients with IBS typically have a good prognosis, as IBS is not evidenced to be associated with the development of a serious long-term physical disease.[85] Although no lasting physiological harms to the bowel are evidenced to be caused by IBS, the psychosocial impacts of IBS symptoms and the brian-gut sensitivity relationship can greatly impact a sufferer's quality of life.[86]

Comprehensive review evidence supports depression and anxiety being greater burdens to IBS patients compared to healthy controls.[87] Evidence indicates that people with a prolonged history of IBS are less likely to have symptom improvement and have increased reporting of mood disorders, health anxiety, and neuroticism. Morbidity rates of panic disorder and agoraphobia are significantly higher in people with IBS compared to those without IBS.[13]

When comparing subtypes, IBS-D and IBS-M are shown to have a poorer prognosis in terms of quality of life.[88]

# References

1. Quigley EM, Fried M, Gwee KA, *et al.* (2016) World Gastroenterology Organisation Global Guidelines Irritable Bowel Syndrome: A global perspective (update: September 2015). *J Clin Gastroenterol.* **50(9):** 704–713.
2. National Institute for Health and Care Excellence (NICE). (2017) Irritable bowel syndrome in adults: Diagnosis and management (CG61). In: *National Institute for Health and Care Excellence.* United Kingdom.
3. Drossman DA. (2016) Functional gastrointestinal disorders: History, pathophysiology, clinical features and Rome IV. *Gastroenterology.* **150 (6):** 1262–79.e2.
4. Chey WD, Kurlander J, Eswaran S. (2015) Irritable bowel syndrome: A clinical review. *JAMA.* **313(9):** 949–958.
5. Ringel Y, Williams RE, Kalilani L, Cook SF. (2009) Prevalence, characteristics, and impact of bloating symptoms in patients with irritable bowel syndrome. *Clin Gastroenterol Hepatol.* **7(1):** 68–72.

6. Engsbro AL, Simren M, Bytzer P. (2012) Short-term stability of subtypes in the irritable bowel syndrome: Prospective evaluation using the Rome III classification. *Aliment Pharmacol Ther.* **35(3):** 350–359.

7. Saito YA, Locke GR, Talley NJ, *et al.* (2000) A comparison of the Rome and Manning criteria for case identification in epidemiological investigations of irritable bowel syndrome. *Am J Gastroenterol.* **95(10):** 2816–2824.

8. Lovell RM, Ford AC. (2012) Global prevalence of and risk factors for irritable bowel syndrome: A meta-analysis. *Clin Gastroenterol Hepatol.* **10(7):** 712–21.e4.

9. Okeke EN, Ladep NG, Adah S, *et al.* (2009) Prevalence of irritable bowel syndrome: A community survey in an African population. *Ann Afr Med.* **8(3):** 177–180.

10. Dapoigny M, Bellanger J, Bonaz B, *et al.* (2004) Irritable bowel syndrome in France: A common, debilitating and costly disorder. *Eur J Gastroenterol Hepatol.* **16(10):** 995–1001.

11. Sperber AD, Dumitrascu D, Fukudo S, *et al.* (2017) The global prevalence of IBS in adults remains elusive due to the heterogeneity of studies: A Rome Foundation working team literature review. *Gut.* **66(6):** 1075–1082.

12. Schmulson MJ, Drossman DA. (2017) What is new in Rome IV. *J Neurogastroenterol Motil.* **23(2):** 151–163.

13. Kumano H, Kaiya H, Yoshiuchi K, *et al.* (2004) Comorbidity of irritable bowel syndrome, panic disorder, and agoraphobia in a Japanese representative sample. *Am J Gastroenterol.* **99(2):** 370–376.

14. Vandvik PO, Wilhelmsen I, Ihlebaek C, Farup PG. (2004) Comorbidity of irritable bowel syndrome in general practice: A striking feature with clinical implications. *Aliment Pharmacol Ther.* **20(10):** 1195–1203.

15. Taylor DC, Kosinski M, Reilly K, Lindner L. (2014) Comparison of the burden of IBS with constipation on health-related quality of life (HRQoL), work productivity, and health care utilization to asthma, migraine, and rheumatoid arthritis in the US, UK, and France. *Value Health.* **17(7):** A371–2.

16. Maxion-Bergemann S, Thielecke F, Abel F, Bergemann R. (2006) Costs of irritable bowel syndrome in the UK and US. *Pharmacoeconomics.* **24(1):** 21–37.

17. Soubieres A, Wilson P, Poullis A, *et al.* (2015) Burden of irritable bowel syndrome in an increasingly cost-aware National Health Service. *Frontline Gastroenterol.* **6(4):** 246–251.

18. Buono JL, Carson RT, Flores NM. (2017) Health-related quality of life, work productivity, and indirect costs among patients with irritable bowel syndrome with diarrhea. *Health Qual Life Outcomes.* **15(1):** 35.

19. Zhang F, Xiang W, Li CY, Li SC. (2016) Economic burden of irritable bowel syndrome in China. *World J Gastroenterol.* **22(47):** 10450–10460.

20. Flik CE, Laan W, Smout AJ, *et al.* (2015) Comparison of medical costs generated by IBS patients in primary and secondary care in the Netherlands. *BMC Gastroenterol.* **15:** 168.

21. Saito YA, Petersen GM, Larson JJ, *et al.* (2010) Familial aggregation of irritable bowel syndrome: A family case-control study. *Am J Gastroenterol.* **105(4):** 833–841.

22. Wojczynski MK, North KE, Pedersen NL, Sullivan PF. (2007) Irritable bowel syndrome: A co-twin control analysis. *Am J Gastroenterol.* **102(10):** 2220–2229.

23. Makker J, Chilimuri S, Bella JN. (2015) Genetic epidemiology of irritable bowel syndrome. *World J Gastroenterol.* **21(40):** 11353–11361.

24. Whitehead WE, Crowell MD, Robinson JC, *et al.* (1992) Effects of stressful life events on bowel symptoms: Subjects with irritable bowel syndrome compared with subjects without bowel dysfunction. *Gut.* **33(6):** 825–830.

25. Whitehead WE, Palsson O, Jones KR. (2002) Systematic review of the comorbidity of irritable bowel syndrome with other disorders: What are the causes and implications? *Gastroenterology.* **122(4):** 1140–1156.

26. Hayes P, Corish C, O'Mahony E, Quigley EM. (2014) A dietary survey of patients with irritable bowel syndrome. *J Hum Nutr Diet.* **27 (Suppl 2):** 36–47.

27. Lubrano E, Iovino P, Tremolaterra F, *et al.* (2001) Fibromyalgia in patients with irritable bowel syndrome. An association with the severity of the intestinal disorder. *Int J Colorectal Dis.* **16(4):** 211–215.

28. Ford AC, Talley NJ. (2011) Mucosal inflammation as a potential etiological factor in irritable bowel syndrome: A systematic review. *J Gastroenterol.* **46(4):** 421–431.

29. Porter CK, Gormley R, Tribble DR, *et al.* (2011) The incidence and gastrointestinal infectious risk of functional gastrointestinal disorders in a healthy US adult population. *Am J Gastroenterol.* **106(1):** 130–138.

30. Kaji M, Fujiwara Y, Shiba M, *et al.* (2010) Prevalence of overlaps between GERD, FD and IBS and impact on health-related quality of life. *J Gastroenterol Hepatol.* **25(6):** 1151–1156.

31. Barbara G, Zecchi L, Barbaro R, *et al.* (2012) Mucosal permeability and immune activation as potential therapeutic targets of probiotics in irritable bowel syndrome. *J Clin Gastroenterol.* **46 Suppl:** S52–5.

32. Moloney RD, Johnson AC, O'Mahony SM, *et al.* (2016) Stress and the microbiota-gut-brain axis in visceral pain: Relevance to irritable bowel syndrome. *CNS Neurosci Ther.* **22(2):** 102–117.

33. Cashman MD, Martin DK, Dhillon S, Puli SR. (2016) Irritable bowel syndrome: A clinical review. *Curr Rheumatol Rev.* **12(1):** 13–26.

34. Tornblom H, Van Oudenhove L, Sadik R, *et al.* (2012) Colonic transit time and IBS symptoms: What's the link? *Am J Gastroenterol.* **107(5):** 754–760.

35. Greenwood-Van Meerveld B, Johnson AC, Grundy D. (2017) Gastrointestinal physiology and function. *Handb Exp Pharmacol.* **239:** 1–16.

36. Sikander A, Rana SV, Prasad KK. (2009) Role of serotonin in gastrointestinal motility and irritable bowel syndrome. *Clin Chim Acta.* **403(1–2):** 47–55.

37. Cremon C, Carini G, Wang B, *et al.* (2011) Intestinal serotonin release, sensory neuron activation, and abdominal pain in irritable bowel syndrome. *Am J Gastroenterol.* **106(7):** 1290–1298.

38. Farzaei MH, Bahramsoltani R, Abdollahi M, Rahimi R. (2016) The role of visceral hypersensitivity in irritable bowel syndrome: Pharmacological targets and novel treatments. *J Neurogastroenterol Motil.* **22(4):** 558–574.

39. Camilleri M, Lasch K, Zhou W. (2012) Irritable bowel syndrome: Methods, mechanisms, and pathophysiology. The confluence of increased permeability, inflammation, and pain in irritable bowel syndrome. *Am J Physiol Gastrointest Liver Physiol.* **303(7):** G775–85.

40. Grundy D. (2008) 5-HT system in the gut: Roles in the regulation of visceral sensitivity and motor functions. *Eur Rev Med Pharmacol Sci.* **12 (Suppl 1):** 63–67.

41. Coss-Adame E, Rao SS. (2014) Brain and gut interactions in irritable bowel syndrome: New paradigms and new understandings. *Curr Gastroenterol Rep.* **16(4):** 379.

42. Gaman A, Kuo B. (2008) Neuromodulatory processes of the brain-gut axis. *Neuromodulation.* **11(4):** 249–259.

43. Stasi C, Bellini M, Bassotti G, *et al.* (2014) Serotonin receptors and their role in the pathophysiology and therapy of irritable bowel syndrome. *Tech Coloproctol.* **18(7):** 613–621.

44. Fichna J, Storr MA. (2012) Brain-gut interactions in IBS. *Front Pharmacol.* **3:** 127.

45. Jones MP, Dilley JB, Drossman D, Crowell MD. (2006) Brain gut connections in functional GI disorders: Anatomic and physiologic relationships. *Neurogastroenterol Motil.* **18(2):** 91–103.

46. Chang JY, Talley NJ. (2011) An update on irritable bowel syndrome: From diagnosis to emerging therapies. *Curr Opin Gastroenterol.* **27(1):** 72–78.

47. Choudhury BK, Shi XZ, Sarna SK. (2009) Norepinephrine mediates the transcriptional effects of heterotypic chronic stress on colonic motor function. *Am J Physiol Gastrointest Liver Physiol.* **296(6):** G1238–47.

48. Winston JH, Xu GY, Sarna SK. (2010) Adrenergic stimulation mediates visceral hypersensitivity to colorectal distension following heterotypic chronic stress. *Gastroenterology.* **138(1):** 294–304.e3.

49. Palsson OS, Whitehead WE, van Tilburg MAL, *et al.* (2016) Development and validation of the Rome IV diagnostic questionnaire for adults. *Gastroenterology.* **150(6):** 1481–1491.

50. Manning AP, Thompson WG, Heaton KW, Morris AF. (1978) Towards positive diagnosis of the irritable bowel. *Br Med J.* **2(6138):** 653–654.

51. Kruis W, Thieme C, Weinzierl M, *et al.* (1984) A diagnostic score for the irritable bowel syndrome: Its value in the exclusion of organic disease. *Gastroenterology.* **87(1):** 1–7.

52. Drossman DA, Richter JE, Talley NJ, *et al.* (1994) The functional gastrointestinal disorders: Diagnosis, pathophysiology and treatment. Degnon Associates, McLean, Virginia.

53. Drossman DA, Corazziari E, Talley NJ, *et al.* (2000) Rome II. The functional gastrointestinal disorders. diagnosis, pathophysiology and treatment: A multinational consensus. Degnon Associates, McLean, Virgina.

54. Drossman DA, Corazziari E, Delvaux M, *et al.* (2006) Rome III: The functional gastrointestinal disorders. Degnon Associates, McLean, Virgina.

55. Lewis SJ, Heaton KW. (1997) Stool form scale as a useful guide to intestinal transit time. *Scand J Gastroenterol.* **32(9):** 920–924.

56. Spiller R, Aziz Q, Creed F, *et al.* (2007) Guidelines on the irritable bowel syndrome: Mechanisms and practical management. *Gut.* **56(12):** 1770–1798.

57. Clouse RE, Mayer EA, Aziz Q, *et al.* (2006) Functional abdominal pain syndrome. *Gastroenterology.* **130(5):** 1492–1497.

58. Halder SL, Locke GR 3rd, Schleck CD, *et al.* (2007) Natural history of functional gastrointestinal disorders: A 12-year longitudinal population-based study. *Gastroenterology.* **133(3):** 799–807.

59. Suarez FL, Savaiano DA, Levitt MD. (1995) A comparison of symptoms after the consumption of milk or lactose-hydrolyzed milk by people with self-reported severe lactose intolerance. *N Engl J Med.* **333(1):** 1–4.

60. Agreus L, Svardsudd K, Nyren O, Tibblin G. (1995) Irritable bowel syndrome and dyspepsia in the general population: Overlap and lack of stability over time. *Gastroenterology.* **109(3):** 671–680.

61. Hammer J, Eslick GD, Howell SC, *et al.* (2004) Diagnostic yield of alarm features in irritable bowel syndrome and functional dyspepsia. *Gut.* **53(5):** 666–672.

62. Guclu M, Pourbagher A, Serin E, *et al.* (2006) Ultrasonographic evaluation of gallbladder functions in patients with irritable bowel syndrome. *J Gastroenterol Hepatol.* **21(8):** 1309–1312.

63. El-Salhy M, Gundersen D. (2015) Diet in irritable bowel syndrome. *Nutr J.* **14**: 36.

64. Johannesson E, Ringstrom G, Abrahamsson H, Sadik R. (2015) Intervention to increase physical activity in irritable bowel syndrome shows long-term positive effects. *World J Gastroenterol.* **21(2):** 600–608.

65. Aucoin M, Lalonde-Parsi MJ, Cooley K. (2014) Mindfulness-based therapies in the treatment of functional gastrointestinal disorders: A meta-analysis. *Evid Based Complement Alternat Med.* 140724.

66. Camilleri M. (2009) Do the symptom-based, Rome criteria of irritable bowel syndrome lead to better diagnosis and treatment outcomes? The con argument. *Clin Gastroenterol Hepatol.* **8(2):** 129.

67. Gastroenterological Society of Australia. (2006) Irritable bowel syndrome — Clinical update. In: *Digestive Health Foundation*, 2nd ed. Digestive Health Foundation, Sydney, Australia.

68. Weinberg DS, Smalley W, Heidelbaugh JJ, Sultan S. (2014) American Gastroenterological Association Institute Guideline on the pharmacological management of irritable bowel syndrome. *Gastroenterology.* **147(5):** 1146–1148.

69. Fukudo S, Kaneko H, Akiho H, *et al.* (2015) Evidence-based clinical practice guidelines for irritable bowel syndrome. *J Gastroenterol.* **50(1):** 11–30.

70. Longstreth GF. (2005) Definition and classification of irritable bowel syndrome: Current consensus and controversies. *Gastroenterol Clin North Am.* **34(2):** 173–187.

71. McKee DP, Quigley EM. (1993) Intestinal motility in irritable bowel syndrome: Is IBS a motility disorder? Part 1. Definition of IBS and colonic motility. *Dig Dis Sci.* **38(10):** 1761–1772.

72. Creed F. (2006) How do SSRIs help patients with irritable bowel syndrome? *Gut.* **55(8):** 1065–1067.

73. Bohn L, Storsrud S, Tornblom H, *et al.* (2013) Self-reported food-related gastrointestinal symptoms in IBS are common and associated with more severe symptoms and reduced quality of life. *Am J Gastroenterol.* **108(5):** 634–641.

74. Staudacher HM, Whelan K, Irving PM, Lomer MC. (2011) Comparison of symptom response following advice for a diet low in fermentable carbohydrates (FODMAPs) versus standard dietary advice in patients with irritable bowel syndrome. *J Hum Nutr Diet.* **24(5):** 487–495.

75. Whelan K, Martin LD, Staudacher HM, Lomer MCE. (2018) The low FODMAP diet in the management of irritable bowel syndrome: An evidence-based review of FODMAP restriction, reintroduction and personalisation in clinical practice. *J Hum Nutr Diet.* **31(2):** 239–255.

76. Johannesson E, Simren M, Strid H, *et al.* (2011) Physical activity improves symptoms in irritable bowel syndrome: A randomized controlled trial. *Am J Gastroenterol.* **106(5):** 915–922.

77. Ford AC, Quigley EM, Lacy BE, *et al.* (2014) Efficacy of prebiotics, probiotics, and synbiotics in irritable bowel syndrome and chronic idiopathic constipation: Systematic review and meta-analysis. *Am J Gastroenterol.* **109(10):** 1547–1561; quiz 6, 62.

78. Khanna R, MacDonald JK, Levesque BG. (2014) Peppermint oil for the treatment of irritable bowel syndrome: A systematic review and meta-analysis. *J Clin Gastroenterol.* **48(6):** 505–512.

79. Fukudo S, Suzuki J. (1987) Colonic motility, autonomic function, and gastrointestinal hormones under psychological stress on irritable bowel syndrome. *Tohoku J Exp Med.* **151(4):** 373–385.

80. Saha L. (2014) Irritable bowel syndrome: Pathogenesis, diagnosis, treatment, and evidence-based medicine. *World J Gastroenterol.* **20(22):** 6759–6773.

81. Talley NJ. (2003) Pharmacologic therapy for the irritable bowel syndrome. *Am J Gastroenterol.* **98(4):** 750–758.

82. Brandt LJ, Chey WD, Foxx-Orenstein AE, *et al.* (2009) An evidence-based position statement on the management of irritable bowel syndrome. *Am J Gastroenterol.* **104(Suppl 1):** S1–35.

83. Xing JH, Soffer EE. (2001) Adverse effects of laxatives. *Dis Colon Rectum.* **44(8):** 1201–1209.
84. Mazzawi T, El-Salhy M. (2017) Effect of diet and individual dietary guidance on gastrointestinal endocrine cells in patients with irritable bowel syndrome (Review). *Int J Mol Med.* **40(4):** 943–952.
85. Harvey RF, Mauad EC, Brown AM. (1987) Prognosis in the irritable bowel syndrome: A 5-year prospective study. *Lancet.* **1(8539):** 963–965.
86. The American Gastroenterological Association. (2016) *IBS: A Guide to Irritable Bowel Syndrome.* AGA Institute, Bethesda, USA.
87. Lee C, Doo E, Choi JM, *et al.* (2017) The increased level of depression and anxiety in irritable bowel syndrome patients compared with healthy controls: Systematic review and meta-analysis. *J Neurogastroenterol Motil.* **23(3):** 349–362.
88. Singh P, Staller K, Barshop K, *et al.* (2015) Patients with irritable bowel syndrome-diarrhea have lower disease-specific quality of life than irritable bowel syndrome-constipation. *World J Gastroenterol.* **21(26):** 8103–8109.

# 2

# Irritable Bowel Syndrome in Chinese Medicine

## OVERVIEW

In Chinese medicine (CM), irritable bowel syndrome (IBS) is referred to by its most predominant symptoms: *xie xie* 泄泻 (diarrhoea), *bian mi* 便秘 (constipation) or *fu tong* 腹痛 (abdominal pain). Treatment with CM may improve IBS symptoms and prevent recurrence. This chapter reviews key CM guidelines, textbooks and published standards in discussing CM terminology, aetiology and pathogenesis, and syndrome principles for IBS. Various IBS treatment and prevention regimes are also described, including Chinese herbal medicine, acupuncture and other CM therapies.

## Introduction

Irritable bowel syndrome (IBS) is a modern disease term and is not specifically mentioned in ancient Chinese medical literature. In Chinese medicine (CM), IBS is identified and diagnosed according to predominant symptoms experienced by the patient, including *xie xie* 泄泻 (diarrhoea), *bian mi* 便秘 (constipation) and *fu tong* 腹痛 (abdominal pain).[1] In classical CM medical texts such as *Nan Jing* 难经 (c. 220), symptoms and signs of IBS with predominant diarrhoea (IBS-D), including abdominal pain and diarrhoea, especially after eating, have been described. Symptoms and signs of IBS with predominant constipation (IBS-C) were described in *Yi Yuan* 医原 (c. 1861) as "pain in the intestines, [which] can be reduced after defecation, tenesmus, stool difficulty, and that a lack of smooth *qi* movement can cause constipation".

Although the contemporary understanding of IBS reflects a combination of these symptoms, clinically, CM syndromes of Spleen-Stomach weakness and Liver stagnation dominate the pathogenesis and treatment of IBS.[2,3]

## Aetiology and Pathogenesis

In CM, the IBS condition is understood to be mainly related to dysfunction in the Large Intestine, Liver, Spleen and Kidney organs.[2] According to CM theory, IBS aetiology can vary; however, disturbance in the Spleen and Stomach is considered to be the main cause.[3]

Weak Spleen-Stomach, *pi wei xu ruo* 脾胃虚弱, or long-term disease damaging the Spleen function, *jiu bing shang pi* 久病伤脾, can lead to IBS. Dietary irregularities, *yin shi bu jie* 饮食不节, such as too much cold or oily food, irregular meal times, and consuming too much or too little food can also damage the Spleen and Stomach, *sun shang pi wei* 损伤脾胃.[4] Emotional upsets, *qing zhi bu sui* 情志不遂, can cause Liver *qi* stagnation, *gan qi yu jie* 肝气郁结, and if prolonged, Liver *qi* stagnation can then invade the Spleen, *jiu ze heng ni fan pi* 久则横逆犯脾. If the disease is prolonged or goes untreated, *ri jiu shi zhi* 日久失治, the condition can progress to damage the Spleen as well as the Kidney, *sun shang pi shen* 损伤脾肾, and an IBS-like disease begins.

Disruptions to any of the mentioned CM processes can impede or cause the Spleen's transportation function to fail, *pi shi jian yun* 脾失健运. Impediment to its transportation function can result in dampness, damp-heat, phlegm and Blood stasis, food retention, or other types of accumulation.[1] This abnormal accumulation can then lead to the development of a complex deficiency-excess pattern and the lingering of IBS.[2]

Accumulation can also cause Liver stagnation, and its subsequent invasion to the Spleen can impede the Spleen function, and so its *qi* can fail to rise upward, *pi shi shu xie* 肝失疏泄, *heng ni fan pi* 横逆犯脾, and *pi qi bu sheng* 脾气不升. Failure of the Spleen *qi* to rise results in the IBS symptom of diarrhoea. The constrained Liver and Spleen *qi* can also cause the bowel *qi* to fail to bear downwards, *fu qi tong jiang bu li* 腹气通降不利. and lead to symptoms of abdominal pain and bloating. During these abnormal CM processes, *chang fu chuan dao shi si* 肠腑传导失司, if there is a disruption to the transmission of intestinal *qi*, then IBS symptoms of constipation occur, alternating with diarrhoea.[1]

According to CM theory, Liver stagnation and Spleen deficiency, *gan yu pi xu* 肝郁脾虚, are the most recognised IBS pathogenesis.[1,2] Generally, Spleen-Stomach weakness, *pi xu wei ruo* 脾胃虚弱, is understood to be the root cause of IBS, with emotional upsets contributing as both a major causative factor and a symptom aggravator.

## Syndrome Differentiation and Treatments

During the early stage of IBS, excess-type syndromes are more predominant, but if the condition persists and becomes chronic, then deficiency-type syndromes become predominant. For treatment, a practitioner should identify whether the patient's main syndrome is a complex of deficiency and excess, or cold and heat. The primary treatment focus is on harmonising the Liver and Spleen *qi*, and the secondary goals are to warm the Kidneys and strengthen the Spleen.[5]

In recent years, there has been progress in understanding IBS CM syndrome differentiation and therapy. In 2005, the *Integrated Traditional Chinese and Western Medicine Diagnosis and Treatment Strategy for Irritable Bowel Syndrome (Draft)* was published.[6] Through revision, *Consensus Opinion of Integrated Traditional Chinese and Western Medicine Diagnosis and Treatment Strategy for Irritable Bowel Syndrome* was then published in 2011.[7] The two guidelines differentiated IBS syndromes into (1) Liver depression and *qi* stagnation, *gan yu qi zhi* 肝郁气滞, (2) Liver *qi* invading the Spleen, *gan qi cheng pi* 肝气乘脾, (3) Spleen-Stomach weakness syndrome, *pi wei xu ruo* 脾胃虚弱, (4) cold-heat complex syndrome, *han re jia za*

寒热夹杂, and (5) large intestinal heat and fluid deficiency, *da chang zao re* 大肠燥热.

In 2008, the China Association of Chinese Medicine (CACM) published *Chinese Medicine Clinical Diagnosis and Treatment Strategy for Irritable Bowel Syndrome*.[8] In the same year, the CACM Spleen and Stomach Branch drafted another guideline, *Consensus Opinion of Traditional Chinese Medicine Diagnosis and Treatment Strategy for Irritable Bowel Syndrome (Draft)* and, after modification, *Consensus Opinion of Traditional Chinese Medicine Diagnosis and Treatment Strategy for Irritable Bowel Syndrome* was published in 2010.[3] In 2017, the most recent version, *Consensus Opinion of Specialists of Traditional Chinese Medicine Diagnosis and Treatment Strategy for Irritable Bowel Syndrome* was published.[1] This current guideline separates the CM syndromes by IBS subtype and provides clearer guidance on IBS treatment. These will be discussed later in the chapter.

In addition to these guidelines to assist in standardising IBS treatment, the State Administration of Traditional Chinese Medicine of the People's Republic of China, since 2010, has collaborated with many CM hospitals to develop guides for IBS diagnosis and treatment. Publication of these collaborative guides has included a guide for IBS-D, *22 Professional 95 Diseases of Chinese Medicine Diagnosis and Treatment Strategy*[9] and a guide for IBS-C, *24 Professional 105 Diseases of Chinese Medicine Diagnosis and Treatment Strategy*.[10]

## Chinese Herbal Medicine Treatment for Irritable Bowel Syndrome

Chinese herbal medicine (CHM) treatment for different types of IBS is summarised here. CHM treatments include oral CHM and topical CHM. For IBS, the use of some herbs may be restricted in some countries. In addition, some herbs are restricted under the provisions of the Convention on International Trade in Endangered Species of Wild Fauna and Flora (CITES). Readers are advised to comply with relevant regulations.

## Oral Chinese Herbal Medicine Treatment Based on Syndrome Differentiation

### *Irritable Bowel Syndrome with Predominant Diarrhoea*

*Liver qi stagnation with Spleen deficiency,* 肝郁脾虚证

Clinical manifestations: Diarrhoea after abdominal pain, pain reduces after diarrhoea, easily agitated or angered, hypochondrium fullness, poor appetite, torpid intake, fatigue and lassitude, a pale enlarged tongue with teeth marks and thin white coating, and a fine and string-like pulse.

Treatment principle: Remove Liver stagnation and strengthen the Spleen.

Formula: *Tong xie yao fang* 痛泻要方.[1]

Herbs: *Bai zhu* 白术, *bai shao* 白芍, *fang feng* 防风, *chen pi* 陈皮.

Main actions of herbs: *Bai zhu* dry dampness to strengthen the Spleen; *bai shao* to pacify the Liver to relax tension and relieve pain; *fang feng* to inhibit the Liver and relax the Spleen; and *chen pi* to regulate *qi* and invigorate the Spleen. All herbs act together to harmonise the Liver and Spleen.

Chinese patent medicine: *Tong xie ning ke li* 痛泻宁颗粒.[2]

*Spleen and Stomach deficiency or Spleen deficiency with dampness,* 脾胃虚弱证/脾虚湿盛证

Clinical manifestations: Sometimes sloppy stool, sometimes diarrhoea, stool with mucus, dull abdominal pain, diarrhoea encumbrance with pain or increased diarrhoea when fatigued or cold, distension after eating, gastric fullness, lassitude and poor appetite, fatigue and weak limbs, sallow complexion, a pale tongue body with teeth marks and greasy white coating, and a weak pulse.[1,7]

Treatment principle: Tonify the Spleen and replenish *qi*, resolve dampness and stop diarrhoea.

Formula: Modified *Shen ling bai zhu san* 参苓白术散.[7]

Herbs: *Dang shen* 党参, *chao bai zhu* 炒白术, *fu ling* 茯苓, *bai shao* 白芍, *shan yao* 山药, *chao bian dou* 炒扁豆, *lian zi* 莲子, *yi yi ren* 薏苡仁, *sha ren* 砂仁, *chao chen pi* 炒陈皮, *mu xiang* 木香, *gan cao* 甘草.

Main actions of herbs: *Dang shen, chao bai zhu, fu ling* and *gan cao* tonify the Spleen and Stomach *qi*; *chao bian dou, yi yi ren, shan yao* and *lian zi* assist *chao bai zhu* to strengthen the Spleen to drain dampness and stop diarrhoea; *sha ren* aromatically invigorates the Spleen; *bai shao* and *mu xiang* soothe the Liver and regulate *qi*; and *chao chen pi* regulates *qi* and invigorates the Spleen. All herbs act together to fortify the Spleen and replenish *qi*, resolve dampness, and stop diarrhoea.

Chinese patent medicines: *Shen ling bai zhu ke li* 参苓白术颗粒, *Bu pi yi chang wan* 补脾益肠丸.[7]

## *Spleen and Kidney yang deficiency,* 脾肾阳虚证

Clinical manifestations: Abdominal pain and diarrhoea after waking, abdominal pain relieved by heat, cold sensation in body and extremities, sore and weakness in the lower back and knees, poor appetite, a pale enlarged tongue body with greasy white coating, and a fine and sunken pulse.

Treatment principle: Warm and tonify Spleen and Kidney.

Formula: *Fu zi li zhong tang* 附子理中汤 combined with *Si shen wan* 四神丸.[1]

Herbs: *Fu zi* 附子, *ren shen* 人参, *gan jiang* 干姜, *gan cao* 甘草, *bai zhu* 白术, *bu gu zhi* 补骨脂, *rou dou kou* 肉豆蔻, *wu zhu yu* 吴茱萸, *wu wei zi* 五味子.

Main actions of herbs: *Ren shen* and *bai zhu* fortify the Spleen and replenish *qi*; *fu zi, gan jiang, bu gu zhi, rou dou kou* and *wu zhu yu* warm the Kidney and Spleen; *wu wei zi* astringes the intestines and stops diarrhoea, and together with *gan cao*, they warm and tonify the Spleen and Kidney.

Chinese patent medicines: *Gu ben yi chang pian* 固本益肠片,[3] *Si shen wan* 四神丸.[7]

## Dampness-heat in the Spleen and Stomach, 脾胃湿热证

Clinical manifestations: Dull abdominal pain, diarrhoea with urgency or sense of incomplete evacuation, smelly stool, a sensation of heat around the anus, oppression in the chest, dry mouth without thirst, bitter taste in the mouth and foul mouth odour, a red tongue body with greasy yellow coating, and a slippery and rapid pulse.

Treatment principle: Clear heat and drain dampness.

Formula: *Ge gen huang qin huang lian tang* 葛根黄芩黄连汤.[1]

Herbs: *Ge gen* 葛根, *huang qin* 黄芩, *huang lian* 黄连, *gan cao* 甘草.

Main actions of herbs: *Ge gen* clears heat and raises the middle *qi* to stop diarrhoea; *huang qin* and *huang lian* clear heat and dry dampness to stop diarrhoea; and *gan cao* harmonises the middle *qi*. All herbs act together to clear heat, drain dampness and stop diarrhoea.

Chinese patent medicine: *Feng liao chang wei kang ke li* 枫蓼肠胃康颗粒.[3]

## Complex cold-heat syndrome 寒热错杂证

Clinical manifestations: Sometimes sloppy stools, sometimes diarrhoea, abdominal pain prior to diarrhoea that is relieved after defecation, bloating and borborygmus, a bitter taste in the mouth or foul mouth odour, aversion to cold, symptoms aggravated by a cold, pale tongue body with thin yellow coating, and a fine and string-like pulse or slippery and string-like pulse.

Treatment principle: Balance cold and heat, tonify and warm the middle *jiao*.

Formula: *Wu mei wan* 乌梅丸.[1]

Herbs: *Wu mei* 乌梅, *xi xin* 细辛, *gan jiang* 干姜, *huang lian* 黄连, *fu zi* 附子, *dang gui* 当归, *huang bai* 黄柏, *gui zhi* 桂枝, *ren shen* 人参, *hua jiao* 花椒.

Main actions of herbs: *Wu mei* astringes the intestines and stops diarrhoea; *huang lian* and *huang bai* clear heat and dry dampness; *xi xin*, *gan jiang*, *fu zi*, *gui zhi* and *hua jiao* warm the middle *qi* and dissipate cold; *dang gui* moistens dryness and harmonises the Blood; and *ren shen* strengthens the Spleen and replenishes *qi*. All herbs act together to balance the cold and heat, and tonify and warm the middle *qi*.

## Irritable Bowel Syndrome with Predominant Constipation

### Liver qi stagnation 肝郁气滞证

Clinical manifestations: Constipation and difficulty passing stool, fullness and moving pain in the chest, hypochondrium and abdomen, easily agitated and angered, oppression in the chest, frequent belching, borborygmus and flatulence, a dark red tongue body with thin white coating, and a string-like pulse.

Treatment principle: Soothe the Liver and regulate *qi*, move *qi* to remove stagnation.

Formula: Modified *Liu mo tang* 六磨汤.[7]

Herbs: *Chen xiang* 沉香, *guang mu xiang* 广木香, *bin lang pian* 槟榔片, *wu yao* 乌药, *zhi shi* 枳实, *sheng da huang* 生大黄, *yu jin* 郁金, *hou pu* 厚朴.

Main actions of herbs: *Sheng da huang, zhi shi* and *bin lang pian* purge to remove accumulation, remove stagnation, and relax the bowels; *chen xiang, guang mu xiang, wu yao* and *yu jin* soothe the Liver and move *qi* to relieve stagnation; and *hou pu* moves *qi* to relieve stagnation. All herbs act together to strengthen the action of relaxing the bowels.

Chinese patent medicine: *Si mo tang kou fu ye* 四磨汤口服液.[3]

### Heat accumulating in the Stomach and Large Intestine, 胃肠积热证

Clinical manifestations: Difficulty passing stool, dry stool with mucus, abdominal pain or distention, weight loss, dry mouth with foul mouth odour, dizziness, a red tongue body with dry yellow coating, and a fine and rapid pulse.

Treatment principle: Purge heat, moisten the Intestines and relax the bowels.

Formula: *Ma zi ren wan* 麻子仁丸.[1]

Herbs: *Huo ma ren* 火麻仁, *xing ren* 杏仁, *bai shao* 白芍, *da huang* 大黄, *hou pu* 厚朴, *zhi shi* 枳实.

Main actions of herbs: *Huo ma ren* moistens the Intestines and relaxes the bowels; *xing ren* directs *qi* downward and moistens the Intestines; *bai shao* nourishes *yin* and harmonises nutrients; *da huang* purges heat and relaxes the bowels; and *hou pu* and *zhi shi* move *qi* to remove stuffiness and fullness in the abdomen. All herbs act together to purge heat, move *qi*, moisten the Intestines, and relax the bowels.

Chinese patent medicines: *Ma ren wan* 麻仁丸, *Ma ren run chang wan* 麻仁润肠丸.[3]

## Spleen and Kidney *yang* Deficiency, 脾肾阳虚证

Clinical manifestations: Difficulty passing stools, stools may be dry, pain from abdominal cold can be reduced with heat, profuse clear urine, cold extremities, a pale tongue body with white coating, and a slow and sunken pulse.

Treatment principle: Warm the Kidney and Spleen, moisten the bowels.

Formula: *Ji chuan jian* 济川煎.[1]

Herbs: *Dang gui* 当归, *niu xi* 牛膝, *rou cong rong* 肉苁蓉, *ze xie* 泽泻, *sheng ma* 升麻, *zhi qiao* 枳壳.

Main actions of herbs: *Dang gui* tonifies the Blood and moistens dryness to relax the bowels; *niu xi* tonifies the Liver and Kidney; *rou cong rong* warms the Kidney and lower back, replenishes Kidney essence, and relaxes the bowels; *ze xie* induces diuresis to clear Kidney turbidity; *sheng ma* raises *yang* to relax the bowels; and *zhi qiao* directs *qi* downward to relax the bowels. All herbs act together to warm the Kidney and replenish its essence, moisten the Intestines, and relax the bowels.

Chinese patent medicines: *Bian mi tong* 便秘通, *Cong rong tong bian kou fu ye* 苁蓉通便口服液.[10]

## Lung *qi* and Spleen *qi* Deficiency, 肺脾气虚证

Clinical manifestations: Stool is difficult to pass but not excessively hard, straining during defecation with sweating and shortness of breath, abdominal pain prior to defecation, weakness after defecation, lassitude of spirit and not wanting to speak, a pale tongue body with white coating, and a weak pulse.

Treatment principle: Tonify *qi* and moisten the Intestines.

Formula: *Huang qi tang* 黄芪汤.[1]

Herbs: *Huang qi* 黄芪, *chen pi* 陈皮, *bai mi* 白蜜, *huo ma ren* 火麻仁.

Main actions of herbs: *Huang qi* tonifies the Spleen and Lung *qi*; *bai mi* and *huo ma ren* moisten the intestines and relax the bowels; and *chen pi* regulates *qi*. All herbs act together to tonify the Spleen and Lung *qi,* moisten the Intestines, and relax the bowels.

Chinese patent medicine: *Qi rong run chang kou fu ye* 芪蓉润肠口服液.[1]

A summary of oral CHM treatment for IBS-D and IBS-C is presented in Table 2.1.

## Topical Chinese Herbal Medicine Treatment

Topical CHM therapies include CHM enema, CHM topical application, CHM foot baths, and others. Commonly used topical therapies for IBS are CHM topical application and CHM enema.

CHM topical application: Topical treatment should be applied to CV8 *Shenque* 神阙. When treating a deficiency syndrome pattern, *dang gui* 当归, *sheng ma* 升麻 and *dang shen* 党参 can be used. When the syndrome is an excess pattern, *da huang* 大黄 and *mu dan pi* 牡丹皮 can be administered. Topical application to CV8 *Shenque* 神阙 can be administered for two to four hours daily, for seven days.[1]

CHM enema: When there is severe constipation, such as abdominal pain, abdominal distension or no stool for a long period that is causing the patient distress, *xuan ming fen* 玄明粉 and *fan xie ye* 番泻叶 or *da huang* 大黄 can be applied. Decoct *fan xie ye* 番泻叶 or soak *da huang* 大黄in boiling water, and then add *xuan ming fen*

**Table 2.1. Summary of Oral Chinese Herbal Medicines for Irritable Bowel Syndrome**

| Subtype | Syndrome Differentiation | Treatment Principle | Formula |
|---|---|---|---|
| IBS-D | Liver *qi* stagnation with Spleen deficiency 肝郁脾虚证 | Calm the Liver and tonify the Spleen 抑肝扶脾 | Tong xie yao fang 痛泻要方[1] |
| | Spleen and Stomach deficiency or Spleen deficiency with dampness 脾胃虚弱证/脾虚湿盛证 | Strengthen the Spleen and replenish *qi*, resolve dampness and stop diarrhoea 健脾益气/健脾益气，化湿止泻 | Modified *Shen ling bai zhu san* 参苓白术散[7] |
| | Spleen and Kidney *yang* deficiency 脾肾阳虚证 | Warm and tonify Spleen and Kidney *yang* 温补脾肾 | *Fu zi li zhong tang* 附子理中汤 combined with *Si shen wan* 四神丸[1] |
| | Dampness-heat in the Spleen and Stomach 脾胃湿热证 | Clear heat and drain dampness 清热利湿 | *Ge gen huang qin huang lian tang* 葛根黄芩黄连汤[1] |
| | Cold-heat complex syndrome 寒热错杂证 | Balance cold and heat, tonify and warm the middle *qi* 平调寒热，益气温中 | *Wu mei wan* 乌梅丸[1] |
| IBS-C | Liver *qi* stagnation 肝郁气滞证 | Soothe the Liver and regulate *qi*, move *qi* to remove stagnation 疏肝理气，行气导滞 | Modified *Liu mo tang* 六磨汤[7] |
| | Heat accumulation in the Stomach and Intestines 胃肠积热证 | Dispel heat via purgation, moisten the Intestines and relax the bowels 泄热清肠，润肠通便 | *Ma zi ren wan* 麻子仁丸[1] |
| | Spleen and Kidney *yang* deficiency 脾肾阳虚证 | Warm and moisten to relax the bowels 温润通便 | *Ji chuan jian* 济川煎[1] |
| | Lung *qi* and Spleen *qi* deficiency 肺脾气虚证 | Tonify *qi* and moisten the Intestines 益气润肠 | *Huang qi tang* 黄芪汤[1] |

Abbreviations: IBS-C: irritable bowel syndrome with predominant constipation; IBS-D: irritable bowel syndrome with predominant diarrhoea.

玄明粉, stir until it is completely dissolved, and then use the liquid for an enema.

## Acupuncture Therapies and Other Chinese Medicine Therapies

Acupuncture can also be used for the treatment of IBS. Clinically, acupuncture point selection is based on the IBS subtype and its CM syndrome.[1,10] Commonly used acupoints for IBS are summarised below.

**Acupuncture points for irritable bowel syndrome with diarrhoea:** Main points: ST36 *Zusanli* 足三里, ST25 *Tianshu* 天枢, SP6 *Sanyinjiao* 三阴交; treat deficiency by tonification and excess with purgation.

**Spleen deficiency with dampness:** Supplementary points BL20 *Pishu* 脾俞, LR13 *Zhangmen* 章 门 may be selected.

**Spleen and Kidney *yang* deficiency:** Supplementary points of BL23 *Shenshu* 肾俞, GV4 *Mingmen* 命门, CV4 *Guanyuan* 关元 can be selected and administered acupuncture or moxibustion.

**Gastric stuffiness and poor appetite:** Supplementary point of SP4 *Gongsun* 公孙 can be selected.

**Liver *qi* stagnation:** Supplementary points of BL18 *Ganshu* 肝俞, LR2 *Xingjian* 行间 can be selected.

**Acupuncture points for irritable bowel syndrome with constipation:** To tonify deficiency and purge excess, select BL25 *Dachangshu* 大肠俞, ST25 *Tianshu* 天枢, TE6 *Zhigou* 支沟, ST40 *Fenglong* 丰隆, and when there is a cold syndrome, combine acupuncture with moxibustion.

**Intestinal dryness:** Supplementary points of LI4 *Hegu* 合谷, LI11 *Quchi* 曲池 can be added.

***Qi* stagnation:** Using a purgation needling method, supplementary points of CV12 *Zhongwan* 中脘, LR2 *Xingjian* 行间 can be added.

**Spleen *qi* deficiency:** Acupuncture of supplementary points of BL20 *Pishu* 脾俞, BL21 *Weishu* 胃俞 can be added.

**Spleen and Kidney *yang* deficiency:** Moxibustion supplementary points CV8 *Shenque* 神阙 and CV6 *Qihai* 气海.

## Ear Acupuncture

Ear acupuncture can assist to improve symptoms of constipation. Some useful ear points for IBS include: CO4 *Wei* (Stomach) 胃, CO7 *Dachang* (Large intestine) 大肠, CO6 *Xiaochang* (Small intestine) 小肠, HX2 *Zhichang* (Rectum) 直肠, AH6a *Jiaogan* (Sympathetic) 交感, AT4 *Pizhixia* (Subcortex) 皮质下, and CO17 *Sanjiao* (Triple Energizer) 三焦. These points can be stimulated for three minutes on each ear, ten times per day. Three to four points should be selected for each treatment course.[10]

## Other Chinese Medicine Therapies for Irritable Bowel Syndrome

Other CM therapies such as massage and electromagnetic heat treatment (*te ding dian ci bo pu zhi liao yi* 特定电磁波谱治疗仪) may also assist to relieve IBS symptoms. Clinically, when using massage for IBS, points that regulate the Spleen and Stomach functions can be selected and manipulated by rubbing or kneading these points.[9, 10]

A summary of acupuncture and other CM therapies for IBS-D and IBS-C can be found in Table 2.2.

## Other Irritable Bowel Syndrome Management Strategies

### Therapy to Manage Emotions

Emotional disturbances can have an impact on IBS symptoms and the exacerbation of symptoms during episodes of emotional tension or depression. Therapy for IBS should also address these emotions to ensure they remain balanced.[2, 5]

### Diet Therapy

A regular, healthy and balanced diet is beneficial for the management of IBS. Patients should avoid overconsuming fatty, cold and

**Table 2.2. Summary of Acupuncture Therapies and Other Chinese Medicine Therapies for Irritable Bowel Syndrome**

| Subtype | Syndrome/ Symptoms | Acupuncture Points/Body Area | Other CM Therapies |
|---|---|---|---|
| IBS-D | All syndrome types | ST36 *Zusanli* 足三里, ST25 *Tianshu* 天枢, SP6 *Sanyinjiao* 三阴交 | Not described |
| | Spleen deficiency with dampness 脾虚湿盛 | BL20 *Pishu* 脾俞, LR13 *Zhangmen* 章门 | |
| | Spleen and Kidney *yang* deficiency 脾肾阳虚 | BL23 *Shenshu* 肾俞, GV4 *Mingmen* 命门, CV4 *Guanyuan* 关元 | |
| | Gastric fullness and poor appetite 脘痞纳呆 | SP4 *Gongsun* 公孙 | |
| | Liver *qi* stagnation 肝郁 | BL18 *Ganshu* 肝俞, LR2 *Xingjian* 行间 | |
| IBS-C | All syndrome types | BL25 *Dachangshu* 大肠俞, ST25 *Tianshu* 天枢, TE6 *Zhigou* 支沟, ST40 *Fenglong* 丰隆 | CO4 *Wei* (Stomach) 胃, CO7 *Dachang* (Large intestine) 大肠, CO6 *Xiaochang* (Small intestine) 小肠, HX2 *Zhichang* (Rectum) 直肠, AH6a *Jiaogan* (Sympathetic) 交感, AT4 *Pizhixia* (Subcortex) 皮质下, CO17 *Sanjiao* (Triple Energizer) 三焦 |
| | Intestinal dryness 肠燥 | LI4 *Hegu* 合谷, LI11 *Quchi* 曲池 | |
| | *Qi* stagnation 气滞 | CV12 *Zhongwan* 中脘, LR2 Xingjian 行间 | |
| | Spleen *qi* deficiency 脾气虚弱 | BL20 *Pishu* 脾俞, BL21 *Weishu* 胃俞 | |
| | Spleen and Kidney *yang* deficiency 脾肾阳虚 | CV8 *Shenque* 神阙, CV6 *Qihai* 气海 | |

Abbreviations: IBS-C: irritable bowel syndrome with predominant constipation; IBS-D: irritable bowel syndrome with predominant diarrhoea.

fried foods and exclude foods that could be potentially irritating (e.g., coffee, tea, alcohol, beans).[5] To avoid intestinal dysfunction, meals should be regular and consumed in quantities that are easily digested and absorbed.[1,7]

# References

1. 中华中医药学会脾胃病分会. (2017) 肠易激综合征中医诊疗专家共识意见. 中医杂志. **58(18):** 1615–1620.
2. 张声生，沈洪，王垂杰，唐旭东. (2016) *中华脾胃病学*. 人民卫生出版社，北京.
3. 中华中医药学会脾胃病分会. (2010) 肠易激综合征中医诊疗共识意见. *中华中医药杂志*. **25(7):** 1062–1065.
4. 周仲瑛. (2007) *中医内科学(普通高等教育"十二五"国家级规划教材)*. 中国中医药出版社，中国北京.
5. 陈志强，杨关林. (2016) *中西医结合内科学*. 中国中医药出版社，中国北京.
6. 中国中西医结合学会消化系统疾病专业委员会. (2005) 肠易激综合征中西医结合诊治方案(草案). *中国中西医结合消化杂志*. **13(1):** 65–67.
7. 中国中西医结合学会消化系统疾病专业委员会. (2011) 肠易激综合征中西医结合诊疗共识意见. *中国中西医结合杂志*. **31(5):** 587–590.
8. 中华中医药学会. (2008) *中医内科常见病诊疗指南. 西医部分*. 中国中医药出版社，北京.
9. 国家中医药管理局. (2010) 22个专业95个病种中医诊疗方案. 国家中医药管理局医政司.
10. 国家中医药管理局. (2011) 24个专业105个病种中医诊疗方案 (试行). 国家中医药管理局医政司.

# 3

# Classical Chinese Medicine Literature

## OVERVIEW

Classical Chinese medicine literature can provide a rich source of information for the prevention and management of various diseases including conditions like irritable bowel syndrome (IBS). This chapter describes the findings from a systematic search of the *Zhong Hua Yi Dian* 中华医典, based on a selection of search terms identified from classical dictionaries and texts. The 729 citations that were judged possible or likely IBS were analysed to find information about the diagnosis and treatment of IBS-like symptoms in ancient literature.

## Introduction

In modern Chinese medicine (CM), irritable bowel syndrome (IBS) is recognised by the common terms *fu tong* 腹痛 ("abdominal pain"), *xie xie* 泄泻 ("diarrhoea") or *bian mi* 便秘 ("constipation"), with a relationship between abdominal pain and stool habit (e.g., frequency, form). Classical CM texts contain many citations of these terms, and some citations describe the relationship between these IBS-like terms. The *Ling Shu* 灵枢 (c. 221) states "A person has distension in the large intestine, abdominal pain, and borborygmus; if the cold attacks, then he will have diarrhoea"; 《灵枢·胀论篇》曰: "大肠胀者, 肠鸣而痛濯濯, 冬日重感于寒, 则飧泄不化". The *Da Fang Mai* 大方脉 (c. 1795) states that "dry stool can be seen with abdominal pain and bloating"; 《大方脉》曰: "实燥, 即胃实便燥也, 与腹满痛症同见者也". These citations from classical literature provide an opportunity to explore in further detail the historical evidence for CM therapies for IBS-like conditions.

To systematically summarise information from classical and pre-modern medical literature, an electronic search of the *Zhong Hua Yi Dian* (ZHYD) 中华医典 was conducted. The ZHYD consists of more than 1,100 classical Chinese medical books and was searched via CD-ROM form.[1] This collection is currently the largest available and is representative of other large collections of classical and pre-modern Chinese medical literature.[2,3]

# Search Terms

Contemporary texts diagnose IBS based on a sufficient presentation of specific IBS symptoms. Similarly, for the classical literature, IBS search terms were developed based on the most current Rome IV IBS criteria and consisted of "abdominal pain", "diarrhoea" and "constipation".[4] In ancient times, *fu tong* 腹痛 "abdominal pain", *xie xie* 泄泻 "diarrhoea", *bian mi* 便秘 "constipation" and related terms were widely used to denote diseases or symptoms. Therefore, we identified three groups of search terms using *fu tong* 腹痛, *xie xie* 泄泻 and *bian mi* 便秘 and related terms.

## Abdominal Pain Search Terms

The term *fu tong* 腹痛 first appeared in the *Shan Hai Jing* 山海经 and from the *Zhu Bing Yuan Hou Lun* 诸病源候论 (c. 610) onwards used as a disease name.[5,6] Other terms were also used for abdominal pain based on the location and characteristics of the pain. These terms were *rao qi tong* 绕脐痛, *huan qi er tong* 环脐而痛, *fu zhong tong* 腹中痛, *fu leng tong* 腹冷痛, *fu zhong gan tong* 腹中干痛, *fu zhong jiao tong* 腹中绞痛, *fu man tong* 腹满痛, *fu zhong man tong* 腹中满痛, and *fu zhong qie tong* 腹中切痛.

## Diarrhoea Search Terms

The term *xie xie* 泄泻 first appeared in the *Tai Ping Sheng Hui Fang* 太平圣惠方 (c. 992) from the Song dynasty. The *San Yin Ji Yi Bing*

*Zheng Fang Lun* 三因极一病证方论 (c. 1174) was the first book that presented a separate chapter on *xie xie* 泄泻.[7] Before this, there were various related terms, including *dong xie* 洞泄, *sun xie* 飧泄, *tang xie* 溏泄, *ru xie* 濡泄, *wu xie* 鹜溏, *hou xie* 后泄, *da chang xie* 大肠泄, *pi xie* 脾泄, *shui gu zhu xia* 水谷注下, and *xia li* 下利.

## Constipation Search Terms

In classical literature, there was no commonly used term for constipation. However, many constipation-like terms were cited, including the term *bi* 闭, which was first cited as a symptom in the *Yin Yang Shi Yi Mai Jiu Jing* 阴阳十一脉灸经, and *da bian mi* 大便秘, which first appeared in the *Lei Zheng Huo Ren Shu* 类证活人书. The term *bian mi* 便秘 was first used as a disease term in the *Zhong Hua Yi Xue Za Zhi* 中华医学杂志 in 1919.[5,8] Other terms that describe constipation included *da bian nan* 大便难, *bi se* 秘涩, *da bian bu tong* 大便不通, *yang jie* 阳结, *yin jie* 阴结, *pi yue* 脾约, *bian bi* 便闭, *bu da bian* 不大便, *da bian jie* 大便结, *da bian gan zao* 大便干燥, *ge chang bu bian* 鬲肠不便, *shi jiong zhi hou* 时窘之后, *da bian bu li* 大便不利, *da bian ying* 大便硬, *bu geng yi* 不更衣, *feng mi* 风秘, *re mi* 热秘, *leng mi* 冷秘, *xu mi* 虚秘, and *shi mi* 实秘.

## Other Terms

First mentioned in the *Dan Xi Xin Fa* 丹溪心法 (c. 1481), the term *tong xie* 痛泻 describes the concomitant symptoms of abdominal pain and diarrhoea, and their relationship.[5] This term is closely related to the modern disease IBS, although it is not used as a disease name in classical texts. For these IBS-related terms, dictionaries, medical nomenclature, guidelines, journal articles, and theses were consulted to determine a group of suitable Chinese terms for further search in the ZHYD.[5-14] From these sources, along with an investigation of clinical texts for historical usage of IBS-like terms, a comprehensive list of 104 IBS-related classical search terms was developed.

These 104 search terms were tested in a limited pre-search of the ZHYD to assess their accuracy in identifying citations of interest in relation to IBS. A consultation process involving clinical and methodology experts then reviewed these results. The initial list of classical search terms was subsequently reduced from 104 to 21 terms, consisting only of terms considered to be suitable for a comprehensive search of the ZHYD.

The search terms considered to be most relevant to the IBS condition were split into four categories: abdominal pain, diarrhoea, constipation, and a combination of abdominal pain with either diarrhoea or constipation (Table 3.1).

**Table 3.1. Terms Used to Identify Classical Literature Citations**

| Pinyin Abdominal Pain Search Term | Chinese Search Term | Possible Translation/Meaning |
|---|---|---|
| **Abdominal Pain** | | |
| *Fu tong/Fu zhong tong* | 腹痛/腹中痛 | Abdominal pain |
| *Fu man tong/Fu zhong man tong* | 腹满痛/腹中满痛 | Abdominal pain and fullness |
| *Rao qi tong* | 绕脐痛 | Pain around the umbilicus |
| **Diarrhoea** | | |
| *Xie 1/Xie 2/Li/Zhu xia* | 泄/泻/利/注下 | Diarrhoea |
| *Tang* | 溏 | Sloppy stool |
| **Constipation** | | |
| *Mi/ Bian bi/Da bian bu tong/ Yang jie/Yin jie* | 秘/便闭/大便不通/阳结/阴结 | Constipation |
| *Da bian nan* | 大便难 | Difficulty passing stool |
| *Bu da bian* | 不大便 | No stool |
| *Pi yue* | 脾约 | Splenic constipation |
| **Abdominal Pain and Diarrhoea/constipation** | | |
| *Tong xie 1/Tong xie 2* | 痛泻/痛泄 | Abdominal pain and diarrhoea |
| *Tong mi* | 痛秘 | Abdominal pain and constipation |

# Procedures for Data Search, Data Coding and Data Analysis

Each search term was entered into the ZHYD search field: abdominal pain search terms (Group A search terms) were combined with diarrhoea search terms (Group B search terms) or constipation search terms (Group C search terms), and combinations of abdominal pain search terms with either diarrhoea or constipation terms (Group D search terms) were searched independently.

All search results were downloaded into an Excel spreadsheet, and by summing the search results, the total number of identified hits was calculated (Fig. 3.1). Duplicate results identified by multiple search terms were removed. Codes were then allocated based on the type of citation identified, the book it was identified in, and the

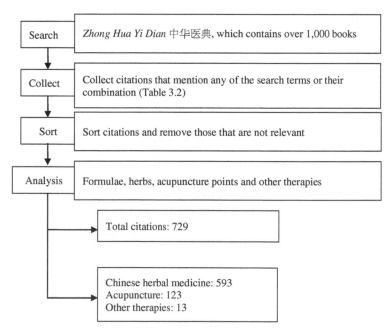

**Fig. 3.1.** Classical literature citations.

dynasty when it was published, according to the procedures described by May and colleagues.[2] Books published after 1949 were excluded.

A "citation" was defined as a distinct passage of text referring to one or more of the mentioned search terms, including treatment for an IBS-like disorder and/or a definition or description of the aetiology or pathogenesis of the condition. When an extended passage referred to multiple treatments, each treatment was recorded and presented as a separate citation.

After removing duplicates, exclusion criteria were applied to remove citations considered to be unrelated to IBS; these included citations not related to IBS, CM dictionary citations, and pharmaco-peia-type entries not related to the treatment of IBS. Citations were also excluded if they did not include a type of CM treatment or provided only a single herb without a description of its use.

Based on the Rome IV IBS diagnosis criteria, the following screening criteria were applied to identify citations unlikely to refer to IBS. This was where the cited condition was:

- Found in infants;
- Related to obstetrics and/or gynaecology;
- Characterised by an acute or sudden onset;
- Related to a surgical procedure; and
- Not IBS-related (such as tumours, intestinal obstruction, liver disease or parasites).

After the screening process, the final dataset consisted only of citations with descriptions of CM treatments (Chinese herbal medicine (CHM), acupuncture and related therapies, or other CM therapies) and considered potentially to refer to IBS. Citations that mentioned abdominal pain and diarrhoea and/or constipation together were considered "possible" IBS citations, regardless of whether they mentioned bloating, stool urgency, borborygmus or tenesmus. Following the Rome IV criteria, citations describing a relationship between abdominal pain and diarrhoea or constipation, as well as a duration of disease longer than three months, were judged and categorised as the group of citations "most likely to be IBS".[4]

Citations judged "possible" and "most likely" to be IBS citations were grouped according to their CM intervention. Data is presented for the frequencies of identified formulae, herbs and/or acupuncture points for "possible" and "most likely" IBS.

## Search Results

A total of 31,244 citations were obtained from the search of the 21 selected IBS terms (Table 3.2). *Li* 利 combined with various terms had the greatest number of hits (11,193), followed by *Xie* 泻 combined with various terms (9,492). When looking at two-word combinations, the terms that had the greatest number of hits were the combination of *fu tong* 腹痛 and *xie 2* 泻 (9136, 29.24%), followed by the

**Table 3.2. Hit Frequencies by Search Term**

| Search Terms | Fu tong 腹痛 | Fu zhong tong 腹中痛 | Fu man tong 腹满痛 | Fu zhong man tong 腹中满痛 | Rao qi tong 绕脐痛 | Hit Frequency (n, %) |
|---|---|---|---|---|---|---|
| Li 利 | 9,081 | 1,478 | 450 | 72 | 112 | 11,193 (35.82%) |
| Xie 2 泻 | 9,136 | 237 | 90 | 6 | 23 | 9,492 (30.38%) |
| Xie 1 泄 | 5,797 | 338 | 79 | 6 | 38 | 6,258 (20.03%) |
| Mi 秘 | 947 | 39 | 15 | 3 | 4 | 1,008 (3.23%) |
| Tang 溏 | 680 | 43 | 28 | 0 | 19 | 770 (2.46%) |
| Bu da bian 不大便 | 179 | 19 | 194 | 9 | 208 | 609 (1.95%) |
| Tong xie 2 痛泄 | N/A | N/A | N/A | N/A | N/A | 587 (1.88%) |
| Tong xie 1 痛泻 | N/A | N/A | N/A | N/A | N/A | 370 (1.18%) |
| Bian bi 便闭 | 272 | 11 | 26 | 1 | 1 | 311 (1.00%) |

*(Continued)*

45

**Table 3.2.** (*Continued*)

| Search Terms | Fu tong 腹痛 | Fu zhong tong 腹中痛 | Fu man tong 腹满痛 | Fu zhong man tong 腹中满痛 | Rao qi tong 绕脐痛 | Hit Frequency (n, %) |
|---|---|---|---|---|---|---|
| Da bian bu tong 大便不通 | 200 | 3 | 19 | 2 | 3 | 227 (0.73%) |
| Da bian nan 大便难 | 121 | 42 | 28 | 7 | 5 | 203 (0.65%) |
| Zhu xia 注下 | 116 | 1 | 6 | 0 | 0 | 123 (0.39%) |
| Yin jie 阴结 | 31 | 4 | 2 | 3 | 0 | 40 (0.13%) |
| Tong mi 痛秘 | N/A | N/A | N/A | N/A | N/A | 30 (0.096%) |
| Yang jie 阳结 | 12 | 1 | 1 | 4 | 0 | 18 (0.058%) |
| Pi yue 脾约 | 4 | 1 | 0 | 0 | 0 | 5 (0.016%) |
| Hit Frequency (n, %) | 26,576 (85.06%) | 2,217 (7.10%) | 938 (3.00%) | 113 (0.36%) | 413 (1.32%) | 31,244 (100%) |

Note: N/A terms did not require combined searches, as they are single phrases.

combination of *fu tong* 腹痛 and *li* 利 (9081, 29.06%) and the combination of *fu tong* 腹痛 with *xie 1* 泄 (5797, 18.55%). The numbers of other single-term and combined-term hits were significantly lower, and for some term combinations, there were no citation hits (Table 3.2).

## Citations Related to Irritable Bowel Syndrome

After reviewing all citations, 307 citations were considered relevant to IBS but did not include CM treatment information, and 729 citations were considered suitable for further analysis (Fig. 3.1).

Among the citations that included CM treatment information, 593 citations mentioned CHM formulae as a treatment for IBS, including 512 citations referring to IBS with predominant diarrhoea (IBS-D), 80 referring to IBs with predominant constipation (IBS-C), and one referring to IBS with mixed bowel habits (IBS-M). Acupuncture-related therapies were mentioned in 123 citations, with 13 mentioning treatment for both IBS-D and IBS-C. Other CM therapies were included in 13 citations — six were associated with IBS-D and seven with IBS-C. Among the included citations, 150 citations were case studies — 137 relating to IBS-D and 13 relating to IBS-C.

Using the judgement criteria for "possible" or "most likely" IBS-relevant citations, 729 citations were classified as "possible" IBS. Of these, 18 were classified as "most likely IBS"; all of the "most likely" IBS citations referred to IBS-D treatment with CHM.

## Definitions, Etiology and Pathogenesis

During the search of classical CM literature, there were no citations that directly corresponded to modern IBS diagnosis criteria. CM refers to IBS according to its most prominent symptoms, such as painful diarrhoea *tong xie 1* 痛泻, *tong xie 2* 痛泄, or painful constipation *tong mi* 痛秘.

When considering the clinical manifestations of IBS in classical texts, some citations described symptoms that resemble those of IBS. For instance, the *Nan Jing* 难经 (c. 220) mentioned "diarrhoea caused by the large intestine is indicated by its occurrence after eating, white stool along with borborygmus and pain"; 《难经·五十七难》中"大肠泄者，食已窘迫·大便色白，肠鸣切痛". Gong Ting Xian in the Ming dynasty wrote in the *Wan Bing Hui Chun* 万病回春 (c. 1587) that "diarrhoea caused by diet would present with diarrhoea with extreme abdominal pain, reduced after defecation and the pulse is string-taut"; 明代《万病回春》记载: "食积泻者, 腹疼甚而泻, 泻后痛减, 脉弦是也". The *Yi Yuan* 医原 (c. 1861, by Shi Shou Tang, Qing dynasty) described symptoms of IBS as "pain in the intestinal tract [that] can be reduced after defecation, tenesmus, stool difficulty, and a lack of smooth *qi* movement can cause constipation"; 《医原·燥气论》曰 "肠中切痛, 痛而后行, 里急后重, 艰涩不通, 行后稍止, 气机终觉不利, 糟粕又或结为燥粪".

Some citations also described potential IBS-like aetiology and pathogenesis, and these citations were much more frequently identified for IBS-D than for IBS-C. In order to find the aetiology and pathogenesis of IBS-C-like symptoms, descriptions in citations involving formulae were also considered for evaluation.

## Definitions and Etiology of Irritable Bowel Syndrome with Predominant Diarrhoea

An irregular diet, emotional upsets, and deficiencies of the Spleen, Stomach and Kidneys can all lead to abdominal pain and diarrhoea.

Irregularity in the diet is recognised as aetiology for IBS-D. The *Ming Yi Za Zhu* 明医杂著 (c. 1502, by Wang Lun, Ming dynasty) stated: "A person who has [an] irregular diet and abnormal lifestyle (e.g., poor sleep/wake cycles) causes damages to Spleen and Stomach. The Stomach then has difficulty receiving and the Spleen [has] difficulty transporting. With an original *qi* weakness, it is easy for external pathogens to attack, there is fullness, oppression and accumulation in the abdomen, urinary and faecal stoppage, vomiting, abdominal pain, diarrhoea and dysentery will occur"; 《明医杂著·枳术丸论》云: "人惟饮食不节, 起居不时, 损伤脾胃. 胃损则不能纳, 脾损则不能化, 脾胃俱损, 纳化皆难, 元气斯弱, 百邪易侵, 而饱闷, 痞积, 关格, 吐逆, 腹痛, 泄痢等症作矣". The *Jin Gui Gou Xuan* 金匮钩玄 (c. 1358, by Tu Zhen Hen, Yuan dynasty) also mentioned that "extreme abdominal pain with diarrhoea, and the pain can reduce after diarrhoea" is caused by food accumulation; 《金匮钩玄·泄泻》云: "腹痛甚而泻, 泻后痛减者, 是食积也". Dietary irregularities can damage the Spleen and Stomach, leading to abnormal Spleen and Stomach transportation functions and diarrhoea.

The effect of emotional disturbance is described in the *Gu Jin Ming Yi Hui Cui* 古今名医汇粹 (c. 1675, by Luo Mei, Qing dynasty), which states that "anger can damage Liver wood and make it stagnated, causing Spleen earth *qi* to sink. From this, there is then vomiting, bloating, diarrhoea, abdominal pain, and difficulty with diet"; 《古今名医汇粹》云: "以怒伤而木郁无伸, 致侵脾土气陷, 为呕为胀, 为泄为痛, 为饮食不行, 此伤阳".

The *Tai Ping Sheng Hui Fang* 太平圣惠方 (c. 992, by Wang Huai Yin, Song and Jin dynasties) states that "Spleen deficiency causes cold, then *yin qi* grows, causing bloating and fullness in the chest and abdomen, food cannot be digested, with belching and acid regurgitation. There is vomiting after eating, *qi* counterflows, cholera, abdominal pain and borborygmus, constant diarrhoea, heavy limbs, anxiety, misophonia and a weak pulse"; 《太平圣惠方 • 治脾虚补脾诸方》云: "夫脾者. 位居中央. 王于四季. 受水谷之精气. 化气血以荣华. 周养身形. 灌溉脏腑者也. 若虚则生寒. 寒则阴气盛. 阴气盛则心腹胀满. 水谷不消. 喜噫吞酸. 食则呕吐. 气逆. 霍乱. 腹痛肠鸣. 时自泄利. 四肢沉重. 常多思虑. 不欲闻人声. 多见饮食不足. 诊其脉沉细软弱者. 是脾虚之候也". This citation describes the pathogenesis of Spleen *yang* deficiency leading to abdominal pain and diarrhoea.

The *Yi Guan Bian* 医贯砭 (c. 1741, Xu Ling Tai, Qing dynasty) states that *Ba wei wan* 八味丸 can treat the symptoms caused by Spleen-Kidney *yang* deficiency; 《医贯砭》: 八味丸 治命门火衰, 不能生土, 致脾胃虚寒, 饮食少思, 大便不实, 下元衰惫, 脐腹疼痛, 夜多漩溺等证. From the *Bu Ju Ji* 不居集 (c. 1739, by Wu Chen, Qing dynasty), it can be surmised that there is potential for the syndrome of Kidney deficiency and heat accumulation in the Spleen to be IBS-related. It states: "The person who has Spleen and Kidney related diarrhoea for more than ten years has symptoms of pre-dawn abdominal pain with diarrhoea, frequent toilet visits (seven to eight times per day), symptoms of tiredness, lack of appetite, etc."; 《不居集 • 治案》 "江应宿治一人, 患脾肾泄十余年, 五鼓初必腹痛, 数如厕, 至辰刻共四度, 巳午腹微痛而泄, 凡七八度, 日以为常, 食少倦怠, 嗜卧. 诊得右关滑数，左尺微弦无力. 此肾虚而脾中有积热病也". Li Yong Cui in the *Zheng Zhi Hui Bu* 证治汇补 (c. 1687, Qing dynasty) describes Kidney-related diarrhoea with symptoms resembling modern IBS criteria, including "abdominal pain just before dawn, diarrhoea with a small sound in the abdomen and cold feet"; 《证治汇补 • 泄泻》曰 "肾泄者. 五更腹痛. 微响乃泄. 必兼足冷".

Spleen deficiency and dampness is another potential IBS-D pathogenesis, with the *Za Bing Yuan Liu Xi Zhu* 杂病源流犀烛 (c. 1773, by Shen Jin Ao, Qing dynasty), stating "Spleen deficiency causing stagnation of the water in the body, leading to diarrhoea, abdominal pain, borborygmus and thirst"; 《杂病源流犀烛·泄泻源流》云: "脾受湿不能渗泄, 致伤阑门元气, 不能分别水谷, 并入大肠而成泻, 故口渴, 肠鸣, 腹痛, 小便赤涩, 大便反快, 是泄固由于湿矣".

## Definitions and Etiology of Irritable Bowel Syndrome with Predominant Constipation

The search of classical texts revealed only a few descriptions of aetiology and pathogenesis that resemble IBS-C (abdominal pain with constipation). Numerous citations describe the single IBS-C symptoms of abdominal pain or constipation. Among the citations describing abdominal pain with constipation, the most frequently mentioned aetiology was the stagnation of dampness, food or a pathogen, and the most frequently mentioned pathogenesis was stagnation in *qi* movement.

In the *You Yu Zhai Yi Hua* 友渔斋医话 (c. 1812, by Huang Kai Jun, Qing dynasty), it is mentioned that food accumulation can cause "abdominal pain, bloating, fullness, constipation and tenesmus"; 《友渔斋医话·上池涓滴一卷》: "伤饮食则病腹痛胀满, 痞闷不安, (脾气滞碍.) 大便或闭或泄, 里急后重, (湿热郁结.)".

In the *Jian Ming Yi Gou* 简明医彀 (c. 1629, by Sun Zhi Hong, Ming dynasty), a citation describes the pathogenesis that heat stagnation can cause "abdominal pain, fullness and hard abdomen that is heavier when pressed, constipation and thirst"; 《简明医彀·腹痛》: "时痛时止, 腹满坚实, 按之愈痛, 口渴, 大便秘结, 脉洪数者, 实热也". Stagnation of dampness is cited in the *Cao Cang Zhou Yi An* 曹沧洲医案 (c. 1924) written by Cao Cang Zhou in the Mingguo period to cause "stagnation of *qi* movement" and that subsequent "abdominal pain and constipation" should be treated by purgation; 《曹沧洲医案·肝脾门》: "湿滞气机胶结, 脘腹痛, 大便闭. 法当疏导下之".

In the *Ye Shi Yi An Cun Zhen* 叶氏医案存真 (c. 1832, by Ye Tian Shi, Qing dynasty), there is a description of a lack of fluid in the Large Intestine leading to symptoms of "abdominal pain with three to four days between defecation that can be reduced with pressure, along with cold limbs and phlegm"; 《叶氏医案存真 • 卷三》云 "痛而喜按属虚, 痰多肢冷, 是脾厥病. 大便三四日一通, 乃津液约束".

The *Cao Cang Zhou Yi An* 曹沧州医案 (c. 1924, by Cao Cang Zhou, Minguo period) describes an IBS-C-like syndrome as "dampness stagnation and *qi* movement stagnation"; 民国 《曹沧州医案 • 肝脾门》 中有一案"左 湿滞气机胶结, 脘腹痛, 大便闭. 法当疏导下之".

# Treatment with Chinese Herbal Medicine

Chinese herbal formulae were the most common therapies for IBS, accounting for 593 citations (81.3%) of the total analysed citations. These 593 citations were then further analysed based on the likely IBS subtype they were referring to. Citations related to IBS-D, IBS-C or IBS-M, are presented separately. For each subtype, where possible, two pools of studies — "possible" IBS and "likely" IBS — are presented, followed by the most frequently cited formulae and herbs for each pool. Where an included citation does not specify the ingredients of a CHM formula, a search was done within the book to identify the formula ingredients and, if available, these CHM ingredients are included in the analyses.

## Chinese Herbal Medicine for Irritable Bowel Syndrome with Predominant Diarrhoea

A total of 512 of the included citations mention CHM treatment for IBS-D, including 18 citations judged "likely" IBS-D. These 512 citations were identified from 153 different books, with 132 of the citations describing clinical treatment cases and all citing the use of an oral form of CHM.

## Frequency of Treatment Citations by Dynasty for Irritable Bowel Syndrome with Predominant Diarrhoea

Books produced in the Ming (c. 1369–1644) (50%) and Qing dynasties (c. 1645–1911) revealed the largest portion of citations (83.4%).

Table 3.3 presents the distribution of citations with treatment information by dynasty. Among the 153 books citing CHM treatments for IBS-D, those with the largest number of citations are: *Pu Ji Fang* 普济方 (c. 1406, n = 48 citations), *Ji Yang Gang Mu* 济阳纲目 (c. 1626, n = 25), *Zheng Zhi Zhun Sheng* 证治准绳 (c. 1602, n = 22), *Za Bing Guang Yao* 杂病广要 (c. 1853, n = 15), and *Lin Zheng Zhi Nan Yi An* 临证指南医案 (c. 1746, n = 12). Eight included citations are from texts published during an unclear period and 20 citations are from texts published in Japan.

The earliest citation related to IBS-D treatment was found in the *Tai Ping Sheng Hui Fang* 太平圣惠方 (c. 992, by Wang Huai Yin, Song and Jin dynasties). The texts include six citations from three different chapters, four of which refer to watery diarrhoea. The earliest citations to describe IBS-D-like clinical treatment cases are in the *Ming Yi Za Zhu* 明医杂著 (c. 1502, by Wang Lun, Ming dynasty). The text includes two cases citing the use of the following CHM: *Ba wei wan* 八味丸 or *Liu jun zi tang jia wei* 六君子汤加味. The most recent case reports are from a text — the *Shao Lan Sun Yi An* 邵兰荪医案 — published during the Minguo period (c. 1912–1949),

**Table 3.3. Dynastic Distribution of Chinese Herbal Medicine Treatment Citations for Irritable Bowel Syndrome with Predominant Diarrhoea**

| Dynasty | No. of Treatment Citations |
|---|---|
| Before Tang Dynasty (before 618) | 0 |
| Tang and 5 Dynasties (618–960) | 0 |
| Song and Jin Dynasties (961–1271) | 33 |
| Yuan Dynasty (1272–1368) | 12 |
| Ming Dynasty (1369–1644) | 256 |
| Qing Dynasty (1645–1911) | 171 |
| Ming Guo/Republic of China (1912–1949) | 12 |
| Others | 20 (Japan)*; 8 (Unclear publication dynasty) |
| Total | 512 |

*CM books published in Japan

which mentions two citations of unnamed CHM formulae, both for the dampness-heat syndrome.

## Most Frequent Formulae in "Possible" Irritable Bowel Syndrome with Predominant Diarrhoea Citations

All but one citation described an oral form of CHM. Four formulae used a single herb, including a topical formula, while others had multiple ingredients. Of the 414 treatment citations describing CHM for IBS-D, 171 CHM formulae are described with distinct names. A total of 98 citations described a combination of herbs without providing a formula name.

The CHM formula *Tong xie yao fang* 痛泻要方 was the most frequently cited (n = 18). The formula name was first cited in the *Yi Xue Zheng Zhuan* 医学正传 (c. 1515, by Yu Bo, Ming dynasty), though this same combination of ingredients was cited earlier but without any attribution. It was found that the same formula combination of herbs was cited using differing names. Fifteen citations named this formulation *Tong xie yao fang* 痛泻要方, two cited the formula name as *Bai zhu shao yao san* 白术芍药散, and one named the formulation as *Fang feng shao yao tang* 防风芍药汤.

Four other CHM formulae were cited by classical texts at least 10 times: *Wei ling tang* 胃苓汤 (n = 16), *Wen pi tang* 温脾汤 (n = 13), *Li zhong tang* 理中汤 (n = 13), and *Sheng yang chu shi tang* 升阳除湿汤 (n = 11) (Table 3.4).

## Most Frequent Herbs in "Possible" Irritable Bowel Syndrome with Predominant Diarrhoea Citations

Seven citations from the 512 "possible" IBS-D citations did not describe formulae ingredients. As details of their ingredients were unclear, they were excluded from herb frequency analyses. There were 3,784 ingredients in the included 505 citations detailing 181 different herbs. Only one of the included formulae cited topical herb use, describing the use of *suan* 蒜, which was not used in the oral formulae.

**Table 3.4. Most Frequent Formulae in Possible Irritable Bowel Syndrome with Predominant Diarrhoea Citations**

| Formula Name | Herb Ingredients | No. Citations (Per Formula Name) |
|---|---|---|
| *Tong xie yao fang/ Bai zhu shao yao san/Fang feng shao yao tang* 痛泻要方/白术芍药散/防风芍药汤 | *Bai zhu* 白术, *bai shao* 白芍, *chen pi* 陈皮, *fang feng* 防风 (*Yi Xue Zheng Zhuan* 医学正传, c. 1515) | 18 (15/2/1) |
| *Wei ling tang* 胃苓汤 | *Chen pi* 陈皮, *hou pu* 厚朴, *cang zhu* 苍术, *gan cao* 甘草, *ze xie* 泽泻, *zhu ling* 猪苓, *bai zhu* 白术, *fu ling* 茯苓, *rou gui* 肉桂, *sheng jiang* 生姜, *da zao* 大枣 (*Yi Fang Xuan Yao* 医方选要, c. 1495) | 16 |
| *Wen pi tang* 温脾汤 | *Hou pu* 厚朴, *gan jiang* 干姜, *gan cao* 甘草, *rou gui* 肉桂, *fu zi* 附子, *da huang* 大黄 (*Pu Ji Ben Shi Fang* 普济本事方, c. 1132) | 13 |
| *Li zhong tang* 理中汤 | *Ren shen* 人参, *gan jiang* 干姜, *bai zhu* 白术, *gan cao* 甘草 (*Shi Yi De Xiao Fang* 世医得效方, c. 1345) | 13 |
| *Sheng yang chu shi tang* 升阳除湿汤 | *Sheng ma* 升麻, *chai hu* 柴胡, *fang feng* 防风, *shen qu* 神曲, *ze xie* 泽泻, *zhu ling* 猪苓, *cang zhu* 苍术, *chen pi* 陈皮, *gan cao* 甘草, *mai ya* 麦芽 (*Ren Zhai Zhi Zhi Fang Lun* (*Fu Bu Yi*) 仁斋直指方论 (附补遗), c. 1264) | 11 |
| *Si shen wan* 四神丸 | *Bu gu zhi* 补骨脂, *rou dou kou* 肉豆蔻, *wu wei zi* 五味子, *wu zhu yu* 吴茱萸, *sheng jiang* 生姜, *da zao* 大枣 (*Ming Yi Zhi Zhang* 明医指掌, c. 1579) | 10 |
| *Fu zi li zhong tang* (*Fu zi bu zhong tang*) 附子理中汤 (附子补中汤) | *Ren shen* 人参, *bai zhu* 白术, *gan cao* 甘草, *gan jiang* 干姜, *fu zi* 附子 (*Mi Chuan Zheng Zhi Yao Jue Ji Lei Fang* 秘传证治要诀及类方, c. 1443) | 10 |
| *Liu jun zi tang jia jian* 六君子汤加减 | *Ren shen* 人参, *bai zhu* 白术, *fu ling* 茯苓, *gan cao* 甘草, *ban xia* 半夏, *chen pi* 陈皮, *sha ren* 砂仁, *mu xiang* 木香 (*Ming Yi Za Zhu* 明医杂著, c. 1502) | 10 |

**Table 3.4.** (*Continued*)

| Formula Name | Herb Ingredients | No. Citations (Per Formula Name) |
|---|---|---|
| *Da yi han wan* 大己寒丸 | *Bi ba* 荜茇, *gan jiang* 干姜, *rou gui* 肉桂, *gao liang jiang* 高良姜 (*Yi Xue Yuan Li* 医学原理, c. 1539) | 8 |
| *Zhu yu duan xia wan* 茱萸断下丸 | *Ai ye* 艾叶, *sha ren* 砂仁, *fu zi* 附子, *rou dou kou* 肉豆蔻, *wu zhu yu* 吴茱萸, *chi shi zhi* 赤石脂, *gan jiang* 干姜 (*Shi Zhai Bai Yi Xuan Fang* 是斋百一选方, c. 1196) | 7 |
| *Ba wei wan* 八味丸 | *Shu di huang* 熟地黄, *shan zhu yu* 山茱萸, *shan yao* 山药, *mu dan pi* 牡丹皮, *fu ling* 茯苓, *ze xie* 泽泻, *rou gui* 肉桂, *fu zi* 附子 (*Ming Yi Za Zhu* 明医杂著, c. 1502) | 7 |

Note:

— In classical literature, formulae with the same name can vary in their ingredients, and the same combination of ingredients may have different names. In this data, formulae with the same name that have variations in a few ingredients are grouped together, while those with large herbal ingredient variations are separated. Also, formulae with the same ingredients but different names are grouped together.

— Formula ingredients are based on the earliest book within the group of included citations.

— The use of some herbs/ingredients may be restricted in some countries or under the provisions of CITES. Readers are advised to comply with relevant regulations.

Variations of *Zingiber officinale* (Willd.) Rosc (n = 312) were the most commonly cited: *gan jiang* 干姜 (n = 195), *sheng jiang* 生姜 (n = 64), and *jiang* 姜 (n = 53). These herbs all have a common action to warm the middle. Other herbs with middle-warming activity were also frequently cited, including *gui* 桂 (n = 122), *fu zi* 附子 (n = 111), and *wu zhu yu* 吴茱萸 (n = 63) (Table 3.5).

Used for regulating *qi*, *chen pi/qing pi* 陈皮/青皮 (n = 236) was the next most frequently cited herb. *Mu xiang* 木香 (n = 127), another *qi* regulating herb, was also frequently cited.

Other frequently cited herbs include those that fortify the Spleen and dry dampness, such as *bai zhu* 白术 (n = 191), *fu ling* 茯苓 (n = 186), *sha ren* 砂仁 (n = 73), and *cang zhu* 苍术 (n = 68); herbs that move *qi* and resolve dampness, such as *hou pu* 厚朴 (n = 133) and

**Table 3.5. Most Frequent Herbs in Possible Irritable Bowel Syndrome with Predominant Diarrhoea Citations**

| Herb Name | Scientific Name | No. Citations (Per Herb Name) |
|---|---|---|
| Gan jiang/sheng jiang/jiang 干姜/生姜/姜） | *Zingiber officinale* (Willd.) Rosc. | 312 (195/64/53) |
| Chen pi/qing pi/ju hong/ju he/ju ye/ju bai 陈皮/青皮/橘红/橘核/橘叶/橘白 | *Citrus reticulata* Blanco | 236 (187/39/7/1/1/) |
| Gan cao 甘草 | *Glycyrrhiza* spp. | 221 |
| Bai zhu 白术 | *Atractylodes macrocephala* Koidz. | 191 |
| Fu ling/chi fu li/fu shen/fu ling pi 茯苓/赤茯苓/茯神/茯苓皮 | *Poria cocos* (Schw.) Wolf | 186 (158/20/4/4) |
| Hou pu 厚朴 | *Magnolia officinalis* Rehd. et Wils. | 133 |
| Mu xiang 木香 | *Aucklandia lappa* Decne. | 127 |
| Rou gui/gui zhi 肉桂/桂/桂枝 | *Cinnamomum cassia* Presl | 122 (100/14/8) |
| Fu zi/wu tou 附子/乌头 | *Aconitum carmichaeli* Debx. | 115 (111/4) |
| Ren shen 人参 | *Panax ginseng* C.A. Mey. | 109 |
| Bai shao/chi shao 白芍/赤芍 | *Paeonia lactiflora* Pall. | 94 (92/2) |
| Rou dou kou 肉豆蔻 | *Myristica fragrans* Houtt | 87 |
| Ze xie 泽泻 | *Alisma orientalis* (Sam.) Juzep. | 78 |
| Da zao 大枣 | *Ziziphus jujuba* Mill. | 75 |
| Sha ren 砂仁 | *Amomum villosum* Lour. | 73 |
| Huang lian 黄连 | *Coptis chinensis* Franch | 73 |
| Cang zhu 苍术 | *Atractylodes lancea* (Thunb.) DC. | 68 |
| Shen qu/jian qu/yun qu/xia tian qu 神曲/建曲/芸曲/霞天曲 | Massa Medicata Fermentata | 67 (61/4/1/1) |
| Ban xia 半夏 | *Pinellia ternata* (Thunb.) Breit. | 65 |
| Wu zhu yu 吴茱萸 | *Evodia rutaecarpa* (Juss.) Benth. | 63 |

Note: The use of some herbs such as *fu zi* 附子 may be restricted in some countries. Readers are advised to comply with relevant regulations.

*ze xie* 泽泻 (n = 78); and herbs that induce diuresis to drain dampness/astringe the intestines and stop diarrhoea, such as *rou dou kou* 肉豆蔻 (n = 87), *he zi/he li le pi* 诃子/诃黎勒皮 (n = 47), and *wu wei zi* 五味子 (n = 24).

The functions of *bai shao* 白芍 for emolliating the liver function and *fang feng* 防风 for expelling wind are commonly prescribed in modern CM clinical IBS therapy. The search of classical texts confirms that they were also historically and commonly used in IBS-D treatments, with *bai shao* 白芍 cited 92 times and *fang feng* 防风 45 times.

## Most Frequent Formulae from "Most Likely" Irritable Bowel Syndrome with Predominant Diarrhoea Citations

In total, 18 citations, including 16 clinical case reports, were assessed as "most likely" IBS-D citations. Fourteen citations mentioned a total of seven different formulae, with the other four citations all describing a combination of herbs but not detailing a formula name. All cited formulae were described as oral formulations.

From the searched classical texts, *Ba wei wan* 八味丸 (n = 4) was the most frequently cited formula. This formula was first cited in the *Jin Gui Yao Lue* 金匮要略 (c. 206). Used for Kidney deficiency, *Ba wei wan* 八味丸 contains *fu zi* 附子, *gui zhi* 桂枝/*rou gui* 肉桂, *shu di huang* 熟地黄, *shan zhu yu* 山茱萸, *ze xie* 泽泻, *mu dan pi* 牡丹皮, *shan yao* 山药, and *fu ling* 茯苓 (Table 3.6). Another common formula, *Si shen wan* 四神丸, is also Kidney-related but is used specifically for kidney *yang* deficiency.

## Most Frequent Herbs from "Most likely" Irritable Bowel Syndrome with Predominant Diarrhoea Citations

In the "most likely" IBS-D citations, 118 herb ingredients were cited. Their ingredients consist of 41 different herbs, with a number of herb function groups noted to be more frequently cited than others. The herbal group most commonly cited was herbs that warm the middle, such as *rou gui* 肉桂 (n = 8), *fu zi* 附子 (n = 6), *jiang* 姜 (n = 5),

**Table 3.6.  Most Frequent Formulae in Most Likely Irritable Bowel Syndrome with Predominant Diarrhoea Citations**

| Formula Name | Herb Ingredients | No. Citations |
|---|---|---|
| *Ba wei wan* 八味丸 | *Shu di huang* 熟地黄, *shan zhu yu* 山茱萸, *shan yao* 山药, *mu dan pi* 牡丹皮, *fu ling* 茯苓, *ze xie* 泽泻, *rou gui* 肉桂, *fu zi* 附子 (*Ming Yi Za Zhu* 明医杂著, c. 1502) | 4 |
| *Si shen wan* 四神丸 | *Bu gu zhi* 补骨脂, *rou dou kou* 肉豆蔻, *wu wei zi* 五味子, *wu zhu yu* 吴茱萸, *sheng jiang* 生姜, *da zao* 大枣 (*Ming Yi Zhi Zhang* 明医指掌, c. 1579) | 3 |
| *Huang lian zhi shi wan* 黄连枳实丸 | *Huang lian* 黄连, *zhi shi* 枳实 (*Gu Jin Yi An An* 古今医案按, c. 1778, reference from *Ming Yi Lei An* 名医类案) | 2 |
| *Huang lian zhi zhu wan* 黄连枳术丸 | *Huang lian* 黄连, *zhi shi* 枳实, *bai zhu* 白术 (*Bu Ju Ji* 不居集, c. 1739, reference from *Ming Yi Lei An* 名医类案) | 2 |
| *La gui ba dou wan* 蜡匮巴豆丸 | *Ba dou* 巴豆, *la* 蜡 (*Xu Ming Yi Lei An* 续名医类案, c. 1770, reference from *Ben Cao Gang Mu* 本草纲目) | 1 |
| *Tian kan tang* 填坎汤 | *Shan zhu yu* 山茱萸, *fu ling* 茯苓, *ba ji tian* 巴戟天, *rou gui* 肉桂, *che qian zi* 车前子, *wu wei zi* 五味子, *ren shen* 人参, *qian shi* 芡实, *bai zhu* 白术 (*Bian Zheng Lu* 辨证录, c. 1687) | 1 |
| *Wu shen dan* 五神丹 | *Shu di huang* 熟地黄, *shan zhu yu* 山茱萸, *wu wei zi* 五味子, *bu gu zhi* 补骨脂, *rou gui* 肉桂 (*Bian Zheng Lu* 辨证录, c. 1687) | 1 |

Note:

— In classical literature, formulae with the same name can vary in their ingredients, and the same combination of ingredients may have different names. In this data, formulae with the same name but with variation in a few ingredients are grouped together, while formulae with significant ingredient variations are separated. Also, formulae with the same ingredients but different names are grouped together.

— Formula ingredients are based on the earliest book within the group of included citations.

— The use of some herbs/ingredients may be restricted in some countries or under the provisions of CITES. Readers are advised to comply with relevant regulations.

and *wu zhu yu* 吴茱萸 (n = 3) (Table 3.7). Herbs that function to tonify the Spleen and dry dampness were also common, such as *fu ling* 茯苓 (n = 6) and *bai zhu* 白术 (n = 5), as well as herbs that tonify the Spleen and replenish *qi*, such as *da zao* 大枣 (n = 5), *shan*

**Table 3.7. Most Frequent Herbs from Most Likely Irritable Bowel Syndrome with Predominant Diarrhoea Citations**

| Herb Name | Scientific Name | No. Citations (Per Herb Name) |
|---|---|---|
| Rou gui 肉桂 | *Cinnamomum cassia* Presl | 8 |
| Fu ling/fu shen 茯苓/茯神 | *Poria cocos* (Schw.) Wolf | 6 (5/1) |
| Fu zi 附子 | *Aconitum carmichaeli* Debx. | 6 |
| Bu gu zhi 补骨脂 | *Psoralea corylifolia* L. | 6 |
| Shan zhu yu 山茱萸 | *Cornus officinalis* Sieb. et Zucc. | 6 |
| Jiang/sheng jiang 姜/生姜 | *Zingiber officinale* (Willd.) Rosc. | 5 (3/2) |
| Mu dan pi 牡丹皮 | *Paeonia suffruticosa* Andr. | 5 |
| Shu di huang 熟地黄 | *Rehmannia glutinosa* Libosch. | 5 |
| Da zao 大枣 | *Ziziphus jujuba* Mill. | 5 |
| Wu wei zi 五味子 | *Schisandra chinensis* (Turcz.) Baill. | 5 |
| Bai zhu 白术 | *Atractylodes macrocephala* Koidz. | 5 |
| Ze xie 泽泻 | *Alisma orientalis* (Sam.) Juzep. | 4 |
| Shan yao 山药 | *Dioscorea opposita* Thunb. | 4 |
| Bai shao 白芍 | *Paeonia lactiflora* Pall. | 4 |
| Huang lian 黄连 | *Coptis chinensis* Franch | 4 |
| Zhi shi 枳实 | *Citrus aurantium* L. | 4 |
| Rou dou kou 肉豆蔻 | *Myristica fragrans* Houtt. | 3 |
| Ren shen 人参 | *Panax ginseng* C.A. Mey. | 3 |
| Wu zhu yu 吴茱萸 | *Evodia rutaecarpa* (Juss.) Benth. | 3 |
| Qian shi 芡实 | *Euryale ferox* Salisb. | 2 |
| Sheng ma 升麻 | *Cimicifuga heracleifolia* Kom. | 2 |
| Huang qi 黄芪 | *Astragalus membranaceus* (Fisch.) Bge. var. *mongholicus* (Bge.) Hsiao | 2 |
| Du zhong 杜仲 | *Eucommia ulmoides* Oliv. | 2 |
| Fang feng 防风 | *Saposhnikovia divaricata* (Turcz.) Schischk. | 2 |

Note: The use of some herbs such as *fu zi* 附子 may be restricted in some countries. Readers are advised to comply with relevant regulations.

*yao* 山药 (n = 4), *ren shen* 人参 (n = 3), and *huang qi* 黄芪 (n = 2). Another frequently cited herb group was herbs utilised to tonify the Kidney, such as *Bu gu zhi* 补骨脂 (n = 6), *shan zhu yu* 山茱萸 (n = 6), *shu di huang* 熟地黄 (n = 5), and *du zhong* 杜仲 (n = 2). It was found that herbs that astringe the intestines and stop diarrhoea, such as *wu wei zi* 五味子 (n = 5), *rou dou kou* 肉豆蔻 (n = 3), and *qian shi* 芡实 (n = 2), were also cited.

## Chinese Herbal Medicine for Irritable Bowel Syndrome with Predominant Constipation

A total of 80 of the included classical text citations mentioned CHM treatment for IBS-C, including 13 clinical case reports. One case report described topical CHM for IBS-C, and the remaining case reports described CHM in oral form. The included citations that were "possible" IBS-C citations were identified from 50 different books.

## Frequency of Treatment Citations by Dynasty for Irritable Bowel Syndrome with Predominant Constipation

Overall, the majority of treatment citations (45%) were from Ming dynasty (c. 1369–1644) (33.75%) and Qing dynasty (c. 1645–1911) books. Among the 50 books that cited "possible" IBS-C CHM treatments, the *Za Bing Guang Yao* 杂病广要 (c. 1853), *Yi Xue Zheng Zhuan* 医学正传 (c. 1515), and *Zheng Zhi Zhun Sheng* 证治准绳 (c. 1602) contained the greatest numbers of CHM treatment citations (n = 4 each). These books were published between c. 206 and c. 1942. There were also seven citations extracted from CM books published in Japan (Table 3.8).

Published during the Dong Han dynasty, the earliest IBS-C CHM treatment-related citation was in the *Jin Gui Yao Lue Fang Lun* 金匮要略方论 (c. 206). The earliest IBS-C clinical CHM case report was found in the *Yi Xue Zheng Zhuan* 医学正传 (c. 1515). This citation described one case and presented the use of three different formulae for different stages of the disease.

**Table 3.8.** **Dynastic Distribution of Chinese Herbal Medicine Treatment Citations for Irritable Bowel Syndrome with Predominant Constipation**

| Dynasty | No. Treatment Citations |
| --- | --- |
| Before Tang Dynasty (before 618) | 1 |
| Tang and 5 Dynasties (618–960) | 0 |
| Song and Jin Dynasties (961–1271) | 3 |
| Yuan Dynasty (1272–1368) | 0 |
| Ming Dynasty (1369–1644) | 27 |
| Qing Dynasty (1645–1911) | 36 |
| Ming Guo/Republic of China (1912–1949) | 6 |
| Others | 7 (Japan)* |
| Total | 80 |

*CM books published in Japan

The most recent classical text citation was a case report published during the Ming Guo period, in the book *Zou Yi Zhong Yi An Xin Bian* 邹亦仲医案新编 (c. 1942). It reported a case of *Pi Yue Zheng* 脾约症 treated first with *Pi yue wan* plus *Wen dan tang* 脾约丸合温胆汤 to relieve symptoms, then with *Bu zhong yi qi tang jia jian* 补中益气汤加减 to treat the disease.

## Most Frequent Formulae in "Possible" Irritable Bowel Syndrome with Predominnat Constipation Citations

Of the 80 citations assessed to be "possible" IBS-C, five citations described a combination of herbs (including one topical administration citation) without details of names for these formulations. The remaining 75 citations were all oral CHM and provided detail of 42 different formulae with names.

Classically the most frequently cited IBS-C treatment formula was *Hou pu san wu tang* 厚朴三物汤 (n = 15), with its earliest mention in the *Jin Gui Yao Lue Fang Lun* 金匮要略方论 (c. 206, by Zhang Zhong Jing, Dong Han dynasty) (Table 3.9). The formula *Da cheng qi tang* 大承气汤 was the next most cited (n = 5). Both were used for excess heat syndrome.

**Table 3.9.  Most Frequent Formulae in "Possible" Irritable Bowel Syndrome with Predominnat Constipation Citations**

| Formula Name | Herb Ingredients | No. Citations |
|---|---|---|
| *Hou pu san wu tang* 厚朴三物汤 | *Hou pu* 厚朴, *da huang* 大黄, *zhi shi* 枳实 (*Jin Gui Yao Lue Fang Lun* 金匮要略方论, c. 206) | 15 |
| *Da cheng qi tang* 大承气汤 | *Da huang* 大黄, *hou pu* 厚朴, *zhi shi* 枳实, *mang xiao* 芒硝 (*Yu Ji Wei Yi* 玉机微义, c. 1396) | 5 |
| *Bei ji wan/Bei ji da huang wan* 备急丸/备急大黄丸 | *Da huang* 大黄, *ba dou* 巴豆, *gan jiang* 干姜 (*Yi Xue Zheng Zhuan* 医学正传, c. 1515) | 4 |
| *Mu xiang wan* 木香丸 | *Mu xiang* 木香, *ding xiang* 丁香, *gan jiang* 干姜, *mai ya* 麦芽, *chen pi* 陈皮, *ba dou* 巴豆, *shen qu* 神曲 (*Yi Xue Xin Wu* 医学心悟, c. 1732) | 3 |
| *San huang zhi zhu wan* 三黄枳术丸 | *Huang qin* 黄芩, *huang lian* 黄连, *da huang* 大黄, *shen qu* 神曲, *bai zhu* 白术, *zhi shi* 枳实, *chen pi* 陈皮, *he ye* 荷叶 (*Yi Xue Xin Wu* 医学心悟, c. 1732) | 3 |
| *Zhi shi da huang tang* 枳实大黄汤 | *Zhi shi* 枳实, *da huang* 大黄, *bin liang* 槟榔, *hou pu* 厚朴, *mu xiang* 木香, *gan cao* 甘草 (*Wan Bing Hui Chun* 万病回春, c. 1587) | 3 |
| *Xiao qi xiang wan* 小七香丸 | *Gan song* 甘松, *yi zhi ren* 益智仁, *xiang fu* 香附, *ding xiang* 丁香, *gan cao* 甘草, *sha ren* 砂仁, *e zhu* 莪术, *jiang* 姜 (*Mi Chuan Zheng Zhi Yao Jue Ji Lei Fang* 秘传证治要诀及类方, c. 1443) | 2 |
| *Shen bao wan* 神保丸 | *Mu xiang* 木香, *hu jiang* 胡椒, *ba dou* 巴豆, *quan xie* 全蝎, *zhu sha* 朱砂 (*Wen Yin Ju Hai Shang Xian Fang* 温隐居海上仙方, c. 1216, reference from *Tai Ping Hui Min He Ji Ju Fang* 太平惠民和剂局方) | 2 |
| *Bu zhong yi qi tang jia jian* 补中益气汤加减 | *Ren shen* 人参, *huang qi* 黄芪, *gan cao* 甘草, *bai zhu* 白术, *chen pi* 陈皮, *dang gui* 当归, *sheng ma* 升麻, *chai hu* 柴胡, *da huang* 大黄 (*Cheng Xing Xuan Yi An* 程杏轩医案, c. 1804)<br>*Ren shen* 人参, *huang qi* 黄芪, *gan cao* 甘草, *bai zhu* 白术, *chen pi* 陈皮, *dang gui* 当归, *sheng ma* 升麻, *chai hu* 柴胡, *fu ling* 茯苓, *ban xia* 半夏 (*Zou Yi Zhong Yi An Xin Bian* 邹亦仲医案新编, c. 1942) | 2 |

**Table 3.9.** *(Continued)*

| Formula Name | Herb Ingredients | No. Citations |
|---|---|---|
| *Hou pu qi wu tang* 厚朴七物汤 | *Hou pu* 厚朴, *da huang* 大黄, *zhi shi* 枳实, *gui zhi* 桂枝, *gan cao* 甘草, *sheng jiang* 生姜, *da zao* 大枣 (*Ping Qin Shu Wu Yi Lue* 评琴书屋医略, c. 1865) | 2 |
| *Huo xiang zheng qi san jia jian* 藿香正气散加减 | *Da fu pi* 大腹皮, *bai zhi* 白芷, *fu ling* 茯苓, *zi su* 紫苏, *huo xiang* 藿香, *hou pu* 厚朴, *bai zhu* 白术, *chen pi* 陈皮, *jie geng* 桔梗, *ban xia* 半夏, *gan cao* 甘草, *sheng jiang* 生姜, *da zao* 大枣, *rou gui* 肉桂, *mu xiang* 木香, *da huang* 大黄 (*Yi Zong Bi Du* 医宗必读, c. 1637) | 2 |
| *Zhu hui dan* 逐秽丹 | *Dang gui* 当归, *da huang* 大黄, *gan cao* 甘草, *zhi shi* 枳实, *mu dan pi* 牡丹皮 (*Bian Zheng Lu* 辨证录, c. 1687) | 2 |

Note:
— In classical literature, formulae with the same name can vary in their ingredients, and the same combination of ingredients may have different names. In this data, formulae with the same name but with variation in a few ingredients are grouped together, while formulae with significant ingredient variations are separated. Also, formulae with the same ingredients but different names are grouped together.
— Formula ingredients are based on the earliest book within the group of included citations.
— The use of some herbs/ingredients may be restricted in some countries or under the provisions of CITES. Readers are advised to comply with relevant regulations.

## Most Frequent Herbs from "Possible" Irritable Bowel Syndrome with Predominant Consitipation Citations

Of the 80 included "possible" IBS-C citations, three citations did not provide details on herbal ingredients as they historically have ingredient variations; thus, they were excluded from further analysis. From the herb data in the remaining 77 included citations, a total of 467 ingredients were identified, consisting of 86 different herbs. Only one citation described topical CHM, using *sheng jiang* 生姜, *cong tou* 葱头, *lai fu zi* 莱菔子, *xiang fu* 香附, and salt.

From the searched texts, the most commonly cited herb was *da huang* 大黄 (n = 56), followed by herb variations on *zhi shi* 枳实

*Citrus aurantium* L. (n = 38). These herbs have the actions to purge or move *qi*. Other herbs with a similar moving function were also frequently cited, such as *hou pu* 厚朴 (n = 31), variations on *chen pi* 陈皮 *Citrus reticulata* Blanco (n = 20), *mu xiang* 木香 (n = 18), *bin lang/da fu pi* 槟榔/大腹皮 (n = 12), *ba dou* 巴豆 (n = 10), and *mang xiao* 芒硝 (n = 9).

Herbs with laxative functions were also frequently cited, such as *dang gui* 当归 (n = 12), *tao ren* 桃仁 (n = 9), and *huo ma ren* 火麻仁 (n = 6). Interestingly, herbs that warm the middle, *jiang* 姜 (n = 24), *ding xiang* 丁香 (n = 6), and *gui* 桂 (n = 6), showed up in IBS-D classical search frequency but were also frequently reported in IBS-C related texts. Similarly, herbs that fortify the Spleen for IBS-D such as *bai zhu* 白术 (n = 13) and *fu ling* 茯苓 (n = 10) were also some of the most frequently cited for IBS-C (Table 3.10).

## Chinese Herbal Medicine for Irritable Bowel Syndrome with Mixed Bowel Habits

One citation mentions CHM treatment for "possible IBS-M" and is found in the book *Pu Ji Fang* 普济方 (c. 1406). The citation listed herbal ingredients that match *Hou pu wan* 厚朴丸 (*hou pu* 厚朴, *chen pi* 陈皮, *gan jiang* 干姜, *fu zi* 附子, *da zao* 大枣) and is described for the treatment of Spleen-Stomach deficiency with cold stagnation.

## Discussion of Chinese Herbal Medicine for Irritable Bowel Syndrome

Through a search of the ZHYD, many citations reference CHM treatments that are possibly for IBS. From these citations, it is recognised that they relate more frequently to a condition more like IBS-D than IBS-C. While there were citations assessed to be most likely IBS-D, there was no such certainty identified for citations in relation to IBS-C. The lack of any IBS-C "likely" citations may be due to classical treatments for constipation, predominantly only cited for emergency use, with chronic constipation symptoms less relevant in the texts.

**Table 3.10.   Most Frequent Herbs from "Possible" Irritable Bowel Syndrome with Predominant Constipation Citations**

| Herb Name | Scientific Name | No. Citations |
|---|---|---|
| Da huang 大黄 | *Rheum palmatum* L. | 56 |
| Zhi shi/zhi qiao 枳实/枳壳 | *Citrus aurantium* L. var. *sinensis* Osbeck | 38 (33/5) |
| Hou pu 厚朴 | *Magnolia officinalis* Rehd. et Wils. | 31 |
| Gan jiang/sheng jiang/Jiang 干姜/生姜/姜 | *Zingiber officinale* (Willd.) Rosc. | 24 (10/9/5) |
| Gan cao 甘草 | *Glycyrrhiza* spp. | 22 |
| Chen pi/qing pi 陈皮/青皮 | *Citrus reticulata* Blanco | 20 (18/2) |
| Mu xiang 木香 | *Dolomiaea soulei* (Franch.) Shih | 18 |
| Bai zhu 白术 | *Atractylodes macrocephala* Koidz. | 13 |
| Bin lang/da fu pi 槟榔/大腹皮 | *Areca catechu* L. | 12 (10/2) |
| Fu ling/chi fu ling/fu shen 茯苓/赤茯苓/茯神 | *Poria cocos* (Schw.) Wolf | 12 (10/1/1) |
| Dang gui 当归 | *Angelica sinensis* (Oliv.) Diels | 12 |
| Shen qu 神曲 | Massa Medicata Fermentata | 12 |
| Ba dou 巴豆 | *Croton tiglium* L. | 10 |
| Ban xia 半夏 | *Pinellia ternata* (Thunb.) Breit. | 9 |
| Mang xiao 芒硝 | Sodium sulfate | 9 |
| Tao ren 桃仁 | *Prunus persica* (L.) Batsch | 9 |
| Huang lian 黄连 | *Coptis chinensis* Franch | 7 |
| Shu di huang/sheng di huang 熟地黄/生地黄 | *Rehmannia glutinosa* Libosch. | 7 (4/3) |
| Huo ma ren 火麻仁 | *Cannabis sativa* L. | 6 |
| Ding xiang 丁香 | *Eugenia caryophyllata* Thunb. | 6 |
| Rou gui/gui zhi 肉桂/桂枝 | *Cinnamomum cassia* Presl | 6 (3/3) |

Note: The use of some herbs may be restricted in some countries. Readers are advised to comply with relevant regulations.

By comparison, citations assessed as "possible" IBS-D were required to only meet the criteria for basic abdominal pain and diarrhoea. For instance, *Tong xie yao fang* 痛泻要方 cites the use for only "abdominal pain" and "diarrhoea" without a description of any other IBS-D-like symptoms. For IBS-C-like citations, it is recognised that very little detail was cited specific to the condition. Common CHM citations such as *Hou pu san wu tang* 厚朴三物汤 detailed only the words "abdominal pain" and "constipation". This suggests classical understandings of IBS focused predominantly on the symptoms of abdominal pain, diarrhoea and constipation.

## Irritable Bowel Syndrome with Predominant Diarrhoea

When comparing "possible" and "most likely" IBS-D citations, considerably fewer "most likely" IBS-D citations were identified. Some of this classical text variation may be explained by a lack of description in citations of disease duration. Only a few clinical case citations described details of disease duration, and based on modern IBS diagnosis criteria, this prevented some citations from meeting the "most likely" IBS-D criteria.

The most frequently cited herbs were quite similar between the "possible" and "most likely" IBS-D citations. Herbs frequently cited by both pools predominantly consist of herbs with actions for warming the middle, tonifying the Spleen, and regulating *qi*.

Of clinical interest, there is significant variation identified between frequent formulae included in both IBS-D-like citation groups. For instance, *Si shen wan* 四神丸 is a formula of interest as the formula was cited frequently in both "possible" and "most likely" IBS-D citations. In the book *Zheng Zhi Zhun Sheng* 证治准绳 (c. 1602, by Wang Ken Tang, Ming dynasty), *Si shen wan* 四神丸 was described for use in the Spleen and Stomach deficiency syndrome, with symptoms of "soft stool, poor appetite or diarrhoea and abdominal pain". The formula consists of *rou dou kou* 肉豆蔻, *bu gu zhi* 补骨脂, *wu wei zi* 五味子, *chao wu zhu yu* 炒吴茱萸, *sheng jiang* 生姜, and *hong zao* 红枣: 《证治准绳·类方》"四神丸 治脾胃虚弱, 大便不实, 饮食不思, 或泄泻腹痛等证. 肉豆蔻(二两) 补骨脂(四两) 五味子(二两) 吴茱萸(浸, 炒一两)上为末, 生姜八两, 红枣一百枚, 煮熟取枣肉和末丸, 如桐子大. 每服五七十丸, 空心或食前白汤送下".

Another formula of interest for IBS-D therapy is *Tong xie yao fang* 痛泻要方. This is the most frequently cited formula in the "possible" IBS-D citations. *Tong xie yao fang* 痛泻要方 was proposed by Liu Cao Chuang and first cited in the *Dan Xi Xin Fa* 丹溪心法 (c. 1481, Ming dynasty) but without a name. Published in the Ming Dynasty, the *Yi Xue Zheng Zhuan* 医学正传 (c. 1515, written by Yu Bo) first detailed the name *Tong xie yao fang* 痛泻要方 for the formulation. In the *Yi Xue Zheng Zhuan*, the citation describes its use for "abdominal pain and diarrhoea". The formula consists of *chao bai zhu* 白术 (炒), *chao bai shao* 白芍(炒), *chao chen pi* 陈皮(炒), and *fang feng* 防风, and the citation detailed that it could be administered as a decoction or pill. The citation also detailed modifications of the formula, with the addition of *sheng ma* 升麻 suggested if a person has diarrhoea for an extended period: 《医学正传·泄泻》治痛泄要方(刘草窗) 白术(二两, 炒) 白芍药(二两, 炒) 陈皮(一两五钱, 炒) 防风(一两) 上细切, 分作八服, 水煎或丸服. 久泻, 加升麻六钱. It should be noted that other citations were found using the same ingredients but under different formula names. For instance, in the book *Jing Yue Quan Shu* 景岳全书 (c. 1624, written by Zhang Jing Yue), the same formulation of ingredients is referred to as *Bai zhu shao yao san* 白术芍药散 and is described as being administered as a powder, decoction or pill.

## Irritable Bowel Syndrome with Predominant Constipation

The most frequently cited herbs for IBS-C-like conditions were herbs with actions for purging or moving *qi*. The most frequently cited formula for IBS-C was *Hou pu san wu tang* 厚朴三物汤. The formula was first mentioned in the book *Jin Gui Yao Lue Fang Lun* 金匮要略方论 (c. 206, by Zhang Zhong Jing, Dong Han dynasty) and described for use with symptoms of abdominal pain and constipation. The formulation consists of *hou pu* 厚朴, *da huang* 大黄, and *zhi shi* 枳实:《金匮要略方论》"痛而闭者, 厚朴三物汤主之. 厚朴三物汤方 厚朴(八两) 大黄(四两) 枳实(五枚)上三味, 以水一斗二升, 先煮二味, 取五升, 纳大黄, 煮取三升, 温服一升, 以利为度". While classical texts frequently cite the formula, the description of its use in disease varied. In the *Jin Gui Yao Lue Xin Dian* 金匮要略心典 (c. 1729, written by You Yi, Qing dynasty), *Hou pu san wu tang* 厚朴三物汤 was cited as moving *qi*: "《金匮要略心典》痛而闭. 六腑之气不行矣. 厚朴三物汤" while in the *Jin Gui Yao Lue Qian Zhu* 金匮要略浅注 (c. 1803, by Chen Nianzu, Qing dynasty), it was cited for the "interior excess and *qi* stagnation" syndrome: 《金匮要略浅注》今腹) 痛而 (不发热. 止是大便) 闭者. (为内实气滞之的证也. 通则不痛. 以) 厚朴三物汤主之.

## Irritable Bowel Syndrome with Mixed Bowel Habits

As only one CHM-related citation was identified to meet "possible" IBS-M criteria, this suggests that a transitional disease relationship between diarrhoea and constipation was classically recognised. However, the extent of the classical understanding of this IBS-M-like disease and its treatment was very limited.

## Treatment with Acupuncture and Related Therapies

Acupuncture and related therapy citations for IBS were screened according to the same methods described for CHM citations. After the removal of duplicates, 123 citations referring to acupuncture and related therapies were included. All were classified as "possible" IBS, with none meeting the sufficient criteria to be assessed as "most likely" IBS. Of these included citations, 13 cited both IBS-D-like and IBS-C-like conditions. All citations were analysed and presented according to their IBS subtype.

## Irritable Bowel Syndrome with Predominant Diarrhoea

A total of 91 "possible" IBS-D citations from 25 books described acupuncture and related therapies. Three of these citations were clinical case reports, 79 citations mentioned the location and function of acupuncture points, and the other nine citations referred only to IBS-D-like symptom treatment.

## Frequency of Treatment Citations by Dynasty for Irritable Bowel Syndrome with Predominant Diarrhoea

Among the 25 books containing citations for IBS-D, the *Pu Ji Fang* 普济方 (c. 1406) and *Zheng Fang Liu Ji* 针方六集 (c. 1618) provided the most acupuncture-related citations (n = 10). All books were published between c. 282 and c. 1937, with the majority of these citations from books produced during the Ming dynasty (c. 1369–1644) (51%) (Table 3.11). Six citations are found in CM books published in Japan.

The earliest acupuncture-related treatment citation was in the book *Zhen Jiu Jia Yi Jing* 针灸甲乙经 (c. 282, by Huang Pu Yi). This earliest citation describes the use of ST36 *Zusanli* 足三里 for symptoms of abdominal pain, diarrhoea, bloating and borborygmus: 《针灸甲乙经》 肠中寒, 胀满善噫, 闻食臭, 胃气不足, 肠鸣腹痛泄, 食不化, 心下胀, 三里主之.

The three clinical case citations were identified to be the same case cited in three different books. All cited the use of moxibustion on CV8 *Shenque* 神阙 for symptoms of abdominal pain, sloppy stool and diarrhoea. The earliest of the books citing this clinical case was the *Zhen Jiu Zi Sheng Jing* 针灸资生经 (c. 1220, by Wang Zhi Zhong, Bei Song dynasty).

**Table 3.11. Dynastic Distribution of Treatment Citations for Irritable Bowel Syndrome with Predominant Diarrhoea**

| Dynasty | No. Treatment Citations |
| --- | --- |
| Before Tang Dynasty (before 618) | 1 |
| Tang and 5 Dynasties (618–960) | 3 |
| Song and Jin Dynasties (961–1271) | 15 |
| Yuan Dynasty (1272–1368) | 7 |
| Ming Dynasty (1369–1644) | 46 |
| Qing Dynasty (1645–1911) | 9 |
| Ming Guo/Republic of China (1912–1949) | 4 |
| Others | 6 (Japan)* |
| Total | 91 |

*CM books published in Japan

## Most Frequent Acupuncture and Related Therapy from "Possible" Irritable Bowel Syndrome with Predominant Diarrhoea Citations

From the search of classical texts, 91 citations were identified for IBS-D acupuncture-related therapy and these described 32 different acupuncture points. Of these included citations, some (n = 28) included details on acupuncture points used for IBS-D. 39 citations mentioned acupuncture, 62 citations mentioned moxibustion, and one citation described the use of acupoint application therapy.

The search results showed that CV8 *Shenque* 神阙 (n = 11) was the most frequently cited acupoint for IBS-D. One citation mentioned acupoint application therapy to CV8 *Shenque* 神阙, three citations mentioned a point but without detailing a specific type of therapy, and the remaining seven citations all described the use of moxibustion for the point.

Two citations mentioned that acupuncture on CV8 *Shenque* 神阙 is contraindicated and it should only be moxibustioned, and two citations of CV9 *Shuifen* 水分 mentioned the same contraindication. This data, however, is contradicted by another citation that detailed the use of acupuncture and moxibustion at CV9 *Shuifen* 水分 for IBS-D without mentioning any contraindication. The next most frequently cited acupoints were ST37 *Shangjuxu* 上巨虚 and BL25 *Dachangshu* 大肠俞 (n = 10), with citations detailing both acupuncture and moxibustion for the point (Table 3.12).

**Table 3.12. Most Frequent Acupuncture Points in Possible Irritable Bowel Syndrome with Predominant Diarrhoea Citations**

| Acupuncture Point | No. Citations |
| --- | --- |
| CV8 *Shenque* 神阙 | 11 |
| ST37 *Shangjuxu* 上巨虚 | 10 |
| BL25 *Dachangshu* 大肠俞 | 10 |
| SP14 *Fujie* 腹结 | 7 |
| BL28 *Pangguangshu* 膀胱俞 | 6 |
| ST39 *Xiajuxu* 下巨虚 | 5 |

**Table 3.12.**   (*Continued*)

| Acupuncture Point | No. Citations |
|---|:---:|
| ST25 *Tianshu* 天枢 | 5 |
| SP8 *Diji* 地机 | 5 |
| CV9 *Shuifen* 水分 | 3 |
| KI6 *Zhaohai* 照海 | 3 |
| BL20 *Pishu* 脾俞 | 3 |
| PC6 *Neiguan* 内关 | 3 |
| LU7 *Lieque* 列缺 | 3 |
| SP4 *Gongsun* 公孙 | 3 |
| SP6 *Sanyinjiao* 三阴交 | 3 |
| ST36 *Zusanli* 足三里 | 2 |
| CV12 *Zhongwan* 中脘 | 2 |
| BL60 *Kunlun* 昆仑 | 2 |
| CV4 *Guanyuan* 关元 | 2 |
| CV5 *Shimen* 石门 | 2 |

## Irritable Bowel Syndrome with Predominant Constipation

A total of 45 acupuncture-related citations were assessed as "possible" IBS-C. These included citations from 20 different classical texts, with 41 of these citations mentioning the location and function of at least one acupuncture point.

## Frequency of Treatment Citations by Dynasty for Irritable Bowel Syndrome with Predominant Constipation

Among the 20 identified classical texts, the *Zheng Fang Liu Ji* 针方六集 (c. 1618, n = 6), *Pu Ji Fang* 普济方 (c. 1406), and *Yi Xue Ru Men* 医学入门 (c. 1575) (n = 5) contained the greatest number of IBS-C treatment citations. These books were published between c. 682 and c. 1896, with the majority of the citations from texts produced in the Ming dynasty (c. 1369–1644) (64%) (Table 3.13).

The earliest treatment citation was in the *Qian Jin Yi Fang* 千金翼方 (c. 682, by Sun Si Miao, Tang dynasty), where it mentioned

**Table 3.13.  Dynastic Distribution of Treatment Citations for Irritable Bowel Syndrome with Predominant Constipation**

| Dynasty | No. of Treatment Citations |
|---|---|
| Before Tang Dynasty (before 618) | 0 |
| Tang and 5 Dynasties (618–960) | 2 |
| Song and Jin Dynasties (961–1271) | 7 |
| Yuan Dynasty (1272–1368) | 1 |
| Ming Dynasty (1369–1644) | 29 |
| Qing Dynasty (1645–1911) | 6 |
| Minguo/Republic of China (1912–1949) | 0 |
| Total | 45 |

*Rong wei si xue* 荣卫四穴 for treatment of "possible" IBS-C symptoms of abdominal pain, constipation and inhibited urination: 《千金翼方》大小便不利, 欲作腹痛, 灸荣卫四穴各百壮, 在背脊四面各一寸. The most recent IBS-C classical text citation was in the *Nei Jing Ping Wen* 内经评文 (c. 1896) written by Zhou Xue Hai and published in the Qing dynasty. The citation described the use of ST39 *Xiajuxu* 下巨虚 for small intestinal disease with symptoms of abdominal pain, constipation and other symptoms: 《内经评文》小肠病者. 小腹痛腰脊控睾而痛. 时窘之后. (窘迫于后阴也)当耳前热. 若寒甚若独肩上热甚. 及手小指次指之间热. 若脉陷者. 此其候也. 手太阳病也. 取之巨虚下廉.

## Most Frequent Acupuncture and Related Therapy from Irritable Bowel Syndrome with Predominant Constipation Citations

Included IBS-C citations cited 17 different acupuncture points. From these citations, 30 described the use of acupuncture-related therapies, 23 mentioned acupuncture, and 29 mentioned moxibustion.

The most frequently cited point in the searched classical texts was BL25 *Dachangshu* 大肠俞 (n = 11) and it was described for use with symptoms of pain around the umbilicus, bloating, constipation and inhibited urination: 《针灸逢源》大肠腧 在十六椎下两旁. 开脊

**Table 3.14. Most Frequent Acupuncture Points in Possible Irritable Bowel Syndrome with Predominant Constipation Citations**

| Acupuncture Point | No. Citations |
|---|---|
| BL25 *Dachangshu* 大肠俞 | 11 |
| KI16 *Huangshu* 肓俞 | 7 |
| BL28 *Pangguangshu* 膀胱俞 | 6 |
| ST36 *Zusanli* 足三里 | 5 |
| ST39 *Xiajuxu* 下巨虚 | 3 |
| KI3 *Taixi* 太溪 | 2 |
| BL57 *Chengshan* 承山 | 2 |
| *Rong wei si qi xue* 荣卫四气穴 | 2 |
| ST40 *Fenglong* 丰隆 | 1 |
| BL60 *Kunlun* 昆仑 | 1 |
| LR3 *Taichong* 太冲 | 1 |
| SP3 *Taibai* 太白 | 1 |
| KI8 *Jiaoxin* 交信 | 1 |
| BL58 *Feiyang* 飞扬 | 1 |
| BL56 *Chengjin* 承筋 | 1 |
| CV5 *Shimen* 石门 | 1 |
| KI18 *Shiguan* 石关 | 1 |

中二寸. (针三分灸三壮)治大小便难. 腰痛腹胀. 绕脐切痛. Other frequently cited acupuncture points were KI16 *Huangshu* 肓俞 (n = 7) and BL28 *Pangguangshu* 膀胱俞 (n = 6) (Table 3.14).

## Discussion of Acupuncture and Related Therapies for Irritable Bowel Syndrome

Only a few citations from the searched classical texts mentioned acupuncture-related therapies for IBS-like symptoms. It is recognised from these citations that each acupoint cited has multiple functions, and no particular acupoint citations were found that specifically treated an IBS-like condition.

Among the included citations, 13 mentioned that the acupoints could treat symptoms of both "possible" IBS-D and "possible" IBS-C.

This suggests that these acupuncture points were likely understood in the past to be able to either stimulate or reduce intestinal peristalsis. One of the acupoints identified with this dual action was BL25 *Dachangshu* 大肠俞, a point in citations related to both IBS-D and IBS-C. The *Gu Jin Yi Tong Da Quan* 古今医统大全 (c. 1556, by Xu Chun Pu, Ming dynasty) described that BL25 *Dachangshu* 大肠俞 can be used for symptoms of "bloating, pain around umbilical, borborygmus, diarrhoea, dysentery and stool difficulty": 明代《古今医统大全·足太阳膀胱经穴图》"提出大肠俞主治"脊强不得俯仰, 腰痛, 腹胀, 绕脐痛, 肠鸣肠癖, 泻痢不化, 大便难". Other two acupoints that can treat both IBS-D-like and IBS-C-like conditions are BL28 *Pangguangshu* 膀胱俞 and BL60 *Kunlun* 昆仑.

## Irritable Bowel Syndrome with Predominant Diarrhoea

High-frequency acupoint citations for IBS-D were generally those along the Spleen, Bladder and Stomach Channels, as well as the Conception Vessel.

The earliest description of "possible" IBS-D was in the *Zhen Jiu Jia Yi Jing* 针灸甲乙经 (c. 282, by Huang Pu Yi), which described ST36 *Zusanli* 足三里 to treat symptoms of abdominal pain, diarrhoea, distension and fullness: 《针灸甲乙经》肠中寒, 胀满善噫, 闻食臭, 胃气不足, 肠鸣腹痛泄, 食不化, 心下胀, 三里主之. However, it should be noted these symptoms do not correspond solely with "possible" IBS-D symptoms and may actually reflect the clinical symptoms of gastroesophageal reflux disease. Classically, this suggests that ST36 *Zusanli* 足三里 may have been used as a treatment for symptoms of IBS-D as well as for other gastrointestinal disease symptoms.

In the book *Zhen Jiu Zi Sheng Jing* 针灸资生经 (c. 1220, by Wang Zhi Zhong, Bei Song dynasty), there was a citation of a clinical case of "pain in the umbilical with diarrhoea" resembling modern IBS-D-like criteria. The citation described moxibustion treatment to the umbilicus and suggested that moxibustion to CV8 *Shenque* 神阙 may be beneficial for the treatment of these IBS-D-like symptoms: 《针灸资生经》予旧苦脐中疼. 则欲溏泻. 常以手中

指按之少止. 或正泻下. 亦按之. 则不疼. 它日灸脐中. 遂不疼矣. 后又尝溏利不已. 灸之则止. 凡脐疼者. 宜灸神阙.

There were few "possible" IBS D citations describing the use of more than one point. A rare multipoint citation was in the *Wan Shi Jia Chao Ji Shi Liang Fang* 万氏家抄济世良方 (Ming dynasty). The citation described the treatment of "abdominal cold pain and diarrhoea" symptoms by moxibustion to CV12 *Zhongwan* 中脘, ST25 *Tianshu* 天枢, CV4 *Guanyuan* 关元, and SP6 *Sanyinjiao* 三阴交: 《万氏家抄济世良方》腹中寒痛，泄泻不止: 灸中脘一穴、天枢二穴、关元一穴、三阴交二穴各七壮.

## *Irritable Bowel Syndrome with Predominant Constipation*

Classical texts most frequently cited IBS-C treatment acupoints from along the Bladder, Stomach and Kidney Channels.

It was noted that the book *Pu Ji Fang* 普济方 (c. 1406) described different points for similar IBS-C-like symptoms. For symptoms of "abdominal pain and constipation", the book cited KI18 *Shiguan* 石关 and BL28 *Pangguangshu* 膀胱俞: 《普济方·针灸》治腹痛. 大便难. 穴石关 膀胱俞, while for "abdominal pain with constipation and inhibited urination", the book cited the use of *Rong wei si xue* 荣卫四穴 with moxibustion: 《普济方·针灸》治大小便不利. 欲作腹痛. 灸荣卫四气穴百壮. 穴在背脊四面各一寸. This suggests that attention was paid in the past to the severity of abdominal pain and accompanying symptoms when selecting points for an IBS-C-like condition.

# Treatment with Other Chinese Medicine Therapies

The search of classical texts identified two other CM therapy types that were "possible" IBS: diet therapy and *Qigong* therapy, described by 13 citations. The citations are from 10 books, with the majority of these citations identified from books produced during the Ming dynasty (c. 1369–1644) (n = 6, 46.15%). Of the included citations, six referred to the treatment of IBS-D and seven to the treatment of IBS-C.

The earliest identified citation for "possible" IBS-C was in the *Zhu Bing Yuan Hou Lun* 诸病源候论 (c. 610, by Chao Yuan Fang, Sui dynasty) and referred to *Qigong* therapy for symptom treatment. Six of the seven IBS-C citations described the use of *Qigong* therapy and the remaining citation detailed diet therapy. Of the *Qigong* citations, four described the same *Qigong* therapy as described in the *Pu Ji Fang* 普济方 (c. 1406, by Zhu Di, Ming dynasty). People were instructed to lie in a supine position, straighten both hands, twist their flanks, inhale through their mouths, and exhale through their noses for a total of 10 times: 《普济方》导 引 法 养生方云, 偃卧直, 两手捻左右胁, 除大便难, 腹痛, 腹中寒, 口纳气, 鼻出气, 温气咽之数十, 病愈 (Table 3.15).

The most recent classical citation treatment referred to diet therapy for "possible" IBS-D in the book *Zheng Zhi Zhai Yao* 证治摘要 (c. 1862, Qing dynasty). All six IBS-D citations described diet therapy, with these made up of four different diets. Three citations mention including wheat noodles in the diet, *Qiao mai mian* 荞麦面, with two of these case reports from the books *Ben Cao Dan Fang* 本草单方 (c. 1633, by Miu Xi Yong, Ming dynasty) and *Xu Ming Yi Lei An* 续名医类案 (c. 1770, by Wei Zhi Xiu, Qing dynasty). Another two citations described the use of *Zhan mi gu chang gao* 粘米固肠糕 and *Zhi fu tong xiao gu zhi li zhang da dou fang* 治腹痛消谷止利胀大豆方. The remaining IBS-D citation detailed the use of ginger, *sheng jiang* 生姜, black bean, *dou chi* 豆豉, and pepper, *hu jiao* 胡椒, in soup.

**Table 3.15. Other Chinese Medicine Therapies in Possible Irritable Bowel Syndrome Citations**

| Subtype of IBS | Other Chinese Medicine Therapies | No. Citations |
|---|---|---|
| IBS-D | Diet therapy | 6 |
| IBS-C | Diet therapy | 1 |
| IBS-C | *Qigong* therapy | 6 |
| Total | | 13 |

Abbreviations: IBS-C, irritable bowel syndrome with predominant constipation; IBS-D, irritable bowel syndrome with predominant diarrhoea.

# Classical Literature in Perspective

Historically in CM, the diagnosis of IBS-like conditions was determined according to the predominant symptoms at onset and clinical presentation. There was no specific condition that was consistently cited that matched modern understandings of IBS diagnosis such as the Rome IV criteria.[4] To best match modern IBS criteria when evaluating texts, IBS-like symptoms from classical texts should be combined to reflect the modern IBS condition (i.e., abdominal pain + diarrhoea/constipation). These symptoms are not definitive of an IBS condition citation but provide some assurance that the citation is for an IBS-like condition prior to further analysis of the citation data.

The chronic nature of IBS contributes to further making it difficult when evaluating classical texts. Modern IBS criteria require specific disease/symptom durations. The majority of included classical text citations from the search did not describe the duration of symptoms. This reduces the certainty that the identified classical IBS-like citations match modern IBS criteria.

More included citations described IBS-D-like disease (82.08%) compared to IBS-C-like disease (17.79%). From the classical text aetiology and pathogenesis descriptions of IBS, historically dietary factors were shown to be an important cause of IBS-like disease. Emotional upsets were cited as a cause, with Liver *qi* depression attacking the Spleen identified as a key pathogenesis pathway for the development of IBS-D-like disease. For IBS-C-like conditions, the predominant aetiology and pathogenesis emerging from the search was Liver *qi* depression.

More than 80% of the included citations described CHM treatment; this suggests that classically CHM treatments were the main method for treating IBS-like disease.

Comparing classical text citations with modern clinical guidelines for CHM treatment of IBS, frequently cited classical formulae for IBS-D are still recommended. Used classically, *Tong xie yao fang* 痛泻要方 is recommended in modern guidelines for the treatment of IBS-D with the Liver depression and Spleen deficiency syndrome.[9] *Si shen wan* 四神丸 and *Fu zi li zhong tang* 附子理中汤 are recommended for the Spleen-Kidney *yang* deficiency syndrome.[9]

For IBS-C, the common classical CHM citations do not match those recommended by modern guidelines. Some possible explanations for this difference may be:

i) Classical prescriptions were differentiated for stronger emerging effects than the less severe IBS-C symptoms commonly seen in modern clinical practice.

ii) The compositions of early prescriptions were relatively simple and intended to treat only the constipation symptom without reference to underlying IBS-like causes. Over time, simple CHM prescriptions have evolved and developed more complexity. Formulae such as *Liu mo tang* 六磨汤[10] and *Ma zi ren wan* 麻子仁丸[9], which are recommended by modern guidelines, are predominantly used for constipation and abdominal distension in the classical texts and contain ingredients such as *Hou pu san wu tang* 厚朴三物汤 cited classically.

iii) The IBS classification criteria continue to develop, including the definition of abdominal pain in Rome IV and the removal of abdominal discomfort.[4] This excludes citations not mentioning abdominal pain and fails to include citations containing only abdominal discomfort. There may be citations excluded during the search that used treatments similar to modern guideline recommendations but were not IBS-specific enough to be identified.

Although some frequently cited prescriptions are not referenced in the modern guidelines, the similarity is recognised between the actions of classically cited and modern recommended herbs for IBS. For instance, both classical and modern texts suggest the use of herbs that regulate *qi*, tonify Spleen, warm the middle, dispel dampness, and purge and astringe the intestines.

Although classical texts differ in their cited prescriptions for subtypes of IBS, they commonly cited the need to regulate *qi*, which is in line with current guideline treatment actions for IBS related to the impacts of Liver *qi* depression on the severity of IBS symptoms.[12]

For acupuncture and related therapies for IBS, the results show some classical acupoints (BL25 *Dachangshu* 大肠俞, BL28

*Pangguangshu* 膀胱俞 and BL60 *Kunlun* 昆仑) were cited to benefit both IBS-C-like and IBS-D-like conditions.

The most frequently cited point — BL25 *Dachangshu* 大肠俞 — for "possible" IBS-C was also a recommended point guideline for IBS-C in *Consensus Opinion of Integrated Traditional Chinese and Western Medicine Diagnosis and Treatment Strategy For Irritable Bowel Syndrome* and *24 Professional 105 Diseases of Chinese Medicine Diagnosis and Treatment Strategy*.[10,11]

From the searched texts, CV8 *Shenque* 神阙 was most frequently cited for the treatment of "possible" IBS-D, but current clinical guidelines do not highlight its use at all for IBS-D. In contrast, other frequently cited points such as ST36 *Zusanli* 足三里, ST25 *Tianshu* 天枢, SP6 *Sanyinjiao* 三阴交, BL20 *Pishu* 脾俞, and CV4 *Guanyuan* 关元 are also recommended points for IBS-D in modern guidelines.[10]

Classically, it appears diet therapy and *Qigong* had some benefits for IBS-like conditions. While diet therapy is mentioned by modern guidelines as a preventive therapy for IBS, it is not described as a treatment therapy.[10] Modern guidelines do not mention *Qigong* as a treatment for IBS, and further exploration is needed to assess whether it has any benefit for IBS.

# References

1. Hu R. (2014) *Zhong Hua Yi Dian* (*Encyclopaedia of Traditional Chinese Medicine*, 5th ed.), Hunan Electronic and Audio-Visual Publishing House, Changsha.
2. May BH, Lu Y, Lu CJ, Zhang AL, *et al.* (2013) Systematic assessment of the representativeness of published collections of the traditional literature on Chinese Medicine. *J Altern Complement Med.* **5(19):** 403–409.
3. May BH, Lu CJ, Xue CCL. (2012) Collections of traditional Chinese medical literature as resources for systematic searches. *J Altern Complement Med.* **18(12):** 1101–1107.
4. Drossman DA. (2016) Functional gastrointestinal disorders: History, pathophysiology, clinical features and Rome IV. *Gastroenterology.* **150(6):** 1262–1279.e2.
5. 黄绍刚, 黄穗平. (2014) *专病专科中医古今证治通览*. 中国中医药出版社, 中国北京.

6. 李永红, 严季澜. (2008) 腹痛病名考. *吉林中医药*. **28(6):** 462–464.

7. 杨照坤. (2008) 泄泻病证的古今文献研究与学术源流探讨. 北京中医药大学.

8. 张海鹏. (2008) 便秘病证的古今文献研究与学术源流探讨. 北京中医药大学.

9. 中华中医药学会脾胃病分会. (2017) 肠易激综合征中医诊疗专家共识意见. *中医杂志*. **58(18):** 1615–1620.

10. 中国中西医结合学会消化系统疾病专业委员会. (2011) 肠易激综合征中西医结合诊疗共识意见. *中国中西医结合杂志*. **31(5):** 587–590.

11. 国家中医药管理局. (2011) 24个专业105个病种中医诊疗方案 (试行). 国家中医药管理局医政司.

12. 张声生, 沈洪, 王垂杰, 唐旭东. (2016) *中华脾胃病学*. 人民卫生出版社, 北京.

13. 李经纬, 余瀛鳌, 蔡景峰, *et al.* (2005) *中医大辞典* (第二版). 人民卫生出版社, 中国北京.

14. 林昭庚. (2002) *中西医病名对照*. 人民卫生出版社, 中国北京.

# 4

# Methods for Evaluating Clinical Evidence

## OVERVIEW

This chapter describes the methods used to identify and evaluate a range of Chinese medicine interventions for irritable bowel syndrome in clinical studies. Studies identified through a comprehensive search were assessed against eligibility criteria. A review of the methodological quality of the studies was undertaken using standardised methods. Results from the included studies were evaluated to provide an estimate of the effects of a range of Chinese medicine therapies.

## Introduction

The use of Chinese medicine (CM) for irritable bowel syndrome (IBS) has been well described in contemporary literature and has historical evidence from classical CM literature. There is clinical evidence investigating CM use in clinical studies, and a number of systematic reviews have been published evaluating the efficacy and safety of CM therapies, such as Chinese herbal medicine (CHM), acupuncture, moxibustion and other CM therapies for IBS (see Chaps. 5 and 7).

This chapter describes the methods used to evaluate the clinical studies presented in the following chapters. Studies were evaluated for efficacy and safety following the methods from the *Cochrane Handbook of Systematic Reviews* and examined the efficacy and safety of CM interventions for IBS in clinical studies.[1] Interventions have been categorised as follows:

- Chinese herbal medicine (CHM) (Chap. 5);
- Acupuncture-related and other CM therapies (Chap.7);
- Combination CM therapies (Chap. 8).

References to clinical trials were obtained and assessed by an expert group. Randomised controlled trials (RCTs) and non-randomised controlled clinical trials (CCTs) were evaluated in detail. CCTs were evaluated using the same approach as RCTs and have been described separately. Evidence from non-controlled studies is more difficult to evaluate; therefore, the approach was taken to describe the characteristics of the study, details of the intervention, and any adverse events. References to included studies are indicated by a letter followed by a number. Studies of CHM are indicated by "H" (e.g., H1), studies of acupuncture and related therapies by "A" (e.g., A1), studies of other CM therapies by "O" (e.g., O1), and studies of combinations of CM therapies by "C" (e.g., C1; see Table 4.1).

## Search Strategy

Evidence was searched for in English- and Chinese-language databases, and the methods followed the *Cochrane Handbook of*

**Table 4.1. Chinese Medicine Interventions Included in Clinical Evidence Evaluation**

| Category | Intervention |
|---|---|
| Chinese herbal medicines | Oral CHM, topical CHM |
| Acupuncture and related therapies | Acupuncture, ear acupuncture, ear acupressure, electroacupuncture, moxibustion, transcutaneous electrical nerve stimulation (TENS) |
| Other Chinese medicine therapies | *Ba duan jin* (*Qigong*) therapy八段錦 |
| Combination Chinese medicine | Defined as two or more Chinese medicine interventions from different categories administered together, e.g., CHM plus acupuncture |

Abbreviations: CHM, Chinese herbal medicine.

*Systematic Reviews.*[1] English-language databases were PubMed, Excerpta Medica Database (Embase), Cumulative Index of Nursing and Allied Health Literature (CINAHL), Cochrane Central Register of Controlled Trials (CENTRAL), including the Cochrane Library, and Allied and Complementary Medicine Database (AMED). The Chinese-language databases were China BioMedical Literature (CBM), China National Knowledge Infrastructure (CNKI), Chongqing VIP (CQVIP), and Wanfang. Databases were searched from inception to February 2017. No restrictions were applied. Search terms were mapped to controlled vocabulary (where applicable) in addition to being searched as keywords.

To conduct a comprehensive search of the literature, searches were run according to the study design (reviews, controlled trials, non-controlled studies). This was done for each of the three intervention types (CHM, acupuncture and related therapies, and other CM therapies), resulting in nine searches in each of the nine databases:

1. CHM reviews;
2. CHM controlled trials (randomised and non-randomised);
3. CHM non-controlled studies;
4. Acupuncture and related therapies reviews;
5. Acupuncture and related therapies controlled trials (randomised and non-randomised);
6. Acupuncture and related therapies non-controlled studies;
7. Other CM therapies reviews;
8. Other CM therapies controlled trials (randomised and non-randomised); and
9. Other CM therapies non-controlled studies.

Studies of combination CM therapies were identified through the above searches. In addition to electronic databases, reference lists of systematic reviews and included studies were searched for additional publications. Clinical trials registries were searched to identify ongoing or completed clinical trials, and where required, trial investigators were contacted to obtain data. The searched trial registries were the Australian New Zealand Clinical Trial Registry (ANZCTR), Chinese Clinical Trial Registry (ChiCTR), European Union Clinical Trials Register (EU-CTR), and US National Institutes of Health Register (ClinicalTrials.gov).

Where required, trial investigators were contacted to obtain further information. Trial investigators were contacted by email or telephone and were followed up after two weeks if no reply was received. Where no response was received after one month, any unknown information was marked as not available.

## Inclusion Criteria

- Participants: Study subjects diagnosed with IBS using any of the Rome criteria (I–IV) and who had any IBS subtype, including IBS with predominant constipation (IBS-C), IBS with predominant diarrhoea (IBS-D), IBS with mixed bowel habits (IBS-M), and IBS-unspecified (IBS-U) type.[2–6]
- Interventions: CHM, acupuncture and related therapies, other CM therapies or combination of CM therapies (see Table 4.1); integrative medicine such as CHM plus pharmacotherapy was also investigated.
- Comparators: No treatment or waitlist controls, sham/placebo or conventional treatment recommended in clinical practice guidelines.[7–11] These include muscle relaxants, antispasmodic, tricyclic antidepressants, serotonin-norepinephrine reuptake inhibitors, selective serotonin reuptake inhibitors, probiotics, anticholinergics, anti-diarrhoeal (motility) agents, Cholestyramine, 5-HT3 antagonist mucosal epithelium modifiers, 5-HT4 agonists, laxatives, cognitive behaviour therapy, psychotherapy, hypnotherapy, mindfulness therapy, exercise program, low fermentable oligo-di-monosaccharide and polyol (FODMAP) diet, fibre supplements, and anti-allergic diet.
- Outcome measures: Studies reported at least one of the pre-specified outcome measures (Table 4.2).

Table 4.2.    Pre-specified Outcomes

| Outcome Categories | | Outcome Measures | Scoring |
|---|---|---|---|
| Irritable bowel syndrome (IBS) symptom outcomes | Overall condition severity | Adequate relief[17] | Yes/No (total effective rate), a higher score is better |
| | | IBS Severity Scoring Symptom (IBS-SSS)[18] | Score: 0–500, a lower score is better<br>Total effective rate (TER): Number of cases, a higher score is better |
| | | Birmingham IBS Symptom Questionnaire[19] | 0–55, a lower score is better |
| | Stool form | Bristol Stool Form Scale[20] | 1–7 types<br>Score: Dependent on measure<br>TER: Number of cases, a higher score is better. |
| | Stool form and frequency | Based on guidelines[13,21] | Score: Dependent on the measure, a lower score is better<br>TER: Number of cases, a higher score is better |
| | Frequency of stool movements | Complete Spontaneous Bowel Movement (CSBM) | Times per week, used for IBS-C only, an increasing number is better |
| | | Number per week/per day | An increasing number is better for IBS-C and a decreasing number is better for IBS-D |
| | | Based on guidelines diagnosis and treatment strategy for IBS, 2010[22] or 22 professional 95 diseases of CM diagnosis and treatment strategy, 2010[23] | Score: Dependent on measure, a lower score is better<br>TER: Number of cases, a higher score is better |

*(Continued)*

**Table 4.2.** (*Continued*)

| Outcome Categories | Outcome Measures | Scoring |
|---|---|---|
| Pain/ discomfort/ bloating | Visual Analogue Scale (VAS)[24] | 0–100 mm, a lower score is better |
| | Numerical Rating Scale (NRS)[25] | 0–10, a lower score is better |
| | TER improvement | Number of cases, a higher score is better |
| Health-related quality of life | Short-Form Health Survey (SF-36)[26] | 0–100 per domain, a higher score is better |
| | IBS-Quality of Life (IBS-QOL)[27] | 0–100, score direction dependent on the measure |
| | IBS Quality of Life (IBSQOL)[28] | 0–100, a higher score is better |
| | Other IBS QOL if available[29] | Dependent on the measure |
| Psychological state | Hamilton Anxiety Rating Scale (HAMA)[30] | 0–56, a lower score is better |
| | Hamilton Rating Scale for Depression (HRSD)[31] | Score range dependent on version, a lower score is better |
| | Zung Self-rating Anxiety Scale (SAS)[32] | 25–100, a lower score is better |
| | Zung Self-rating Depression Scale (SDS)[33] | 25–100, a lower score is better |
| | Hospital Anxiety and Depression Scale (HADS)[34] | 0–21 for anxiety, 0–21 for depression, a lower score is better |
| Recurrence rate | Number of cases | A lower score is better |
| Adverse events | Frequency, severity and type of adverse events | |

## Exclusion Criteria

- Study type: Epidemiological studies, studies that compared CM therapy to other CM therapies and duplicated studies reporting the same results;
- Participants: Inflammatory bowel syndrome, obstructive bowel syndrome, chronic idiopathic constipation, opioid-induced constipation;
- Intervention: CM interventions not commonly practised worldwide and CM intravenous interventions;
- Comparators: Control not routinely recommended for chronic cough in international clinical practice guidelines or no treatment control; control therapies that included any type of CM therapy; integrative medicine studies that used different therapies in the intervention group compared to the control group.

## Outcomes

The most recent published regional clinical guidelines and previously published Cochrane systematic reviews were consulted to determine included outcomes. Outcomes were considered and determined by clinical experts and pre-specified prior to study selection.

To date, no objective measurables such as blood tests have been developed to measure the severity of IBS, so clinicians need to rely on patients' subjective reporting when evaluating changes to condition severity. There has been discussion around the need for the development and introduction of a multidimensional outcome measure for IBS that broadly encompasses the IBS health burden.[12] No standardised patient-reported outcome measure for IBS has been widely agreed upon, and a variety of outcome measures are used clinically in research for reporting IBS symptom changes and changes to the quality of life.[13,14]

The Rome group established that IBS severity is a biopsychosocial composite of gastrointestinal symptoms, degree of disability, and illness-related perceptions and behaviours of sufferers.[15] It is well established that psychological and physiological symptoms impact people with IBS, such that when the severity of either changes, so does the other.[16] Clinically, this requires observation and measurement of physical symptoms, psychological symptoms, and quality of life. Outcome measures included for further evaluation, therefore, were outcomes for: (1) clinical symptoms, (2) health-related quality of life and psychological state, (3) longer-term IBS recurrence, and (4) safety (Table 4.2).

# Clinical Symptom Outcomes

## Overall Condition Severity

Adequate relief: A binary yes/no measure of improvement in overall IBS symptoms or a subtype predominant symptom with the end point of "adequate relief" (Rome foundation Committee)[35,36] or "satisfactory relief".[37]

IBS Severity Scoring System (IBS-SSS): Consists of five items, including (1) severity of abdominal pain, (2) frequency of abdominal pain, (3) distension, (4) satisfaction of stool frequency and consistency, and (5) interference with life in general. The response for the frequency of abdominal pain is scored for days with pain in the last 14 days, and then multiplied by 100. Responses for other items are scored using the Visual Analogue Scale (VAS) (0–100) with a maximum score of 100 possible for each question. The total possible score range is 0–500. Increasing score corresponds with increasing IBS severity.[18]

Birmingham IBS Symptom Questionnaire: A self-administered 11-item symptom scale based on Rome II criteria scored on a 6-point Likert scale, with responses for the previous four weeks (0 = "none of the time" to 5 = "all the time"). Increasing scores indicate more severe conditions, and scores from the 11 items can be pooled into three domains for the evaluation of change to specific symptom dimensions (pain = 3 items, constipation = 3 items, and diarrhoea = 5 items).[19]

## Stool Form and Frequency of Stool Movements

The US Food and Drug Administration (FDA) recommends evaluating abnormal defecation in IBS, with consideration given to the form of stool from bowel motions[13] and frequency of bowel motions resulting in stools.[13]

Bristol Stool Form Scale: A scale that provides visual images and written descriptions for the classification of the form of stools. Stools can be classified into one of seven types, with types 3 and 4 recognised as normal stools. Stool types 1 and 2 are recognised to indicate constipation, with type 1 indicating greater severity, and types 5–7 to indicate diarrhoea, with the higher number type indicating greater severity.[20]

Number per week or per day: The total number of bowel movements per day or week.[13]

Complete spontaneous bowel movement (CSBM): A study assessing IBS-C can also present the total number of CSBMs per week when calculating the total number of bowel motions.[13]

Total effective rate (TER) and scores from guidelines: The FDA recommends trials to report some form of TER (or responder rate), with criteria described clearly as to what defines an effective responder.[13]

Effective rates from guidelines: The number of responders defined by criteria detailed clearly in clinical guidelines that describe whether the treatment had any benefits due to the study intervention/control.

Score from guidelines: The total score of a single symptom defined by the criteria detailed clearly in guidelines.

The scoring methods from guidelines can be used for both effective rates and scores for single symptoms.

All included TERs and scores for the frequency of stool motion are used for IBS-D per day frequency and for IBS-C per week frequency. The scoring systems for stool form and the frequency scoring methods for IBS-D and IBS-C are different in different guidelines, as summarised in Table 4.3. However, the cutoff TER in each guideline is the same, and "effective" means at least one level of improvement.

## Pain/Discomfort/Bloating

Visual Analogue Scale (VAS): A measure that uses a 100 mm horizontal line. For measurement of pain, the higher end of this scale is

**Table 4.3.    Treatment Effective Rate for Irritable Bowel Syndrome Subtypes**

| IBS Subtype | Mild | Moderate | Severe | Reference |
|---|---|---|---|---|
| IBS-D | Fewer than 3 movements per day | 4–5 movements per day | More than 6 movements per day | 22, 23 |
| | Stools are shaped and passing 3–4 times per day | Loose stools and passing 5–10 times per day | Watery stools and passing more than 10 times per day | 21 |
| | Stools are a bit loose and passing fewer than 3 times per day | Sloppy stools and passing 4–5 times per day | Diarrhoea with mucus plus passing more than 6 times per day | 38, 39 |
| IBS-C | More than 3 movements per week | One to 2 movements per week | Less than once per week | 22, 23 |
| | Dry stools, not taking much time to defecate, once each 3 days | Dry and some time is needed to defecate, once each 4–6 days | Dry hard stools and needing time to defecate, once each 7 days | 39 |

Abbreviations: IBS-C, irritable bowel syndrome with predominant constipation; IBS-D, irritable bowel syndrome with predominant diarrhoea.

associated with increasing severity of pain, and the lower end is a decrease in reported pain severity. The result on the scale is measured and recorded according to the number of mm along the scale where the response lies.[24]

Numerical Rating Scale (NRS): An 11-point scale (0–10) is the most common; however, other number scales are possible. For pain, an increasing score on the scale is indicative of increasing severity, and a score of zero would indicate there is no pain.[25]

Effective rate: The number of responders is defined by any TER criteria detailing clearly where their cut-offs for effective and ineffective response were, with at least one level of improvement.

# Health-related Quality of Life

Short-Form 36 (SF-36): A 36-item instrument that surveys the quality of life generically based on self reported health status. The items use a combination of Likert and dichotomous "yes/no" scales to come up with scores for eight different domains of health (physical functioning, bodily pain, role limitations due to physical health problems, role limitations due to personal or emotional problems, general mental health, social functioning, vitality, and general health perceptions). The eight domains can be summarised as two measures: A physical component summary scale and a mental component summary scale. Reported health transitions cannot be merged with others or scored. Scoring typically uses one of two methods, the Medical Outcomes Study method or the RAND method.[42] The scoring directions of some Likert scales are reversed, so a scoring key is applied to responses. Each item can have a score of 0 to 100 — a total higher score indicates better health quality. Items in the same domain are then averaged together to create a score for each domain.[26]

Irritable Bowel Syndrome-Quality of Life (IBS-QOL): A 34-item self-reported instrument that measures the quality of life specifically related to IBS. The instrument uses a five-point Likert scale. The value for each item is totalled and averaged for a total score. This score is then converted to a scale of 0 to 100. Subscale scores can be calculated for similar items pooled into one of eight domains (dysphoria, interference with activity, body image, health worry, food avoidance, social reaction, sexual, and relationships).[27] There are different scoring methods in different countries when using this scale, so the score direction depends on the measurement.

Another instrument with a similar name has also been published and is referred to as the Irritable Bowel Syndrome Quality of Life Questionnaire (IBSQOL) rather than IBS-QOL. It is a 30-item scale and also uses a Likert scale with scores transformed to a 0–100 scale, with an increasing value indicating a better quality of life. Item values are grouped into nine domains and the mean score is calculated for each domain (emotional health, mental health, sleep, energy, physical functioning, diet, social role, physical role, and sexual relations).[28]

Other quality-of-life outcome measures for IBS: There are many different scales used to evaluate the quality of life of IBS, as there is no one scale used by consensus. Therefore, we only included scales commonly used clinically in this monograph.[29]

## Psychological State

Hamilton Anxiety Rating Scale (HAMA): A 14-item instrument describing symptoms and measures for anxiety. Each item is scored on a five-point Likert scale (0 = "not present", to 4 = "very severe"). The score for each item is totalled with a maximum possible score of 56 and a minimum of zero. A decreasing score corresponds with decreasing severity of anxiety.[30]

Hamilton Rating Scale for Depression (HRSD): A number of versions of the instrument are available as it has been revised a number of times; the original version contains 17 items, and the others contain 7,[41] 21,[42] 24[43] and 29[44] items. Most versions use the first 17 items when calculating the total score. Each item uses either a three-point or five-point Likert scale, with a decreasing score corresponding with a decreased severity of depression. A total score is calculated and reported for an overall depression rating.[31]

Zung Self-rating Anxiety Scale (SAS): A 20-item self-administered instrument measuring anxiety levels. It uses a four-point Likert scale from 1 ("none" or "a little of the time") to 4 ("most of the time"). An index for the SAS is derived by dividing the sum of the values (raw scores) obtained on the 20 items by the maximum possible score of 80, converting to a decimal and multiplying by 100. A total score can range 25–100, with increasing score corresponding with an increasing severity of anxiety.[32]

Zung Self-rating Depression Scale (SDS): A 20-item self-administered instrument measuring depression status. It uses a four-point Likert scale from 1 ("a little of the time") to 4 ("most of the time"). An index for the SDS was derived by dividing the sum of the values (raw scores) obtained on the 20 items by the maximum possible score of 80, converting to a decimal and multiplying by 100. A total score can range from 25 to 100, with an increasing score corresponding with the increasing severity of depression.[33]

Hospital Anxiety and Depression Scale (HADS): A 14-item instrument consisting of two sections. The first section contains seven items related to anxiety, and the second section, seven items related to depression. Each item is scored on a four-point Likert scale (0–3), with higher numbers on the scale indicating higher symptom frequency. Scores for each of the two sections can range from 0 to 21. Higher scores indicate higher levels of distress from anxiety or depression.[34]

## Recurrence Rate

Calculation of the recurrence rate can vary depending on the severity of the included participant cohort, and there is no recognised standard method for IBS, although some guidelines provide guidance.[13,45]

## Adverse Events

Information about the nature, severity and number of adverse events can assist in the assessment of the safety of an intervention in the study population.[46]

## Risk of Bias Assessment

The risk of bias was assessed for RCTs using the Cochrane Collaboration's tool.[1] In clinical trials, bias can be categorised as selection bias, performance bias, detection bias, attrition bias, and reporting bias. Each domain is assessed to determine whether the bias is of a "low", "high" or "unclear" risk. A "low" risk of bias indicates that bias is unlikely, while a "high" risk indicates plausible bias, which seriously weakens confidence in the results. An unclear bias indicates a lack of information or uncertainty over potential bias and raises some doubt about the results. The risk of bias assessment is verified by two persons, and disagreements are resolved by discussion or consultation with a third person.

The risk of bias is categorised using the following six domains:

- Sequence generation: The method used to generate the allocation sequence is given in sufficient detail to allow an assessment of whether it should produce comparable groups. "Low" risk of bias refers to a random number table or computer random generator. "High" risk of bias includes studies that describe non-random sequence generation such as an odd or even date of birth or date of admission.
- Allocation concealment: The method used to conceal the allocation sequence is given in enough detail to determine whether intervention allocations could have been foreseen before or during enrolment. "Low" risk of bias includes central randomisation or sealed envelopes, and "high" risk of bias includes open random sequence, etc.
- Blinding of participants and personnel: Measures used to describe whether the study participants and personnel were blind to the intervention received. In addition, information relating to whether the blinding was effective is also assessed. Studies that ensure blinding of participants and personnel are at "low" risk of bias. If a study is not blind or incompletely blind, it is at a "high" risk of bias.
- Blinding of outcome assessors: Measures used to describe whether the outcome assessors were blind to the knowledge of which intervention a participant received. In addition, information relating to whether the blinding was effective is also assessed. Studies that ensure the blinding of outcome assessors are at "low" risk of bias. If a study is not blind or incompletely blind, it is at a "high" risk of bias.
- Incomplete outcome data: Completeness of outcome data for each main outcome, including dropouts, exclusions from the analysis with numbers missing in each group, and reasons for dropouts and exclusions. Studies with a "low" risk of bias include all outcome data or, if there is missing data, it is unlikely to relate to the true outcome or is balanced between groups. Studies at "high" risk of bias have unexplained missing data.

- Selective reporting: The study protocol is available and the pre-specified outcomes are included in the report. Studies with a published protocol that also include all pre-specified outcomes in their reports are at "low" risk of bias. Studies at "high" risk of bias do not include all pre-specified outcomes, or the outcome data is reported incompletely.

## Statistical Analyses

Frequency of CM syndromes, CHM formulae, herbs and acupuncture points reported in included studies are presented using descriptive statistics. CM syndromes reported in two or more studies are presented. The 10 most frequently reported CHM formulae and 20 most frequently reported herbs are presented where used in at least two studies, although for CHM formulae this was not always possible. The top 10 acupuncture points used in two or more studies are presented where available. Where data was limited, reports of single CM syndromes or acupuncture points are provided as a guide for the reader.

Definitions of statistical tests and results are described in the glossary. Dichotomous data is reported as the risk ratio (RR) with a 95% confidence interval (CI), while continuous data is reported as the mean difference (MD) or standardised mean difference (SMD) with a 95% CI. For dichotomous data, when the RR is greater than 1 and the upper and lower values of the 95% CI are both greater than 1, this indicates that we can be 95% certain that there is a difference between the groups and the true effect lies within these CIs. The same is true for values less than 1. In such cases, we say there is a "significant difference" between the groups. For continuous data, when the MD is greater than zero and both the upper and lower values of the 95% CI are greater than zero, we also say there is a "significant difference" between the groups. The same is true on the negative side of the scale.[1] For all analyses, RR or MD and a 95% CI are reported, together with a formal test for heterogeneity using the $I^2$ statistic. An $I^2$ score greater than 50% was considered to indicate substantial heterogeneity.[1]

Sensitivity analyses were undertaken to explore potential sources of heterogeneity based on a "low" risk of bias for one of the risk of bias domains, sequence generation. Where possible and appropriate, planned subgroup analyses are included, along with CM syndromes, CM formulae, and comparator type. Available case analysis with a random effects model was used in all analyses. The random effects model was used to take into account the clinical heterogeneity likely to be encountered within and between included studies and the variation in treatment effects between included studies.

## Assessment Using Grading of Recommendations Assessment, Development and Evaluation

The Grading of Recommendations Assessment, Development and Evaluation (GRADE) approach was used.[47] The GRADE approach summarises and rates the quality of evidence in systematic reviews using a structured process for presenting evidence summaries. The results are presented in summary-of-findings tables.

A panel of experts was established to evaluate the quality of evidence. The panel included the systematic review team, CM practitioners, integrative medicine experts, research methodologists, and conventional medicine physicians. The experts were asked to rate the clinical importance of key interventions from CHM, acupuncture therapies and other CM therapies, as well as comparators and outcomes. Results were collated and based on the rating scores and subsequent discussion, and a consensus on the content for the summary-of-findings tables was achieved.

The quality of evidence for each outcome was rated according to five factors outlined in the GRADE approach. The quality of evidence may be rated based on:

- Limitations in study design (risk of bias);
- Inconsistency of results (unexplained heterogeneity);
- Indirectness of evidence (interventions, populations and outcomes important to the patients with the condition);

- Imprecision (uncertainty about the results);
- Publication bias (selective publication of studies).

These five factors are additive and a reduction in more than one factor will reduce the quality of the evidence for that outcome. The GRADE approach also includes three domains that can be rated up, including a large magnitude of an effect, dose-response gradient, and effect of plausible residual confounding. However, these three domains relate to observational studies, including cohort, case-control, and before-after and time-series studies. GRADE summaries in this monograph only include RCTs; therefore, these three domains were not assessed.

Treatment recommendations can also be assessed using the GRADE approach, but due to the diverse nature of CM practice, treatment recommendations are not included with the summary of findings. Therefore, the reader should interpret the evidence with reference to the local practice environment. It should also be noted that the GRADE approach requires judgements about the quality of evidence and some subjective assessment. However, the experience of the panel members suggests these judgements are reliable and transparent representations of the quality of evidence.

The GRADE levels of evidence are grouped into four categories:

1) "High" quality evidence: We are very confident that the true effect lies close to that of the estimate of the effect.
2) "Moderate" quality evidence: We are moderately confident in the effect estimate — the true effect is likely to be close to the estimate of the effect, but there is a possibility that it is substantially different.
3) "Low" quality evidence: Our confidence in the effect estimate is limited — the true effect may be substantially different from the estimate of the effect.
4) "Very low" quality evidence: We have very little confidence in the effect estimate — the true effect is likely to be substantially different from the estimate of effect.

# References

1. Higgins JPT, Green S (eds.). (2011). *Cochrane Handbook for Systematic Reviews of Interventions*, Version 5.1.0. The Cochrane Collaboration. www.cochrane-handbook.org
2. Drossman DA, Thompson WG, Talley NJ, *et al.* (1990) Identification of sub-groups of functional gastrointestinal disorders. *Gastroenterology Int.* **3(4):** 159–172.
3. Drossman DA, Richter JE, Talley NJ, *et al.* (1994) The functional gastro-intestinal disorders: Diagnosis, pathophysiology and treatment. Degnon Associates, McLean, Virginia.
4. Drossman DA, Corazziari E, Talley NJ, *et al.* (2000) Rome II. The functional gastrointestinal disorders. Diagnosis, pathophysiology and treatment: A multinational consensus. Degnon Associates, McLean, Virginia.
5. Drossman DA, Corazziari E, Delvaux M, *et al.* (2006) Rome III: The functional gastrointestinal disorders. Degnon Associates, McLean, Virginia.
6. Drossman DA. (2016) Functional gastrointestinal disorders: History, pathophysiology, clinical features and Rome IV. *Gastroenterology.* **150(6):** 1262–1279.e2.
7. Gastroenterological Society of Australia. (2006) Irritable bowel syndrome — clinical update. In: *Digestive Health Foundation*, 2nd ed. Digestive Health Foundation, Sydney, Australia.
8. Spiller R, Aziz Q, Creed F, *et al.* (2007) Guidelines on the irritable bowel syndrome: Mechanisms and practical management. *Gut.* **56(12):** 1770–1798.
9. National Institute for Health and Care Excellence (NICE). (2008) Irritable bowel syndrome in adults: Diagnosis and management (CG61). In: *NICE.* United Kingdom. Updated: February 2015.
10. Weinberg DS, Smalley W, Heidelbaugh JJ, Sultan S. (2014) American Gastroenterological Association Institute guideline on the pharmacological management of irritable bowel syndrome. *Gastroenterology.* **147(5):** 1146–1148.
11. Fukudo S, Kaneko H, Akiho H, *et al.* (2015) Evidence-based clinical practice guidelines for irritable bowel syndrome. *J Gastroenterol.* **50(1):** 11–30.

12. Spiegel B, Strickland A, Naliboff BD, *et al.* (2008) Predictors of patient-assessed illness severity in irritable bowel syndrome. *Am J Gastroenterol.* **103(10):** 2536–2543.

13. Center for Drug Evaluation and Research (CDER). (2012) Guidance for industry irritable bowel syndrome — clinical evaluation of drugs for treatment. In: *Food and Drug Administration.* US Department of Health and Human Services, Silver Spring, MA.

14. Wong RK, Drossman DA. (2010) Quality of life measures in irritable bowel syndrome. *Expert Rev Gastroenterol Hepatol.* **4(3):** 277–284.

15. Drossman DA, Chang L, Bellamy N, *et al.* (2011) Severity in irritable bowel syndrome: A Rome Foundation working team report. *Am J Gastroenterol.* **106(10):** 1749–1759, quiz 60.

16. Levy RL, Olden KW, Naliboff BD, *et al.* (2006) Psychosocial aspects of the functional gastrointestinal disorders. *Gastroenterology.* **130(5):** 1447–1458.

17. Spiegel B, Camilleri M, Bolus R, *et al.* (2009) Psychometric evaluation of patient-reported outcomes in irritable bowel syndrome randomized controlled trials: A Rome Foundation report. *Gastroenterology.* **137(6):** 1944–1953.e1–e3.

18. Francis CY, Morris J, Whorwell PJ. (1997) The irritable bowel severity scoring system: A simple method of monitoring irritable bowel syndrome and its progress. *Aliment Pharmacol Ther.* **11(2):** 395–402.

19. Roalfe AK, Roberts LM, Wilson S. (2008) Evaluation of the Birmingham IBS symptom questionnaire. *BMC Gastroenterol.* **8:** 30.

20. Lewis SJ, Heaton KW. (1997) Stool form scale as a useful guide to intestinal transit time. *Scand J Gastroenterol.* **32(9):** 920–924.

21. 李乾构, 周学文, 单兆伟. (2006) *中医消化病诊疗指南*. 中医药出版社, 中国北京.

22. 中华中医药学会脾胃病分会. (2010) 肠易激综合征中医诊疗共识意见. *中华中医药杂志*. **25(7):** 1062–1065.

23. 国家中医药管理局. (2010) 22个专业95个病种中医诊疗方案. 国家中医药管理局医政司.

24. Ohnhaus EE, Adler R. (1975) Methodological problems in the measurement of pain: A comparison between the verbal rating scale and the visual analogue scale. *Pain.* **1(4):** 379–384.

25. Jensen MP, Karoly P, Braver S. (1986) The measurement of clinical pain intensity: A comparison of six methods. *Pain.* **27(1):** 117–126.

26. Ware JE, Jr., Sherbourne CD. (1992) The MOS 36-item short-form health survey (SF-36). I. Conceptual framework and item selection. *Med Care.* **30(6):** 473–483.

27. Patrick DL, Drossman DA, Frederick IO, *et al.* (1998) Quality of life in persons with irritable bowel syndrome: Development and validation of a new measure. *Dig Dis Sci.* **43(2):** 400–411.

28. Hahn BA, Kirchdoerfer LJ, Fullerton S, Mayer E. (1997) Evaluation of a new quality of life questionnaire for patients with irritable bowel syndrome. *Aliment Pharmacol Ther.* **11(3):** 547–552.

29. Lee J, Lee EH, Moon SH. (2016) A systematic review of measurement properties of the instruments measuring health-related quality of life in patients with irritable bowel syndrome. *Qual Life Res.* **25(12):** 2985–2995.

30. Hamilton M. (1959) The assessment of anxiety states by rating. *Br J Med Psychol.* **32(1):** 50–55.

31. Hamilton M. (1960) A rating scale for depression. *J Neurol Neurosurg Psychiatry.* **23:** 56–62.

32. Zung WW. (1971) A rating instrument for anxiety disorders. *Psychosomatics.* **12(6):** 371–379.

33. Zung WW, Richards CB, Short MJ. (1965) Self-rating depression scale in an outpatient clinic. Further validation of the SDS. *Arch Gen Psychiatry.* **13(6):** 508–515.

34. Snaith RP. (2003) The Hospital Anxiety and Depression Scale. *Health Qual Life Outcomes.* **1(1):** 29.

35. Mangel AW, Hahn BA, Heath AT, *et al.* (1998) Adequate relief as an endpoint in clinical trials in irritable bowel syndrome. *J Int Med Res.* **26(2):** 76–81.

36. Camilleri M, Mangel AW, Fehnel SE, *et al.* (2007) Primary endpoints for irritable bowel syndrome trials: A review of performance of endpoints. *Clin Gastroenterol Hepatol.* **5(5):** 534–540.

37. Kellow J, Lee OY, Chang FY, *et al.* (2003) An Asia-Pacific, double blind, placebo controlled, randomised study to evaluate the efficacy, safety, and tolerability of tegaserod in patients with irritable bowel syndrome. *Gut.* **52(5):** 671–676.

38. 危北海, 陈治水, 张万岱, 中国中西医结合学会消化系统疾病专业委员会. (2004) 胃肠疾病中医证候评分表. *世界华人消化杂志.* **12(11):** 2701–2703.

39. 中国中西医结合学会消化系统疾病专业委员会. (2011) 胃肠疾病中医证候评分表. *中国中西医结合消化杂志*. **1:** 66–68.

40. RAND Health. (nd) 36-Item Short Form Survey (SF-36) scoring instructions RAND Corporation. http://www.rand.org/health/surveys_tools/mos/36-item-short-form/scoring.html Cited: 2018.

41. McIntyre R, Kennedy S, Bagby RM, Bakish D. (2002) Assessing full remission. *J Psychiatry Neurosci.* **27(4):** 235–239.

42. Hamilton M. (1980) Rating depressive patients. *J Clin Psychiatry.* **41(12 Pt 2):** 21–24.

43. Pan S, Liu ZW, Shi S, *et al.* (2017) Hamilton rating scale for depression-24 (HAM-D24) as a novel predictor for diabetic microvascular complications in type 2 diabetes mellitus patients. *Psychiatry Res.* **258:** 177–183.

44. Williams JB. (1988) A structured interview guide for the Hamilton Depression Rating Scale. *Arch Gen Psychiatry.* **45(8):** 742–747.

45. Glynn RJ, Buring JE. (1996) Ways of measuring rates of recurrent events. *BMJ.* **312(7027):** 364–367.

46. Lineberry N, Berlin JA, Mansi B, *et al.* (2016) Recommendations to improve adverse event reporting in clinical trial publications: A joint pharmaceutical industry/journal editor perspective. *Br Med J.* **355:** i5078.

47. Schunemann H, Brozek J, Guyatt G, *et al.* (2013) GRADE handbook for grading quality of evidence and strength of recommendations. The GRADE Working Group. www.guidelinedevelopment.org/handbook

# 5

# Clinical Evidence for Chinese Herbal Medicine

## OVERVIEW

This chapter provides a synopsis of the clinical studies of Chinese herbal medicine (CHM) for irritable bowel syndrome (IBS) with an evaluation of the available clinical evidence. Previous systematic reviews are qualitatively described. Randomised controlled trials and non-randomised controlled clinical trials are systematically reviewed, and meta-analyses are applied to evaluate the efficacy and safety of CHM for IBS. In addition, non-controlled studies were identified as supplementary. These provide an overview of the interventions used as a treatment for IBS.

## Introduction

Chinese herbal medicine (CHM) in the management of irritable bowel syndrome (IBS) has been evaluated in numerous clinical studies. CHM interventions typically employ multi-herb ingredient formulae handed down from ancient China or made up according to Chinese medicine (CM) theory by contemporary CM clinical physicians. CHMs are commonly orally administered with a variety of preparation types, including decoctions, powder capsules, pills and granules for IBS patients. CHMs can also be administered as enemas to IBS patients. The efficacy and safety of CHMs in the management of IBS patients in relation to global or single symptoms, quality of life, and psychological care were assessed and are presented in this chapter.

## Previous Systematic Reviews

From a comprehensive search of the literature, several systematic reviews evaluating CHM for IBS were identified.

A Cochrane systematic review published in 2006 evaluated 75 randomised controlled trials (RCTs) of general herbal medicine alone or with conventional medicine in 7,957 people for IBS, compared to a placebo or conventional therapy.[1] CHM RCTs included both standardised and individualised formulae. CHM improved global IBS symptoms compared to a placebo; however, the quality of the studies was low.[1]

In 2016, a systematic review compared the treatment effect of CHM to a placebo or pharmacotherapy for people with IBS according to the Rome III criteria.[2] The review included 24 RCTs with 2,477 participants.[2] Results showed that compared to control treatments, CHM treatment was superior at improving IBS symptom scores, total effective rate (TER), and recurrence rate. However, the included studies were of low quality and presented publication bias; therefore, their authors advised that the results from these studies need to be interpreted with caution.

Another review in 2008 included 22 RCTs in 1,279 people and also investigated general herbal medicines, but the majority of the included studies (20/22) utilised CHMs. The review concluded that general herbal medicine was effective for reducing IBS symptoms; however, the quality of the included reviews was low.[3] In 2006, Bian and colleagues reported on a systematic review of IBS that included 12 RCTs totalling 1,125 people, but only included studies utilising the formulation *Tong xie yao fang* 痛泻要方. However, this systematic review only reported the meta-analysis result of the total rate of recovery plus improvement, which was an unverified composite outcome. It concluded that *Tong xie yao fang* 痛泻要方 treatment tended to improve IBS symptoms compared to conventional therapy; however, the quality of the studies was low.[4]

Three systematic reviews evaluated the effects of CHM for tonifying the Spleen.[5–7] One systematic review published in 2016 compared the effects of CHM for regulating the Liver and tonifying the Spleen to pinaverium bromide for people with IBS according to the Rome III criteria. The review included 20 RCTs and 1,836 participants. Results showed that using the CM syndrome differentiation in "regulating the Liver and tonifying the Spleen" was superior to pinaverium bromide in improving the clinical effective rate with a low risk ratio (RR).[7] Two systematic reviews compared the effects of "regulating the Liver and tonifying the Spleen" to pharmacotherapy.[5,6] In 2011, Huang and colleagues reported on people with IBS-D based on the Rome II criteria, including 5 RCTs (535 participants); results favoured CM treatments based on the treatment effective rate (TER).[6] Another review by Hou and colleagues in 2016 included people with IBS-D based on the Rome II and Rome III criteria. Results showed that using the CHM treatment was superior to pharmacotherapy in improving the clinical effective rate with a low RR. However, the included studies were of low quality and presented publication bias; therefore, their authors advised that results need to be confirmed by more rigorous research.[5]

Two reviews evaluated CHM for IBS-D; one included seven studies in 954 people only utilising the *Shugan jianpi zhixie* 疏肝健脾止泻 therapy. This 2015 review found that the *Shugan jianpi zhixie* 疏肝健脾止泻 therapy improved IBS symptoms compared to a placebo; however, the sample sizes in the included studies were small, and heterogeneity was high.[8] The other IBS-D systematic review in 2016 included 14 RCTs of 1,551 people and found that, compared to a placebo, CHM improved IBS symptoms.[9]

Two reviews included CHM RCTs for IBS-C, one including 19 RCTs of 1,510 people, but only for studies that were targeted at dispersing or regulating Liver *qi*, based on the efficacy, cure rate, RR and adverse events (AEs). The review by Li and colleagues in 2013 found that CHM was significantly more effective than conventional therapy for IBS-C, but the quality of the included studies was low.[10] Another IBS-C review in 2017 included 11 RCTs of 906 people and concluded CHM to be more effective than the serotonin 5-HT4 receptor agonist cisapride and mosapride; however, the included RCTs were of low quality.[11]

A systematic review in 2015 evaluated 72 RCTs of oral CHM combined with conventional therapy for any IBS type in

6,395 people and found that combined treatment with CHM and conventional therapy to be more effective than conventional therapy alone for the global effective rate,[12] although the quality of the included studies was low.

## Identification of Clinical Studies

Comprehensive database searches identified more than 40,000 citations. After removing duplicates, screening remaining citations by titles and abstracts, and excluding citations according to the exclusion criteria (see Chap. 4) by full-text reading, a total of 129 studies (reported in 132 publications) were included. These included 118 RCTs, 2 non-randomised controlled trials (CCTs), and 9 non-controlled studies. RCTs and CCTs were grouped according to study design and comparison and included in the systematic review and meta-analysis. Information from non-controlled studies was summarised, including the characteristics of the study, details of the intervention and any AEs. Non-controlled studies were not included in the quantitative analysis. Figure 5.1 shows the study selection process.

## Irritable Bowel Syndrome with Predominant Diarrhoea

A total of 112 studies using CHM for IBS-D were found that met our inclusion criteria, including 103 RCTs (H1–H101, H111, H112), one CCT (H102), and 8 non-controlled studies (H103–H110). The included CHM preparations included oral CHM and CHM used as enemas for IBS-D.

### Oral Chinese Herbal Medicine

Oral CHM was investigated in 101 RCTs (H1–H101), one CCT (H102) and 8 non-controlled studies (H103–H110). Eight RCTs had multiple arms — three (H1, H2, H3) had multiple intervention arms

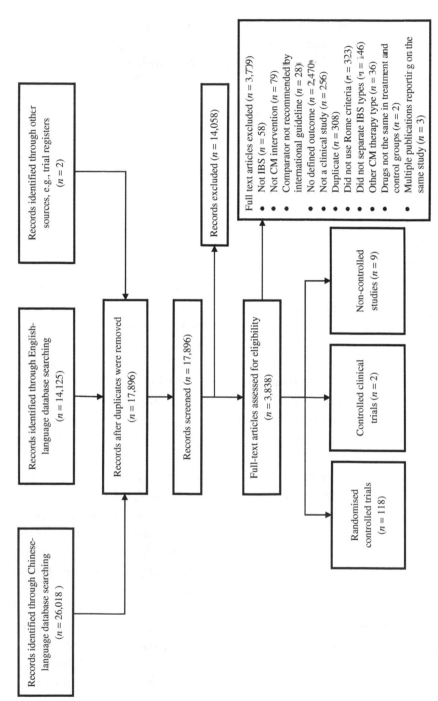

**Fig. 5.1.** Flow chart of study selection process: Chinese herbal medicine.

with two or more different CHM arms, two (H4, H5) had multiple intervention arms with one CHM arm and one integrative medicine arm, one (H6) had multiple control arms with one conventional medicine arm and one placebo arm, another (H7) had one placebo arm and one conventional medicine plus a placebo arm, and the remaining RCT (H8) had multiple interventions and control arms. Studies with multiple intervention groups were extracted and analysed in pairwise comparisons between all possible pairs of intervention groups; pairs that shared the same group were not included in the same meta-analysis.

## Randomised Controlled Trials of Oral Chinese Herbal Medicine

In total, there were 8,909 participants in 101 RCTs (H1–H101) meeting the inclusion criteria that evaluated CHM for IBS-D patients. Of these, four studies were multi-arm studies, with three of them (H9, H10, H11) with one arm utilising CHM alone with results presented in this chapter; the other arms are included in this chapter and/or Chap. 8 ("Clinical Evidence for Combination Therapies"), while another study (H12) with one arm utilising CHM plus sham Transcutaneous Electrical Acupuncture Stimulation (TEAS) vs. placebo plus sham TEAS has results presented in this chapter, and the other arm is included in Chap. 8.

One study (H8) was conducted in Korea, one (H13) in Bangladesh, one (H14) in Thailand and the others in China. A total of 46 studies were conducted in outpatient departments, 4 in inpatient departments, 35 in both outpatient and inpatient departments, and another study was conducted in both outpatient departments and the community. Thirteen studies only mentioned that they were conducted in hospitals but gave no details, while two other studies did not mention the setting.

The lowest mean age in the RCTs CHM groups was 27 years (H13) and the highest was 57.82 years (H15). For the control groups, the lowest mean age was 30.49 years (H13) and the highest was 56.49 years (H15). The duration of pre-existing IBS in the treatment groups ranged from a mean of 5.78 months (H16) to 9.68 years (H17), and in the control groups from 5.38 months (H16) to 9.73 years (H17). Fifteen studies did not report the IBS duration of participants.

The treatment duration of the studies ranged from two weeks to two months. A total of 27 studies followed up with participants after the treatment was over. One (H9) of these did not mention the follow-up period clearly, while another (H12) did another randomisation and treatment during the follow-up period; the results from the follow-up of these two studies are excluded. Five other studies (H18, H19, H20, H21, H22) presented multiple follow-up periods; we only present the last follow-up in the analysis.

Eighty-two of the RCTs utilised the Rome III criteria for participant inclusion, and 19 RCTs utilised Rome II. CM syndrome differentiation was used in 72 studies. Three studies (H7, H23, H24) treated participants allocated to receive CHM according to individual syndrome differentiation. Sixty-two studies applied specific syndromes as one of their inclusion criteria. The specified syndromes, ordered from high to low frequency, are presented in Table 5.1.

**Table 5.1. Frequently Used Syndromes in Randomised Controlled Trials for Irritable Bowel Syndrome with Diarrhoea**

| Syndrome | No. Studies |
| --- | --- |
| Liver stagnation and Spleen deficiency | 33 |
| Spleen and/or Kidney *yang* deficiency | 9 |
| Spleen deficiency with damp retention | 5 |
| Spleen (and stomach) *qi* weakness | 4 |
| Spleen deficiency with dampness and heat | 4 |
| Dampness-heat in the Spleen and Stomach | 1 |
| Cold-heat complex pattern | 1 |
| Spleen deficiency with dampness and phlegm | 1 |
| Spleen-Kidney *yang* 阳 deficiency with cold and *qi* 气 stagnation | 1 |
| Liver stagnation and Spleen deficiency with insecurity of intestines | 1 |
| Liver stagnation and Spleen deficiency with dampness | 1 |
| Liver stagnation and Spleen deficiency with lack of nourishment of Heart *qi* 气 | 1 |

The 101 RCTs evaluated 79 different formulae and 105 different herbs. Among these formulae, 47 were unnamed or self-named, while the others were traditional formulae (standard and modified) as well as commercial products. Peppermint oil was a single-herb formula tested in one study (H13) and in another (H14), chili and *Wu ling jiao nang* 乌灵胶囊 (commercial products) (H25). The most common multi-herb formula was *Tong xie yao fang* 痛泻要方/痛泻药方, tested in 17 studies (Table 5.2). In addition, many of the self-named and unnamed formulae were derived from *Tong xie yao fang* 痛泻要方 or had similar ingredients.

The largest formula was comprised of 18 herbs (H26), and the average size was 9 herbs. The commonly used herbs were *bai zhu* 白术 (89 studies), *bai shao* 白芍 (71 studies), *fu ling* 茯苓 (63 studies), *chen pi* 陈皮 (60 studies), and *gan cao* 甘草 (58 studies) (Table 5.3). Almost 90% of the included studies used *bai zhu* 白术.

**Table 5.2. Frequently Reported Oral Formulae in Randomised Controlled Trials for Irritable Bowel Syndrome with Diarrhoea**

| Most Common Formulae | No. Studies | Ingredients (Study ID) |
|---|---|---|
| *Tong xie yao fang* (including modified) 痛泻要方（加减） | 17 | *Bai zhu* 白术, *bai shao* 白芍, *fang feng* 防风, *chen pi* 陈皮 |
| *Sheng ling bai zhu san* (including modified) 参苓白术散（加减） | 9 | *Dang shen* 党参, *chao bai zhu* 炒白术, *fu ling* 茯苓, *bai shao* 白芍, *shan yao* 山药, *chao bian dou* 炒扁豆, *lian zi* 莲子, *yi yi ren* 薏苡仁, *sha ren* 砂仁, *chao chen pi* 炒陈皮, *mu xiang* 木香, *gan cao* 甘草 |
| *Si ni san* (including modified) 四逆散（加减） | 6 | *Chai hu* 柴胡, *bai shao* 白芍, *zhi shi* 枳实, *gan cao* 甘草 |
| *Chang ji tai* 肠吉泰 | 5 | *Bai zhu* 白术, *fang feng* 防风, *bai shao* 白芍, *chen pi* 陈皮, *wu mei* 乌梅, *yan hu suo* 延胡索 |
| *Ban xia xie xin tang* 半夏泻心汤 | 2 | *Ban xia* 半夏, *huang qin* 黄芩, *gan jiang* 干姜, *ren shen* 人参, *gan cao* 甘草, *huang lian* 黄连, *da zao* 大枣 |

**Table 5.2.** (*Continued*)

| Most Common Formulae | No. Studies | Ingredients (Study ID) |
|---|---|---|
| *Chang an I hao fang* 肠安 I 号方 | 2 | *Huang qi* 黄芪, *bai zhu* 白术, *bai zhu* 白芍, *fang feng* 防风, *sheng jiang* 生姜, *rou dou kou* 肉豆蔻, *ban xia* 半夏, *mu xiang* 木香, *chen pi* 陈皮, *huang lian* 黄连, *zhi gan cao* 炙甘草 |
| *Chang ji ling* (including modified) 肠激灵（加减） | 2 | *Bai shao* 白芍, *bai zhu* 白术, *fang feng* 防风, *chen pi* 陈皮, *yuan hu* 元胡, *he huan pi* 合欢皮 (H18) <br> *Bai shao* 白芍, *bai zhu* 白术, *yuan hu* 元胡, *fu ling* 茯苓, *suan zao ren* 酸枣仁, *su xin hua* 素馨花 (H19) |
| *Fu zi li zhong tang/Fu zi li zhong wan* (including modified) 附子理中汤/附子理中丸（加减） | 2 | *Fu zi* 附子, *ren shen* 人参, *gan jiang* 干姜, *gan cao* 甘草, *bai zhu* 白术 |
| *Jia wei huang qi jian zhong tang* (including modified) 加味黄芪建中汤（加减） | 2 | *Huang qi* 黄芪, *gui zhi* 桂枝, *bai shao* 白芍, *sheng jiang* 生姜, *da zao* 大枣, *gan cao* 甘草, *yi tang* 饴糖 |
| *Li zhong tang/Li zhong wan* (including modified) 理中汤/理中丸（加减） | 2 | *Ren shen* 人参, *bai zhu* 白术, *gan jiang* 干姜, *gan cao* 甘草 |
| *Si shen wan* 四神丸 | 2 | *Bu gu zhi* 补骨脂, *rou dou kou* 肉豆蔻, *wu zhu yu* 吴茱萸, *wu wei zi* 五味子 |
| *Tong xie ning ke li* 痛泻宁颗粒 | 2 | *Bai shao* 白芍, *bai zhu* 白术, *qin pi* 青皮, *xai bai* 薤白 |
| *Wen shen jian pi fang* 温肾健脾方 | 2 | *Bu gu zhi* 补骨脂, *rou dou kou* 肉豆蔻, *wu wei zi* 五味子, *wu zhu yu* 吴茱萸, *dang shen* 党参, *bai zhu* 白术, *yu jin* 郁金, *sheng jiang* 生姜, *da zao* 大枣 |

Note:

— Ingredients are referenced to the original studies where possible. If herb ingredients varied across studies, the herb ingredients were sourced from the *Zhong Yi Fang Ji Da Ci Dian* 中医方剂大辞典.

— The use of the herb *fu zi* 附子 may be restricted in some countries. Readers are advised to comply with relevant regulations.

**Table 5.3. Frequently Reported Orally Used Herbs in Randomised Controlled Trials for Irritable Bowel Syndrome with Diarrhoea**

| Most Common Herbs | Scientific Name | Frequency of Use |
|---|---|---|
| Bai zhu 白术 | *Atractylodes macrocephala* Koidz. | 89 |
| Bai shao/chi shao 白芍/赤芍 | *Paeonia lactiflora* Pall. *Paeoniae veitchill* Lynch | 71/1 |
| Fu ling 茯苓 | *Poria cocos* (Schw.) Wolf | 63 |
| Chen pi/qing pi 陈皮/青皮 | *Citrus reticulata* Blanco | 60/2 |
| Gan cao 甘草 | *Glycyrrhiza* spp. | 58 |
| Fang feng 防风 | *Saposhnikovia divaricata* (Turcz.) Schischk. | 47 |
| Dang shen 党参 | *Codonopsis pilosula* (Franch.) Nannf. | 40 |
| Chai hu 柴胡 | *Bupleurum chinense* DC. | 33 |
| Yi yi ren 薏苡仁 | *Coix lacryma-jobi* L. var. *ma-yuen* (Roman.) Stapf | 28 |
| Gan jiang/pao jiang/sheng jiang 干姜/炮姜/生姜 | *Zingiber officinale* (Willd.) Rosc. | 13/8/5 |
| Shan yao 山药 | *Dioscorea opposita* Thunb. | 22 |
| Huang lian 黄连 | *Coptis chinensis* Franch. | 20 |
| Zhi shi 枳实 | *Citrus aurantium* L. | 20 |
| Sha ren 砂仁 | *Amomum villosum* Lour. | 19 |
| Wu mei/lv e mei 乌梅/绿萼梅 | *Prunus mume* (Sieb.) Sieb. & Zucc. | 15/4 |
| Bai bian dou 白扁豆 | *Dolichos lablab* L. | 18 |
| Mu xiang 木香 | *Aucklandia lappa* Decne. | 15 |
| Rou dou kou 肉豆蔻 | *Myristica fragrans* Houtt. | 15 |
| Huang qi 黄芪 | *Astraglus membranaceus* (Fisch.) Beg. var. mongholicus (Bge.) Hsiao | 14 |
| Lian zi/he ye 莲子/荷叶 | *Nelumbo nucifera* Gaertn. | 13/2 |

Note:
The use of some herbs may be restricted in some countries. Readers are advised to comply with relevant regulations.

## Risk of Bias

All 101 studies were described as "randomised"; however, only 53 studies (52%) reported an appropriate method for random sequence generation, and seven studies (6.9%) described a non-random component in sequence generation, i.e., order of visit and were judged as "high" risk of bias for this domain. Only 11 studies (10.9%) reported that opaque envelopes were used to conceal allocation and were judged as "low" risk of bias for the domain of allocation concealment. A total of 14 studies attempted the blinding of participants and personnel and were judged as "low" risk of bias. Blinding of participants and personnel was not achieved in over 80% of the studies, and they were judged as "high" risk of bias for these domains. Few studies explicitly stated that outcome assessors were blind to group allocation, and 86.1% of the studies were judged as an "unclear" risk. Most of the studies (83.2%) did not have missing data, or any missing data was balanced in numbers with similar reasons across groups. Since no protocols of any included studies were identified, there was insufficient information to judge whether the studies reported any outcomes as pre-specified. The overall methodological quality of the included RCTs was low (Table 5.4), and results should be interpreted with caution because none of the studies were free from bias.

## *Outcomes*

All categories of the predefined primary outcomes (see Chap. 4) were reported, while several secondary outcomes, including the Birmingham scale, were not reported in the included clinical studies.

Table 5.4. **Risk of Bias of Randomised Controlled Trials for Irritable Bowel Syndrome with Diarrhoea: Oral Chinese Herbal Medicine**

| Risk of Bias Domain | Low Risk n (%) | Unclear Risk n (%) | High Risk n (%) |
|---|---|---|---|
| Sequence generation | 53 (52.5) | 41 (40.6) | 7 (6.9) |
| Allocation concealment | 11 (10.9) | 0 (0) | 90 (89.1) |
| Blinding of participants | 14 (13.9) | 0 (0) | 87 (86.1) |
| Blinding of personnel | 14 (13.9) | 0 (0) | 87 (86.1) |
| Blinding of outcome assessors | 14 (13.9) | 87 (86.1) | 0 (0) |
| Incomplete outcome data | 84 (83.2) | 12 (11.9) | 5 (4.9) |
| Selective outcome reporting | 0 (0) | 101 (100) | 0 (0) |

n: Number of studies

Single-symptom endpoints, e.g., abdominal pain and related symptoms and stool form, were the most commonly reported outcomes.

In the following sections, the analysis results are presented by outcome measures. Within each outcome, the following groups are compared:

- CHM vs. placebo;
- CHM vs. pharmacotherapy (subgrouped by medicine type);
- CHM + pharmacotherapy vs. pharmacotherapy (subgrouped by medicine type).

Some studies included various combinations of dietary and lifestyle management in all groups. Subgroup analysis was conducted according to additional factors, including different comparator drugs.

## Adequate Relief

Four studies (H8, H27, H28, H29) reported data on adequate relief (AR); all four studies compared CHM to placebo CHM. One study (H8) presented endpoint data in graphs, and thus data from this study could not be analysed. Another study (H29) considered AR to be at least four out of eight weeks, which was different from the other two studies, so this study could not be pooled. This study compared CHM to a placebo and found that CHM was superior by AR (206 participants, RR: 1.68 [1.24, 2.27]).

Two studies (H27, H28; 177 participants) considered AR to be of "symptom relief in the past week"; their pooled result showed that the effects of these two groups were similar (RR: 1.38 [0.46, 4.17], $I^2$ = 91%). The high heterogeneity may be due to the different CHMs used in the studies. One study (H28) also reported follow-up data at eight weeks and showed no difference between the CHM group and the placebo group (RR: 0.93 [0.56, 1.56]).

## Irritable Bowel Syndrome Severity Scoring Symptoms

A total of 26 studies (H1, H3, H7, H12, H20, H21, H22, H24, H27, H29–H44, H90) reported on the IBS Severity Scoring System

(IBS-SSS), including the TER and IBS-SSS score; 18 studies (H1, H3, H7, H12, H20, H21, H22, H24, H27, H29, H31–H38) reported both the TER and IBS-SSS score.

## Total effective rate of IBS-SSS

Nineteen studies (H1, H3, H7, H12, H20, H21, H22, H24, H27, H29–H38) reported the TER for the IBS-SSS; however, one of these (H30) reported incorrect data, so it was excluded from the analysis.

## Chinese herbal medicine vs. placebo

Five studies (H7, H12, H27, H29, H31) compared CHM to a placebo. Results indicated that CHM was superior to the placebo at the end of the treatment for the TER of the IBS-SSS (528 participants, RR: 1.55 [1.32, 1.80], $I^2 = 2\%$).

## Chinese herbal medicine vs. pharmacotherapy

Thirteen studies (H1, H3, H7, H20–H22, H24, H32–H37) compared CHM to pharmacotherapy. Pooled results showed that CHM was superior to pharmacotherapy (RR: 1.22 [1.15, 1.30], $I^2 = 20\%$) (H1, H3, H7, H20, H21, H22, H24, H32, H33, H34, H35, H36, H37). Amongst the subgroups of a different comparator, significant differences were found in the subgroups of trimebutine and pinaverium (see Table 5.5).

## Chinese herbal medicine + probiotics vs. probiotics

One study (H38) compared CHM plus probiotics to probiotics and found that CHM produced an additional effect in the TER of the IBS-SSS (60 participants, RR: 1.27 [1.01, 1.61]).

## Score for IBS-SSS

A total of 22 studies reported an IBS-SSS score; however, two studies (H32, H90) did not report the total IBS-SSS score, so they were excluded from the analysis.

**Table 5.5.  Oral Chinese Herbal Medicine vs. Pharmacotherapy: Total Effective Rate of Irritable Bowel Syndrome Severity Scoring System for Irritable Bowel Syndrome with Predominant Diarrhoea**

| Total/subgroups | No. Studies (Participants) | Effect Size RR [95% CI], $I^2\%$ | Included Studies |
|---|---|---|---|
| Total | 13 (1,454) | 1.22 [1.15, 1.30]*, 20% | H1, H3, H7, H20–H22, H24, H32–H37 |
| Subgroup: pinaverium | 8 (1,092) | 1.19 [1.10, 1.28]*, 21% | H1, H3, H21, H24, H32–H35 |
| Subgroup: trimebutine | 4 (256) | 1.35 [1.17, 1.55]*, 0% | H7, H20, H22, H36 |
| Subgroup: Pinaverium + probiotics | 1 (106) | 1.31 [1.06, 1.61]*, 0% | H37 |

*Statistically significant; see Statistical Analysis, Chap. 4

## Chinese herbal medicine vs. placebo

Six studies compared CHM to a placebo; however, one study (H29) did not present the results at the end of the treatment, so the data was excluded from analysis. The results of the other five studies (H7, H27, H31, H39, H40) indicated that CHM was superior to the placebo at the end of the treatment for the IBS-SSS score (277 participants, MD: −78.13 [−112.81, −43.46], $I^2$ = 81%).

One study (H29) reported follow-up data at eight weeks and the results showed a significant difference between the CHM group and placebo group (138 participants, MD: −60.35 [−86.89, −33.81]).

## Chinese herbal medicine vs. pharmacotherapy

Thirteen studies (H1, H3, H7, H20, H22, H24, H30, H33, H34, H37, H41–H43) reported score data for the IBS-SSS, comparing CHM to pharmacotherapy. Pooled results showed that CHM was superior to pharmacotherapy in improving the IBS-SSS score (MD: −40.90 [−49.02, −32.77], $I^2$ = 58%). Among the subgroups of different comparators, significant differences were found in all the subgroups (see Table 5.6).

**Table 5.6. Oral Chinese Herbal Medicine vs. Pharmacotherapy: Score of Irritable Bowel Syndrome Severity Scoring System for Irritable Bowel Syndrome with Predominant Diarrhoea**

| Total/subgroups | No. Studies (Participants) | MD [95% CI], I²% | Included Studies |
|---|---|---|---|
| Total | 13 (1,419) | −40.90 [−49.02, −32.77]*, 58% | H1, H3, H7, H20, H22, H24, H30, H33, H34, H37, H41–H43 |
| Subgroup: pinaverium | 7 (1,023) | −37.02 [−43.02, −31.03]*, 7% | H1, H3, H24, H30, H33, H34, H41 |
| Subgroup: trimebutine | 4 (230) | −33.18 [−55.84, −10.52]*, 57% | H7, H20, H22, H42 |
| Subgroup: pinaverium + probiotics | 2 (166) | −63.80 [−93.23, −34.38]*, 77% | H37, H43 |
| Follow-up total | 4 (339) | −66.56 [−80.29, −52.83]*, 53% | H3, H20, H22, H43 |
| Subgroup: pinaverium | 1 (156) | −64 [−86.14, −41.86]* | H3 |
| Subgroup: Pinaverium + probiotics | 1 (60) | −78.63 [−90.10, −67.16]* | H43 |
| Subgroup: trimebutine | 2 (123) | −56.27 [−71.57, −40.98]*, 0% | H20, H22 |

*Statistically significant; see "Statistical Analyses" in Chap. 4

Four of the studies (H3, H20, H22, H43) reported follow-up data. Pooled results showed that CHM was superior to pharmacotherapy (MD: −66.56 [−80.29, −52.83], I² = 53%). A significant difference was found in the subgroup, comparing to trimebutine at the follow-up (MD: −56.27 [−71.57, −40.98], I² = 0%) (H20, H22).

## Chinese herbal medicine + pharmacotherapy vs. pharmacotherapy

Two studies (H38, H44) compared CHM plus pharmacotherapy to pharmacotherapy; significant differences were found between the two groups (180 participants, MD: −56.46 [−104.93, −7.99], $I^2$ = 96%).

## Stool Frequency

Twenty-two studies reported data on stool frequency, including the effective rate and score; however, one of the studies (H14) presented the data only in graphs and one (H28) only reported the median at the end of the treatment, so their data was excluded.

### Effective rate of stool frequency

### Chinese herbal medicine vs. pharmacotherapy

Four studies (H36, H75, H79, H80; 402 participants) reported the effective rate of stool frequency recommended by a guideline,[13] comparing CHM to different pharmacotherapy. Pooled results showed that CHM was superior to pharmacotherapy (RR: 1.32 [1.06, 1.66], $I^2$ = 77%). The subgroup of antispasmodic agents also showed a significant difference between two groups (H36, H75) with low heterogeneity (RR: 1.40 [1.18, 1.66], $I^2$ = 0%).

### Stool frequency based on number of times per day

Ten studies (H1, H15, H24, H27, H30, H31, H33, H34, H37, H89) measured stool frequency based on the number of times per day.

### Chinese herbal medicine vs. placebo

Two studies (H27, H31; 118 participants) compared CHM to a placebo; results showed that CHM was superior to the placebo in reducing the stool frequency per day (MD: −0.35 times less per day [−0.61, −0.08], $I^2$ = 0%).

## Chinese herbal medicine vs. pharmacotherapy

Eight studies (H1, H15, H24, H30, H33, H34, H37, H89; 1,033 participants) compared CHM to pharmacotherapy, including antispasmodic agents and probiotics. Pooled results showed that CHM was superior to pharmacotherapy in reducing the stool frequency per day (MD: −0.22 times less per day [−0.38, −0.07], $I^2$ = 63%). The subgroup of pinaverium (H1, H24, H30, H33, H34; 747 participants) also showed a significant difference between two groups with reduced heterogeneity (MD: −0.19 times per day [−0.36, −0.02], $I^2$ = 36%).

## *Stool frequency based on guideline recommendations*

Eight studies (H10, H16, H45–H48, H79, H80) measured stool frequency based on recommendations by *Consensus Opinion of Traditional Chinese Medicine Diagnosis and Treatment Strategy for Irritable Bowel Syndrome.*[13]

## Chinese herbal medicine vs. pharmacotherapy

Seven studies (H10, H16, H45–H47, H79, H80) compared CHM to pharmacotherapy. Pooled results showed that based on guideline recommendations, CHM was superior to pharmacotherapy at reducing stool frequency (MD: −0.50 [−0.85, −0.15], $I^2$ = 99%). Subgroup analysis with antispasmodic agents and pinaverium also showed similar results (Table 5.7).

## Chinese herbal medicine + pharmacotherapy vs. pharmacotherapy

One study (H48; 40 participants) compared CHM as integrative medicine to probiotics. Results showed that CHM produced an additional reduction in stool frequency (MD: −0.90 [−1.27, −0.53]).

**Table 5.7.** **Oral Chinese Herbal Medicine vs. Pharmacotherapy: Score of Stool Frequency Based on Guidelines for Irritable Bowel Syndrome with Predominant Diarrhoea**

| Total/subgroups | No. Studies (Participants) | MD [95% CI], $I^2$% | Included Studies |
|---|---|---|---|
| Total | 7 (502) | −0.50 [−0.85, −0.15]*, 99% | H10, H16, H45, H46, H47, H79, H80 |
| Subgroup: antispasmodic agents | 3 (188) | −0.56 [−1.00, −0.13]*, 96% | H16, H45, H46 |
| Subgroup: pinaverium | 2 (106) | −0.57 [1.09, −0.04]*, 98% | H16, H46 |
| Subgroup: trimebutine + probiotics | 2 (110) | −0.59 [−1.55, 0.36], 79% | H10, H47 |
| Subgroup: others | 2 (204) | −0.35 [−0.74, 0.04], 65% | H79, H80 |

*Statistically significant; see "Statistical Analyses" in Chap. 4.

## Stool Form

A total of 19 studies reported on stool form, including effective rate and score, based on the Bristol scale. When data was presented in graphs (H14) or the median value was only reported (H28) at the end of the treatment, the studies involved were excluded from data analysis.

### Effective rate of stool form

Six studies (H1, H24, H31, H34, H36, H49) reported on the effective rate using stool form based on the Bristol scale; however, one study (H49) reported the data incorrectly and so was excluded from the analysis.

### Chinese herbal medicine vs. placebo

One study (H31; 60 participants) compared CHM to a placebo, showing that CHM was superior to the placebo in improving the effective rate using a stool form based on the Bristol scale (RR: 1.53 [1.09, 2.16]).

## Chinese herbal medicine vs. pharmacotherapy

Four studies (H1, H24, H34, H36) compared CHM to antispasmodic agents. Pooled results showed that CHM was superior to pharmaco-therapy in improving the effective rate using a stool form based on the Bristol scale (RR: 1.16 [1.09, 1.24], $I^2$ = 0%). When CHM was compared to pinaverium, a significant difference was also found between the two groups favouring CHM (RR: 1.15 [1.08, 1.24], $I^2$ = 0%) (H1, H24, H34) (Table 5.8).

### Stool form scores

Eleven studies (H2, H8, H9, H15, H23, H50, H51, H82, H88, H94, H101) reported on the Bristol Stool Form Scale score; one study (H8) scored the stool type according to the Bristol scale from seven to one points, rating a higher score as a better effect, while the others rated a lower score as a better effect.

## Chinese herbal medicine vs. placebo

Two studies (H2, H8) compared CHM to a placebo. One study (H8; 26 participants) rated a higher score as a better effect, showing no significant difference between the two groups (MD: 0.11 [−0.41,

**Table 5.8.** Oral Chinese Herbal Medicine vs. Antispasmodic Agents: Effective Rate of Stool Form Based on Bristol Scale for Irritable Bowel Syndrome with Predominant Diarrhoea

| Total/subgroups | No. Studies (Participants) | RR [95% CI], $I^2$% | Included Studies |
|---|---|---|---|
| Total | 4 (701) | 1.16 [1.09, 1.24]*, 0% | H1, H24, H34, H36 |
| Subgroup: pinaverium | 3 (611) | 1.15 [1.08, 1.24]*, 0% | H1, H24, H34 |

*Statistically significant; see "Statistical Analyses" in Chap. 4

0.63]). The other study (H2; 120 participants) rated a lower score as a better effect, showing that CHM was superior by a score based on the Bristol scale (MD: −0.39 [−0.70, −0.08]).

## Chinese herbal medicine vs. pharmacotherapy

Seven studies (H9, H15, H23, H50, H51, H88, H101) compared CHM to pharmacotherapy, rating a lower score as a better effect. Pooled results showed there were no significant differences between CHM and pharmacotherapy on the stool score based on the Bristol scale (MD: −0.27 [−0.64, 0.10], $I^2$ = 99%). No significant difference was found in the subgroups by type of medicine (Table 5.9).

## Chinese herbal medicine + pharmacotherapy vs. pharmacotherapy

Three studies (H8, H82, H94) compared CHM as integrative medicine to pharmacotherapy. One study (H8) rated a higher score as a

**Table 5.9. Oral Chinese Herbal Medicine vs. Pharmacotherapy: Score of Stool Form Based on Bristol Scale for Irritable Bowel Syndrome with Predominant Diarrhoea**

| Total/subgroups | No. Studies (Participants) | MD [95% CI], $I^2$% | Included Studies |
|---|---|---|---|
| Total | 7 (887) | −0.27 [−0.64, 0.10], 99% | H9, H15, H23, H50, H51, H88, H101 |
| Subgroup: pinaverium | 3 (249) | 0.04 [0.01, 0.07], 0% | H50, H51, H88 |
| Subgroup: probiotics | 2 (237) | −0.38 [−1.09, 0.32], 99% | H15, H101 |
| Subgroup: others | 2 (401) | −0.54 [−1.63, 0.54], 99% | H9, H23 |

*Statistically significant; see "Statistical Analyses" in Chap. 4

better effect, showing no significant difference between the two groups (MD: 0.04 [−0.71, 0.79]). The other two studies (H82, H94) rated a lower score as a better effect, also showing no significant difference between the two groups by a score based on the Bristol scale (n=191, MD:−0.13 [−0.3942, 0.145], $I^2$ = 0%).

## Stool Frequency and Form

A total of 19 studies reported data on stool frequency and form as a single result, with the effective rate and score based on guidelines; the scoring methods of the guidelines were different, so the data was analysed by grouping studies that used the same guidelines (*Guiding Principles of Clinical Research on Traditional Chinese Medicine* (2002), *Guidelines for the Diagnosis and Treatment of Digestive Diseases of Traditional Chinese Medicine* (2006), *Chinese Medicine Syndrome Score for Gastrointestinal Conditions* (2004), and *Chinese Medicine Syndrome Score for Gastrointestinal Conditions* (2010)).[14–17]

### Effective rate based on stool frequency and form

Five studies (H52, H53, H54, H55, H56) reported data on the effective rate based on stool frequency and form as a single result.[14] One study (H52) reported the data incorrectly and was excluded from the analysis.

### Chinese herbal medicine vs. pharmacotherapy

Three studies (H53, H54, H55; 224 participants) compared CHM to pharmacotherapy using *Guiding Principles of Clinical Research on Traditional Chinese Medicine* (2002),[14] showing that CHM had a better effective rate in reducing stool frequency and improving stool form (RR: 1.25 [1.10, 1.42], $I^2$ = 19%).

## Chinese herbal medicine + pharmacotherapy vs. pharmacotherapy

One study (H56) compared CHM plus probiotics to probiotics using *Chinese Medicine Syndrome Score for Gastrointestinal Conditions* (2004) and *Chinese Medicine Syndrome Score for Gastrointestinal Conditions* (2010),[15,16] also showing that CHM produced an additional effect to probiotics for the effective rate using stool frequency and form (RR: 1.28 [1.06, 1.54]).

### *Score of stool frequency and form*

Fourteen studies (H26, H34, H40, H57, H58. H59, H60, H61, H62, H63, H64, H65, H66, H67) reported data on scores for stool frequency and form based on guidelines.

## Chinese herbal medicine vs. placebo

One study (H40) compared CHM to a placebo, showing that based on *Guiding Principles of Clinical Research on Traditional Chinese Medicine* (2002), CHM was superior in reducing stool frequency and form score (MD: −1.15 [−1.62, −0.68]).

## Chinese herbal medicine vs. pharmacotherapy

Ten studies (H34, H57, H58, H59, H60, H61, H62, H63, H64, H67) compared CHM to pharmacotherapy.

One study (H67) reported data based on *Chinese Medicine Syndrome Score for Gastrointestinal Conditions* (2004) and *Chinese Medicine Syndrome Score for Gastrointestinal Conditions* (2010), showing that CHM was superior to trimebutine and montmorillonite powder in reducing stool frequency and form scores (MD: −1.53 [−2.94, −0.12]).

Nine studies (H34, H57, H58, H59, H60, H61, H62, H63, H64) reported data based on *Guiding Principles of Clinical Research on Traditional Chinese Medicine* (2002). Pooled results showed that

**Table 5.10. Oral Chinese Herbal Medicine vs. Pharmacotherapy: Score of Stool Frequency and Form Based on Guidelines for Irritable Bowel Syndrome with Predominant Diarrhoea**

| Total/subgroups | No. Studies (Participants) | MD [95% CI], $I^2$% | Included Studies |
|---|---|---|---|
| Total | 9 (632) | −0.31 [−0.50, −0.12]*, 78% | H34, H57, H58, H59, H60, H61, H62, H63, H64 |
| Subgroup: pinaverium | 3 (236) | −0.20 [−0.47, 0.06], 77% | H34, H57, H58 |
| Subgroup: probiotics | 2 (138) | −0.17 [−0.46, 0.13], 0% | H59, H60 |
| Subgroup: montmorillonite powder | 2 (134) | −0.88 [−2.30, 0.54], 94% | H63, H64 |

*Statistically significant; see "Statistical Analyses" in Chap. 4

CHM was superior to pharmacotherapy in reducing stool frequency and form score (MD: −0.31 [−0.50, −0.12], $I^2$ = 78%). No significant differences were found in the subgroups (Table 5.10).

One study (H61) also reported follow-up data at one month, and results showed that CHM was superior to pinaverium and probiotics (MD: −1.13 [−1.96, −0.30]).

## Chinese herbal medicine + pharmacotherapy vs. pharmacotherapy

Three studies (H26, H65, H66) compared CHM plus antispasmodic agents to antispasmodic agents using *Guiding Principles of Clinical Research on Traditional Chinese Medicine* (2002), with one study using pinaverium and two studies using trimebutine. The pooled results (MD: −0.45 [−0.80, −0.10], $I^2$ = 68%) and results for the subgroup with trimebutine (MD: −0.62 [−1.10, −0.14], $I^2$ = 52%) (H26, H65) showed that CHM produced an additional effect to trimebutine in reducing the scores for stool frequency and form based on *Guiding Principles of Clinical Research on Traditional Chinese Medicine*

(2002) and *Guidelines for the Diagnosis and Treatment of Digestive Diseases of Traditional Chinese Medicine* (2006).

## Abdominal Pain and Related Symptoms

The related symptoms of abdominal pain include bloating and abdominal discomfort. Data for abdominal pain, abdominal pain and bloating, and abdominal pain or discomfort, were pooled for analysis, and subgroup analysis was performed by different symptoms if available.

Thirty studies (H3–H6, H8, H14, H24, H35, H36, H49, H52–H56, H68–H82) met the PICO that reported data on abdominal pain and related symptoms, including the effective rate and score. Ten studies (H6, H49, H52, H54, H56, H68, H69, H70, H71, H72) reported data incorrectly, so they were excluded. One of the remaining studies (H74) reported both the effective rate and score, whereas the other studies only reported one or the other.

### Effective rate for abdominal pain and related symptoms

Sixteen studies (H3–H5, H24, H35, H36, H53, H55, H73–H80) reported on the effective rate for abdominal pain (and bloating/or discomfort). Five studies (H5, H55, H73, H76, H78) reported data on the effective rate based on bloating; however, three (H55, H76, H78) of these reported incorrect data, so they were excluded.

### Chinese herbal medicine vs. pharmacotherapy

All 16 studies (H3–H5, H24, H35, H36, H53, H55, H73–H80) that reported on the effective rate for abdominal pain (and bloating/or discomfort) compared CHM to pharmacotherapy. Pooled results showed that CHM was superior to pharmacotherapy for the effective rate calculated using abdominal pain and related symptoms (RR: 1.17 [1.10, 1.25], $I^2 = 35\%$). Among the subgroups, no significant differences were found between the two groups when compared to trimebutine (RR: 1.19 [0.90, 1.58], $I^2$ = 81%) (H36, H76, H77) or otilonium (RR: 1.23 [0.94, 1.60], $I^2$ = 58%) (H78, H80), while the other comparisons showed that CHM was superior in the effective rate based on abdominal pain and related symptoms (Table 5.11).

Two studies (H5, H73) compared CHM to pinaverium for the effective rate based on bloating; results showed no significant differences between the groups (RR: 1.08 [0.97, 1.21], $I^2$ = 15%).

Table 5.11. Oral Chinese Herbal Medicine vs. Pharmacotherapy: Effective Rate of Abdominal Pain and Related Symptoms for Irritable Bowel Syndrome with Predominant Diarrhoea

| Total/subgroups | No. Studies (Participants) | RR [95% CI], $I^2$% | Included Studies |
|---|---|---|---|
| Total | 16 (1,617) | 1.17 [1.10, 1.25]*, 35% | H3, H4, H5, H24, H35, H36, H55, H73, H74, H75, H76, H77, H78, H53, H79, H80 |
| Subgroup: abdominal pain | 10 (998) | 1.21 [1.09, 1.33]*, 61% | H4, H5, H34, H36, H55, H74, H75, H76, H77, H78 |
| Subgroup: abdominal pain and bloating | 4 (415) | 1.13 [1.01, 1.26]*, 0% | H3, H35, H57, H73 |
| Subgroup: abdominal pain or discomfort | 2 (204) | 1.18 [1.00, 1.40], 36% | H76, H77 |
| Subgroup: pinaverium | 8 (1,014) | 1.17 [1.09, 1.27]*, 15% | H3, H5, H24, H35, H53, H73, H74, H75 |
| Subgroup: trimebutine | 3 (205) | 1.19 [0.90, 1.58], 81% | H36, H76, H77 |
| Subgroup: otilonium | 2 (200) | 1.23 [0.94, 1.60], 58% | H78, H80 |
| Subgroup: probiotics | 2 (110) | 1.27 [1.04, 1.54]*, 0% | H4, H79 |

*Statistically significant; see "Statistical Analyses" in Chap. 4

## Chinese herbal medicine + pharmacotherapy vs. pharmacotherapy

Two studies (H4, H5; 112 participants) reporting on included other arms comparing CHM plus pharmacotherapy to pharmacotherapy. The results showed that there was no significant difference between the groups for the effective rate based on abdominal pain and related symptoms (RR: 1.25 [0.88, 1.76], $I^2 = 75\%$).

One study (H5) compared CHM plus pinaverium to pinaverium alone for the effective rate based on bloating, showing no significant difference between the two groups (RR: 1.08 [0.92, 1.28]).

### *Score for abdominal pain and related symptoms*

A total of five studies (H8, H14, H74, H81, H82) reported scores for abdominal pain and related symptoms. One (H81) did not report data from the end of the treatment, and another (H14) presented data in the form of graphs only; therefore, their data were excluded from the analysis. The remaining three studies (H8, H74, H82) all mentioned that they used the Visual Analogue Scale (VAS) to measure abdominal pain and related symptoms.

## Chinese herbal medicine vs. placebo

One study (H8; 26 participants) compared CHM to a placebo, showing no significant difference between the two groups for discomfort (MD: 2.54 [−9.68, 14.76]), abdominal pain (MD: 3.36 [−9.41, 16.13]), and bloating (MD: −3.08 [−14.21, 8.05]).

## Chinese herbal medicine vs. pharmacotherapy

One study (H74; 64 participants) compared CHM to pinaverium, showing that CHM was superior to pinaverium for abdominal pain and bloating (MD: −10.90 [−16.17, −5.63]).

## Chinese herbal medicine + pharmacotherapy vs. pharmacotherapy

One study (H8; 27 participants) had an arm comparing CHM as integrative medicine to pharmacotherapy for discomfort, showing no significant difference between the two groups for discomfort (MD: 2.28 [−12.52, 17.08]) and bloating (MD: −5.73 [−18.75, 7.29]).

Two studies (H8, H82; 158 participants) compared CHM as integrative medicine to pharmacotherapy for abdominal pain and bloating, showing that CHM produced an additional reduction in abdominal pain and bloating by VAS (MD: −3.59 [−6.21, −0.96], $I^2 = 0\%$).

### *Recurrence Rate*

Eleven studies (H23, H24, H26, H34, H40, H52, H55, H61, H65, H68, H83) reported on rate of recurrence. The recurrence rate is based on the TER in these studies. The definitions of the TER and RR were different in each study. We pooled all data by a comparator to make it possible to analyse the long-term effect of the treatment.

### *Chinese herbal medicine vs. placebo*

One study (H40; 54 participants) compared CHM to a placebo, showing significant difference between the groups for the recurrence rate (RR: 0.23 [0.07, 0.81]).

### *Chinese herbal medicine vs. pharmacotherapy*

Eight studies (H23, H24, H34, H52, H55, H61, H68, H83) compared CHM to pharmacotherapy. Pooled results showed significant difference between the groups by the recurrence rate (RR: 0.50 [0.36, 0.71], $I^2 = 35\%$), and significant differences were found in the subgroups by different medications (Table 5.12).

**Table 5.12.   Oral Chinese Herbal Medicine vs. Pharmacotherapy: Recurrence Rate for Irritable Bowel Syndrome with Predominant Diarrhoea**

| Total/subgroups | No. Studies (Participants) | RR [95% CI], I²% | Included Studies |
|---|---|---|---|
| Total | 8 (710) | 0.50 [0.36, 0.71], 35% | H23, H24, H34, H52, H55, H61, H68, H83 |
| Subgroup: pinaverium | 3 (459) | 0.67 [0.50, 0.91], 19% | H24, H34, H68 |
| Subgroup: antidiarrheal agents + others | 4 (162) | 0.37 [0.22, 0.61], 0% | H52, H55, H61, H83 |

## Chinese herbal medicine + pharmacotherapy vs. pharmacotherapy

Two studies (H26, H65; 123 participants) compared CHM plus trimebutine to trimebutine, showing significant differences between the groups by the recurrence rate (RR: 0.44 [0.21, 0.93], I² = 0%).

## Irritable Bowel Syndrome Quality of Life

Twenty-three studies reported data on several IBS quality-of-life scales; six studies (H8, H27, H29, H34, H84, H86) reported both the total score and scores of the subscales.

## Total score for irritable bowel syndrome quality of life

Ten studies (H8, H13, H27, H29, H35, H44, H53, H84, H85, H86) mentioned the reporting of the total score for IBS quality of life scales; however, one study (H13) did not present data and was not included in the analysis. Four studies (H34, H53, H84, H85) did not report the total scores within the scale range (see Chap. 4 for the ranges); therefore, their data was excluded from the analysis. Another study (H8) used the scale incorrectly, so the data from this study was excluded. One study (H86) used a scale with 42 items and three domains without any reference, and the scale could not be found;

also, the scale used in this study was unclear, and thus its data was excluded from the analysis.

## Chinese herbal medicine vs. placebo

Two studies (H27, H29) compared CHM to a placebo, rating a lower score as a better effect; however, one study (H29) did not present the result at the end of the treatment and the data was excluded. Another study (H27) showed no significant difference between the two groups for the total score of IBS quality of life (MD: −5.32 [−16.68, 6.04]).

## Chinese herbal medicine + pinaverium vs. pinaverium

One study (H44; 120 participants) compared CHM plus pinaverium to pinaverium, rating a higher score as a better effect, on the quality of life scale, showing that CHM produced an additional improved effect of quality of life (MD: 14.30 [10.13, 18.47]).

## *Scores for subscales of irritable bowel syndrome quality of life*

Nineteen studies reported data on scores for subscales; however, two studies (H7, H8) did not transfer the data into 100 points, and three studies (H26, H84, H87) used the wrong scoring methods, so their data were excluded from the analysis. Six studies (H32, H34, H37, H88, H89, H90) did not report scores within the scale range (see Chap. 4 for the ranges), so their data was excluded from analysis. Two studies (H11, H91) mixed two scales, and it was unclear which scale was used, so their data was excluded from the analysis. One study (H86) used a scale with 42 items and three domains without a reference, and the scale could not be found, so data from this study was also excluded from the analysis. This left 5 of the 19 studies included in the analysis.

## Chinese herbal medicine vs. placebo

Two studies (H27, H29) compared CHM to a placebo, rating a lower score as a better effect; however, one of the studies (H29) did not

**Table 5.13.  Oral Chinese Herbal Medicine vs. Placebo: Score Sub-scales of Irritable Bowel Syndrome Severity Scoring System for Irritable Bowel Syndrome with Predominant Diarrhoea**

| Domain | No. Studies (Participants) | MD [95% CI] | Included Studies |
|---|---|---|---|
| Dysphoria | 1 (58) | −10.73 [−24.56, 3.10] | H27 |
| Interference with Activity | 1 (58) | −3.61 [−16.75, 9.53] | H27 |
| Body Image | 1 (58) | −4.96 [−16.08, 6.16] | H27 |
| Health Worry | 1 (58) | −0.54 [−13.80, 12.72] | H27 |
| Food Avoidance | 1 (58) | −4.96 [−19.69, 9.77] | H27 |
| Social Reaction | 1 (58) | −4.00 [−15.10, 7.10] | H27 |
| Sexual | 1 (58) | −4.08 [−16.67, 8.51] | H27 |
| Relationships | 1 (58) | −3.12 [−13.80, 7.56] | H27 |

present the result at the end of the treatment, so its data was excluded. The results of another study (H27) showed no significant difference between the two groups for all subscales (Table 5.13).

## Chinese herbal medicine vs. pharmacotherapy

Three studies (H3, H43, H79) compared CHM to different pharmacotherapy. One study (H43) rated a lower score as a better effect, comparing to an antispasmodic agent plus probiotics, reporting data at the end of the treatment and a follow-up after three months. The results showed that CMH was superior to pharmacotherapy for some domains at the end of the treatment (Dysphoria, Interference with Activity) and follow-up (Dysphoria, Interference with Activity, Body Image) (Table 5.14).

The two other studies (H3, H79) rated a higher score as a better effect; one of the studies (H3) also reported data from three months' follow-up. The results showed that CMH was superior to pharmacotherapy for Dysphoria at the end of the treatment and some domains at the end of the follow-up, except Body Image (Table 5.14).

Table 5.14.  Oral Chinese Herbal Medicine vs. Pharmacotherapy: Score Sub-scales of Irritable Bowel Syndrome Severity Scoring System for Irritable Bowel Syndrome with Predominant Diarrhoea

| Domain | Observation Time | No. Studies (Participants) | MD [95% CI], I²% | Included Studies |
|---|---|---|---|---|
| Dysphoria | End of | 1 (60) | −4.47 [−7.77, −1.17]* | H43 |
| | treatment | 2 (167) | 4.88 [0.24, 9.52]*, 2% | H3, H79 |
| | Follow-up | 1 (60) | −5.50 [−9.13, −1.87]* | H43 |
| | | 1 (107) | 11.77 [7.65, 15.89]* | H3 |
| Interference with Activity | End of | 1 (60) | −5.67 [−9.49, −1.85]* | H43 |
| | treatment | 2 (167) | 5.85 [−3.30, 14.99], 63% | H3, H79 |
| | Follow-up | 1 (60) | −5.46 [−9.68, −1.24]* | H43 |
| | | 1 (107) | 8.86 [4.49, 13.23]* | H3 |
| Body Image | End of | 1 (60) | −2.33 [−5.40, 0.74] | H43 |
| | treatment | 2 (167) | −2.35 [−5.61, 0.91], 0% | H3, H79 |
| | Follow-up | 1 (60) | −6.36 [−9.77, −2.95]* | H43 |
| | | 1 (107) | 0.07 [−3.22, 3.36] | H3 |
| Health Worry | End of | 1 (60) | 0.20 [−3.49, 3.89] | H43 |
| | treatment | 2 (167) | 8.21 [−0.94, 17.36], 80% | H3, H79 |
| | Follow-up | 1 (60) | 2.70 [−1.59, 6.99] | H43 |
| | | 1 (107) | 13.81 [10.39, 17.23]* | H3 |
| Food Avoidance | End of | 1 (60) | 0.60 [−3.77, 4.97] | H43 |
| | treatment | 2 (167) | 1.38 [−4.26, 7.01], 0% | H3, H79 |
| | Follow-up | 1 (60) | −0.03 [−4.55, 4.49] | H43 |
| | | 1 (107) | 8.09 [3.13, 13.05]* | H3 |
| Social Reaction | End of | 1 (60) | 2.70 [−0.62, 6.02] | H43 |
| | treatment | 2 (167) | 5.37 [−4.74, 15.48], 68% | H3, H79 |
| | Follow-up | 1 (60) | −1.70 [−5.34, 1.94] | H43 |
| | | 1 (107) | 6.19 [2.63, 9.75]* | H3 |
| Sexual | End of | 1 (60) | −0.33 [−3.40, 2.74] | H43 |
| | treatment | 2 (167) | 1.71 [−1.68, 5.09], 0% | H3, H79 |
| | Follow-up | 1 (60) | −0.90 [−4.42, 2.62] | H43 |
| | | 1 (107) | 5.13 [1.13, 9.13]* | H3 |
| Relationships | End of | 1 (60) | 0.17 [−3.55, 3.89] | H43 |
| | treatment | 2 (167) | −0.13 [−3.59, 3.32], 0% | H3, H79 |
| | Follow-up | 1 (60) | 0.90 [−2.76, 4.56] | H43 |
| | | 1 (107) | 3.58 [0.31, 6.85]* | H3 |

*Statistically significant; see "Statistical Analyses" in Chap. 4

## 36-item Short-form Survey

A total of 13 studies (H9, H17–H19, H21, H24, H28, H61, H92–H96) reported on the 36-Item Short-Form Survey (SF-36). Data on the SF-36 can be presented by each of the eight domains: Physical Functioning (PF), Role Functioning/Physical (RP), Role Functioning/Emotional (RE), Energy, Mental Health (MH), Social Functioning (SF), Bodily Pain (BP), General Health, and Health Change. Another way to present the data is by total scores for the physical component or mental component. Two studies (H92, H93) only reported total scores for SF-36, which the scale does not use, so their data was excluded from the analysis. One study (H94) reported only six out of the eight domains of the scale.

## Chinese herbal medicine vs. placebo

Two studies (H19, H28) compared CHM to a placebo, reporting on the SF-36. One study (H28) reported the total scores for the physical component score (PCS) and mental component score (MCS), showing that there was no significant difference between the two groups at the end of the treatment for either PCS (MD: 2.50 [−1.46, 6.46]) or MCS (MD: 1.20 [−2.49, 4.89]). Similarly, there was no difference at eight weeks' follow-up for both the PCS (MD: 3.40 [−0.60, 7.40]) and MCS (MD: 2.00 [−2.02, 6.02]).

Another study (H19) reported the scores for the eight domains, showing that CHM was superior to the placebo at the end of the treatment for PF (MD: 8.60 [3.49, 13.71]), RP (MD: 13.91 [2.17, 25.65]), BP (MD: 8.92 [0.37, 17.47]), SF (MD: 11.59 [4.28, 18.90]), RE (MD: 16.09 [3.90, 28.28]), and MH (MD: 8.57 [0.94, 16.20]), but no significant difference for GH (MD: 7.02 [−1.35, 15.39]) or VT (MD: 7.13 [−0.78, 15.04]). After six months of follow-up, the results showed that CHM was superior to a placebo for PF (MD: 6.78 [1.99, 11.57]), BP (MD: 16.18 [5.69, 26.67]), GH (MD: 10.60 [3.06, 18.14]), VT (MD: 6.79 [0.10, 13.48]), SF (MD: 16.10 [8.15, 24.05]), RE (MD: 14.16 [3.52, 24.80]), and MH (MD: 17.00 [9.79, 24.21]), but not for RP (MD: 10.71 [−1.02, 22.44]).

## Chinese herbal medicine vs. pharmacotherapy

Eight studies (H9, H17, H18, H21, H24, H61, H95, H96) reported data for the SF-36, comparing CHM to different pharmacotherapy. The pooled results showed that CHM was superior to pharmacotherapy at the end of the treatment for the domains of SF-36, except PF (see Table 5.15). Other significant differences were also found in the subgroups (see Table 5.15).

**Table 5.15.  Chinese Herbal Medicine vs. Pharmacotherapy: SF-36 for Irritable Bowel Syndrome with Predominant Diarrhoea**

| Outcome | Total/subgroups | No. Studies (Participants) | MD [95% CI], I²% | Included Studies |
|---|---|---|---|---|
| Physical Function | Total | 8 (1,308) | 1.54 [-0.43, 3.52], 69% | H9, H17, H18, H21, H24, H61, H95, H96 |
| | Antispasmodic agents | 3 (537) | 1.28 [-0.71, 3.28], 47% | H21, H24, H96 |
| | Antispasmodic agents + other medicines | 4 (459) | 2.04 [-2.90, 6.98], 84% | H17, H18, H61, H95 |
| Role Physical | Total | 8 (1,308) | 3.82 [0.66, 6.97]*, 43% | H9, H17, H18, H21, H24, H61, H95, H96 |
| | Antispasmodic agents | 3 (537) | 6.67 [1.76, 11.58]*, 9% | H21, H24, H96 |
| | Antispasmodic agents + other medicines | 4 (459) | 3.66 [-0.84, 8.17], 36% | H17, H18, H61, H95 |
| Bodily Pain | Total | 8 (1,308) | 4.59 [1.46, 7.73]*, 61% | H9, H17, H18, H21, H24, H61, H95, H96 |
| | Antispasmodic agents | 3 (537) | 4.31 [0.08, 8.54]*, 48% | H21, H24, H96 |
| | Antispasmodic agents + other medicines | 4 (459) | 6.71 [2.55, 10.87]*, 37% | H17, H18, H61, H95 |

*(Continued)*

135

**Table 5.15.** (*Continued*)

| Outcome | Total/subgroups | No. Studies (Participants) | MD [95% CI], I²% | Included Studies |
|---|---|---|---|---|
| General Health | Total | 8 (1,308) | 1.95 [0.26, 3.63]*, 0% | H9, H17, H18, H21, H24, H61, H95, H96 |
| | Antispasmodic agents | 3 (537) | 1.24 [−1.49, 3.97], 0% | H21, H24, H96 |
| | Antispasmodic agents + other medicines | 4 (459) | 3.05 [0.47, 5.63]*, 11% | H17, H18, H61, H95 |
| Vitality | Total | 8 (1,308) | 2.40 [0.79, 4.02]*, 0% | H9, H17, H18, H21, H24, H61, H95, H96 |
| | Antispasmodic agents | 3 (537) | 1.93 [−0.22, 4.09], 0% | H21, H24, H96 |
| | Antispasmodic agents + other medicines | 4 (459) | 4.25 [0.80, 7.71]*, 29% | H17, H18, H61, H95 |
| Social Functioning | Total | 8 (1,308) | 3.44 [0.09, 6.80]*, 67% | H9, H17, H18, H21, H24, H61, H95, H96 |
| | Antispasmodic agents | 3 (537) | 4.92 [2.15, 7.70]*, 0% | H21, H24, H96 |
| | Antispasmodic agents + other medicines | 4 (459) | 2.72 [−4.37, 9.82], 82% | H17, H18, H61, H95 |
| Role Emotional | Total | 8 (1,308) | 5.64 [1.70, 9.59]*, 45% | H9, H17, H18, H21, H24, H61, H95, H96 |
| | Antispasmodic agents | 3 (537) | 4.74 [−1.56, 11.03], 27% | H21, H24, H96 |
| | Antispasmodic agents + other medicines | 4 (459) | 8.52 [3.74, 13.30]*, 14% | H17, H18, H61, H95 |
| Mental Health | Total | 8 (1,308) | 6.09 [2.01, 10.17]*, 77% | H9, H17, H18, H21, H24, H61, H95, H96 |
| | Antispasmodic agents | 3 (537) | 2.86 [0.06, 5.66]*, 0% | H21, H24, H96 |
| | Antispasmodic agents + other medicines | 4 (459) | 9.55 [2.51, 16.60]*, 84% | H17, H18, H61, H95 |

*Statistically significant; see "Statistical Analyses" in Chap. 4

**Table 5.16. Chinese Herbal Medicine vs. Pharmacotherapy: SF-36 for Irritable Bowel Syndrome with Predominant Diarrhoea**

| Outcome | No. Studies (Participants) | MD [95% CI], $I^2$% | Included Studies |
|---|---|---|---|
| Physical Functioning | 5 (921) | 1.16 [−0.39, 2.71], 48% | H9, H18, H21, H24, H61 |
| Role Physical | 5 (921) | 3.47 [−0.00, 6.94]*, 37% | H9, H18, H21, H24, H61 |
| Bodily Pain | 5 (921) | 6.66 [3.79, 9.53]*, 14% | H9, H18, H21, H24, H61 |
| General Health | 5 (921) | 2.27 [−0.51, 5.06], 36% | H9, H18, H21, H24, H61 |
| Vitality | 5 (921) | 2.28 [0.49, 4.08]*, 0% | H9, H18, H21, H24, H61 |
| Social Functioning | 5 (921) | 4.07 [1.43, 6.71]*, 35% | H9, H18, H21, H24, H61 |
| Role Emotional | 5 (921) | 3.06 [−0.15, 6.27], 0% | H9, H18, H21, H24, H61 |
| Mental Health | 5 (921) | 4.58 [1.15, 8.01]*, 59% | H9, H18, H21, H24, H61 |

*Statistically significant; see "Statistical Analyses" in Chap. 4

Five studies (H9, H18, H21, H24, H61) reported data for the long-term effect at the end of follow-up. The results showed that CHM was superior to pharmacotherapy for the long-term effect for BP, VT, SF and MH, but there were no significant differences for RP, GH or RE (see Table 5.16).

## Chinese herbal medicine + pharmacotherapy vs. pharmacotherapy

One study (H94) compared CHM plus antispasmodic agents and probiotics to antispasmodic agents and probiotics in 60 participants; however, it only reported data for six domains, not BP or SF. The results showed that CHM produced an additional effect of VT (MD: 5.30 [0.84, 9.76]) and MH (MD: 6.50 [2.75, 10.25]), but no significant differences between the two groups for PF (MD: 3.50 [−3.03, 10.03]), RP (MD: 3.80 [−5.25, 12.85]), GH (MD: 4.10 [−3.47, 11.67]) or RE (MD: 6.60 [−2.35, 15.55]).

## *Zung Self-rating Anxiety Scale*

Eight studies reported on the Zung Self-rating Anxiety Scale (SAS). One study (H97) presented the data for all participants but did not separate them into two groups, so the data was excluded.

### *Chinese herbal medicine vs. pharmacotherapy*

Six studies (H43, H83, H87, H96, H98, H99) compared CHM to pharmacotherapy. Pooled results showed that there was no significant difference between the two groups (MD: −2.17 [−5.78, 1.44], $I^2$ = 87%), and no significant difference was found in the subgroups (Table 5.17); however, a trend in reduction of the score was observed. One of the studies (H43) reported data for three months' follow-up, showing that CHM was superior to pharmacotherapy in a long-term effect on the SAS score in people with IBS-D (MD: −2.87 [−5.29, −0.45]).

### *Chinese herbal medicine + pharmacotherapy vs. pharmacotherapy*

One study (H44; 120 participants) compared CHM plus pinaverium to pinaverium alone, showing that CHM produced an additional effect by the SAS score (MD: −13.60 [−15.17, −12.03]).

**Table 5.17. Oral Chinese Herbal Medicine vs. Pharmacotherapy: Zung Self-rating Anxiety Scale for Irritable Bowel Syndrome with Predominant Diarrhoea**

| Total/subgroups | No. Studies (Participants) | MD [95% CI], $I^2$% | Included Studies |
|---|---|---|---|
| Total | 6 (420) | −2.17 [−5.78, 1.44], 87% | H43, H83, H87, H96, H98, H99 |
| Subgroup: pinaverium | 3 (240) | −4.88 [−12.15, 2.39], 93% | H87, H96, H98 |
| Subgroup: antispasmodic agents + others | 2 (120) | −0.55 [−3.48, 2.38], 55% | H43, H83 |

## Zung Self-rating Depression Scale

Ten studies reported data for the Zung Self-rating Depression Scale (SDS). One study (H97) presented the data for all participants but did not separate them into two groups, so the data was excluded from the analysis.

### Chinese herbal medicine vs. pharmacotherapy

Seven studies (H43, H75, H83, H87, H96, H98, H99) reported data for the SDS, comparing CHM to pharmacotherapy. Pooled results showed there was no significant difference between the two groups at the end of the treatment (MD: −4.86 [−10.17, 0.44], $I^2$ = 96%). Among the subgroups of different comparators, a significant difference was found in the subgroup of pinaverium (MD: −8.74 [−15.28, −2.20], $I^2$ = 95%) (Table 5.18). One study (H43) reported data for three months' follow-up; its results showed no significant difference between the CHM group and conventional medicine group for the long-term effect on the SDS score (MD: −2.90 [−6.46, 0.66]).

### Chinese herbal medicine + pharmacotherapy vs. pharmacotherapy

Two studies (H25, H44; 173 participants) compared CHM plus different pharmacotherapy to pharmacotherapy. The results showed that

**Table 5.18. Oral Chinese Herbal Medicine vs. Pharmacotherapy: Zung Self-rating Depression Scale for Irritable Bowel Syndrome with Predominant Diarrhoea**

| Total/subgroups | No. Studies (Participants) | MD [95% CI], $I^2$% | Included Studies |
|---|---|---|---|
| Total | 7 (528) | −4.86 [−10.17, 0.44], 96% | H43, H75, H83, H87, H96, H98, H99 |
| Subgroup: pinaverium | 4 (348) | −8.74 [−15.28, −2.20]*, 95% | H87, H96, H98 |
| Subgroup: antispasmodic agents + others | 2 (120) | 0.10 [−2.80, 3.00], 30% | H43, H83 |

*Statistically significant; see "Statistical Analyses" in Chap. 4

CHM produced an additional effect in improving the SDS score in people with IBS-D (MD: −10.66 [−14.51, −6.80], $I^2$ = 84%).

## Hospital Anxiety and Depression Scale

Three studies (H27, H29, H42) reported on the Hospital Anxiety and Depression Scale (HADS); however, one study (H29) did not present the result at the end of the treatment and was excluded from the analysis. The remaining studies all reported total scores for the subscales.

### Chinese herbal medicine vs. placebo

One study (H27, 58 participants) compared CHM to a placebo. There was no significant difference between the two groups for anxiety (MD: 0.20 [−1.85, 2.25]) or depression (MD: 0.69 [−1.07, 2.45]).

### Chinese herbal medicine vs. pharmacotherapy

One study (H42, 64 participants) compared CHM to trimebutine, showing that CHM was superior for anxiety scores (MD: −1.97 [−3.60, −0.34]) and depression scores (MD: −2.37 [−3.61, −1.13]).

## Hamilton Anxiety Rating Scale

### Chinese herbal medicine vs. placebo

One study (H19; 57 participants) reported data for the Hamilton Anxiety Rating Scale (HAMA), comparing CHM to a placebo and showing that CHM was superior to a placebo in reducing the HAMA score (MD: −3.73 [−6.58, −0.88]).

### Chinese herbal medicine + pharmacotherapy vs. pharmacotherapy

One study (H54; 80 participants) compared CHM plus trimebutine to trimebutine, showing that CHM produced an additional effect for the HAMA score (MD: −7.79 [−8.42, −7.16]).

## Hamilton Rating Scale for Depression

*Chinese herbal medicine vs. placebo*

One study (H19; 57 participants) reported data for the Hamilton Rating Scale for Depression (HRSD) using a 17-item scale, comparing CHM to a placebo, showing that CHM was superior to a placebo in improving the HRSD score (MD: −3.69 [−6.67, −0.71]).

## Assessment using Grading of Recommendations Assessment, Development and Evaluation

An assessment of the quality of the evidence from the RCTs was made using Grading of Recommendations Assessment, Development and Evaluation (GRADE). Included studies using Rome III as diagnostic criteria were included for GRADE assessment. Interventions, comparators and outcomes to be included were selected based on a consensus process, as described in Chap. 4. Comparisons of oral CHM versus a placebo, CHM versus pinaverium bromide, and CHM versus probiotics were considered critically important.

The AR, IBS-SSS score, stool frequency, Bristol stool form and AEs were considered the most important outcomes for assessing the effects of CHM on IBS-D symptoms.

Three summary-of-findings tables were prepared for oral CHM:

- Oral CHM versus placebo;
- Oral CHM versus pinaverium bromide; and
- Oral CHM versus probiotics.

## Oral Chinese herbal medicine vs. placebo

The certainty of the evidence for oral CHM as compared to a placebo for treating IBS was "moderate" to "very low" (Table 5.19). Moderate evidence showed that CHM was slightly better than a placebo at achieving AR in IBS-D participants. IBS-SSS TER was better in people with IBS-D ("moderate" certainty) and lower in the IBS-SSS score; however, the results were of "very low" certainty. Stool frequency per

**Table 5.19. GRADE: Oral Chinese Herbal Medicine vs. Placebo for Irritable Bowel Syndrome with Predominant Diarrhoea**

| Outcome; Mean Treatment Duration | Estimated Absolute Effect | | Relative Effect (95% CI) No. RCTs (Participants) | Certainty of Evidence GRADE |
|---|---|---|---|---|
| | Oral CHM | Placebo | | |
| AR 8w | **89** per 100 Difference: 52 more per 100 (95% CI: 55 to 100 more per 100 patients) | **37** per 100 | RR 2.44 [1.50, 3.96] 1 (58) | ⊕⊕⊕○ MODERATE[a] |
| IBS-SSS TER 6.4w | **70** per 100 Difference: 25 more per 100 (95% CI: 59 to 81 more per 100 patients) | **45** per 100 | RR 1.55 [1.32, 1.80] 5 (528) | ⊕⊕⊕○ MODERATE[c,d] |
| IBS-SSS score 6.4w | **109.99** MD: 78.13 lower (95% CI: 112.81 to 43.46 lower) | **188.12** | MD −78.13 [−112.81, −43.46] 5 (277) | ⊕○○○ VERY LOW[b,c,d] |
| Stool frequency per day 6w | **1.445** MD: 0.35 lower (95% CI: 0.61 to 0.08 lower) | **1.795** | MD −0.35 [−0.61, −0.08] 2 (118) | ⊕⊕○○ LOW[a,c] |
| Bristol stool form scale- higher is better 8w | **0.96** MD: 0.11 lower (95% CI: 0.41 to 0.63 lower) | **0.85** | MD 0.11 [−0.41, 0.63] 1 (26) | ⊕⊕○○ LOW[c,d] |
| Bristol stool form scale- lower is better 4w | **4.02** MD: 0.39 lower (95% CI: 0.7 to 0.08 lower) | **4.43** | MD −0.39 [−0.7, −0.08] 1 (120) | ⊕⊕○○ LOW[a,d] |

*Statistically significant result; see "Statistical Analyses" in Chap. 4

Abbreviations: CHM, Chinese herbal medicine; CI, confidence interval; GRADE, Grading of Recommendations Assessment, Development and Evaluation; IBS-SSS, IBS-Severity Scoring System; MD, mean difference; RR, risk ratio; TER, total effective rate; w, weeks.

**Table 5.19.**  (*Continued*)

---

aSmall sample size.
bUnexplained heterogeneity.
cHigh risk of bias from lack of blinding.
dLarge CI.

References:
AR at 8 weeks: H27.
IBSSSS-TER: H7, H12, H27, H29, H31.
IBS-SSS score: H7, H27, H31, H39, H40.
Stool frequency per day score: H27, H31.
Bristol lower is better: H2.
Bristol higher is better: H8.

day was lower in people who received oral CHM ("low" certainty). The Bristol stool form was worse in people with oral CHM when higher scores indicated better results ("low" certainty) and were better in people who received oral CHM when lower scores indicated better results ("low" certainty).

Safety was reported in five RCTs (H7, H27, H29, H31, H39). There were no serious AEs reported, and two studies (H31, H39) did not have any AEs in the oral CHM group or the placebo group. One study (H29) mentioned five cases of AEs in the oral CHM group and three cases of AEs in the placebo group but did not provide further details.

In the oral CHM group, AEs included three cases of common colds, one case of elevated alanine aminotransferase (ALT) and aspartate aminostransferase (AST), and one case of headache and dizziness. In the placebo group, AEs included four cases of common colds and one case of itchiness and swollen eyes.

## Oral Chinese herbal medicine vs. pinaverium bromide

Oral CHM was compared to pinaverium bromide in 13 RCTs (H1, H3, H21, H24, H34, H35, H41, H50, H51, H53, H73, H74, H75) that reported on pre-specified outcomes. The certainty of the evidence was "low" to "very low" (Table 5.20). In IBS-D participants, low-quality evidence showed that CHM was significantly better than pinaverium bromide in improving the IBS-SSS score, TER based on

**Table 5.20.  GRADE: Oral Chinese Herbal Medicine vs. Pinaverium Bromide for Irritable Bowel Syndrome with Predominant Diarrhoea**

| Outcome; Mean Treatment Duration | Estimated Absolute Effect | | Relative Effect [95% CI] No. RCTs (Participants) | Certainty of Evidence GRADE |
|---|---|---|---|---|
| | Oral CHM | Pinaverium Bromide | | |
| IBS-SSS TER 4w | **91** per 100 Difference: 16 more per 100 (95% CI: 83 to 100 more per 100 patients) | **75** per 100 | RR 1.20 [1.10, 1.32]* 6 (986) | ⊕⊕○○ LOW[a,b] |
| IBS-SSS score 4.8w | **101.7** MD: 36.49 lower (95% CI: 43.81 lower to 29.15 lower) | **138.19** | MD −36.49 [−43.84, −29.15]* 5 (887) | ⊕⊕○○ LOW[a,b] |
| Pain effective rate 4.6w | **83** per 100 Difference: 14 more per 100 (95% CI: 78 to 89 more per 100 patients) | **69** per 100 | RR 1.20 [1.10, 1.29]* 7 (948) | ⊕⊕○○ LOW[a,b] |
| Stool frequency per day score 4w | **1.84** MD: 0.08 lower (95% CI: 0.23 lower to 0.07 higher) | **1.92** | MD −0.08 [−0.23, 0.07] 3 (611) | ⊕⊕○○ LOW[a,b] |
| Bristol stool form scale- lower is better 4w | **1.09** MD: 0.04 higher (95% CI: 0.01 higher to 0.07 higher) | **1.05** | MD 0.04 [0.01, 0.07]* 2 (204) | ⊕○○○ VERY LOW[a,b,c] |

*Statistically significant result; see "Statistical Analyses" in Chap. 4

Abbreviations: CHM, Chinese herbal medicine; CI, confidence interval; GRADE, Grading of Recommendations Assessment, Development and Evaluation; IBS-SSS, IBS-Severity Score System; MD, mean difference; RR, risk ratio; TER, total effective rate; w, weeks.

[a]High risk of bias from lack of blinding and allocation concealment.
[b]Large CI.
[c]Small sample size.

References:
IBSSSS-TER: H1, H3, H21, H24, H34, H35.
IBS-SSS score: H1, H3, H24, H34, H41.
Pain effective rate: H3, H24, H35, H53, H73–H75.
Stool frequency per day score: H1, H24, H34.
Bristol lower is better: H50, H51.

IBS-SSS, and pain effective rate. The stool frequency per day was lower in people who received oral CHM ("low" certainty). The Bristol stool form was better in people who received pinaverium when lower scores indicated better results ("low" certainty).

Safety was reported in five RCTs (H34, H41, H53, H73, H74). There were no serious AEs reported, and three studies (H41, H53, H74) did not have any AEs in the oral CHM group or the pinaverium bromide group. One study (H34) mentioned no AEs in the oral CHM group and four cases of AEs in the pinaverium bromide group, including constipation (2 cases), nausea (1 case), and dry mouth (1 case). In one study (H73), one case of dry mouth was reported in the oral CHM group, and one case of nausea was reported in the pinaverium bromide group.

## Oral Chinese herbal medicine vs. probiotics

Oral CHM was compared to pinaverium bromide in four RCTs (H4, H15, H79, H101) that reported on pre-specified important outcomes. The certainty of the evidence was "low" to "very low" (Table 5.21). In IBS-D participants, low evidence showed that CHM was significantly better than probiotics in improving the pain effective rate. The stool frequency per day was lower in people who received oral CHM ("low" certainty), but no significant difference was found between groups. The Bristol stool form was better in people who received oral CHM when lower scores indicated better results ("very low" certainty).

Safety was reported in two RCTs (H4, H79); both studies reported no AEs in both the treatment groups.

## *Randomised Controlled Trial Evidence for Individual Oral Formulae*

In the RCTs, three different formulae were used in multiple studies (two or more) that used the same design and outcome measure(s) and provided data suitable for pooling. The analysis results of these individual formulae are presented in Table 5.22 and summarised as follows.

**Table 5.21. GRADE: Oral Chinese Herbal Medicine vs. Probiotics for Irritable Bowel Syndrome with Predominant Diarrhoea**

| Outcome; Mean Treatment Duration | Estimated Absolute Effect | | Relative Effect [95% CI] No. RCTs (Participants) | Certainty of Evidence GRADE |
|---|---|---|---|---|
| | Oral CHM | Probiotics | | |
| Pain effective rate 4w | **88** per 100 Difference: 17 more per 100 patients (95% CI: 72 to 100 more per 100 patients) | **69** per 100 | RR 1.27 [1.04, 1.54]* 2 (110) | ⊕⊕○○ LOW[a,b] |
| Stool frequency per day score 6w | **1.49** MD: 0.06 lower (95% CI: 0.12 lower to 0) | **1.55** | MD −0.06 [−0.12, 0] 1 (120) | ⊕⊕○○ LOW[a,c] |
| Bristol stool form scale-lower is better 5w | **1.66** MD: 0.38 lower (95% CI: 1.09 lower to 0.32 higher) | **2.04** | MD −0.38 [−1.09, 0.32] 2 (237) | ⊕○○○ VERY LOW[a,b,c,d] |

*Statistically significant result; see "Statistical Analyses" in Chap. 4
Abbreviations: CHM, Chinese herbal medicine; CI, confidence interval; GRADE, Grading of Recommendations Assessment, Development and Evaluation; IBS-SSS, IBS-severity score system; MD, mean difference; RR, risk ratio; TER, total effective rate; w, weeks.

[a]High risk of bias from lack of blinding and allocation concealment.
[b]Large CI.
[c]Small sample size.
[d]High heterogeneity.

References:
Pain effective rate: H4, H79.
Stool frequency per day score: H15.
Bristol lower is better: H15, H101.

## *Chang an I hao fang* 肠安 1号方

*Chang an I hao fang* 肠安 1号方 is a self-named formula used in two studies (H27, H29); the ingredients of the formulae in the studies were not the same, although both studies were conducted by the same group. This may have been with the intention of improving the formula.

**Table 5.22.    Individual Formula Meta-analysis Results for Irritable Bowel Syndrome with Predominant Diarrhoea**

| Intervention | Comparator | No. Studies (Participants) | Outcome (Unit) | Effect Size [95% CI], I²% | Included Studies |
|---|---|---|---|---|---|
| *Chang an I hao fang* 肠安 I 号方 | Placebo | 2 (264) | TER-SSS | 1.44 [0.99, 2.10], 54% | H27, H29 |
| *Chang ji tai* 肠吉泰 | Placebo | 2 (220) | TER-SSS | 1.52 [1.23, 1.88]* | H12, H31 |
| | Pharmacotherapy | 2 (106) | TER-SSS | 1.15 [0.91, 1.44] | H32, H33 |
| | | 2 (136) | Score-SSS | −40.20 [−58.47, −21.93]* | H30, H33 |
| | | 2 (136) | Score-frequency per day | −0.42 [−0.66, −0.17]* | H30, H33 |
| *Tong xie yao fang* 痛泻要方 | Pharmacotherapy | 2 (238) | TER-SSS | 1.22 [1.09, 1.36]* | H3, H21 |
| | | 2 (201) | Score-form Bristol | −0.03 [−0.15, 0.09] | H50, H101 |

Notes: Formulae were selected if there were two or more studies using the same formula.
*Statistically significant; see "Statistical Analyses" in Chap. 4
Abbreviations: 95% CI: 95% confidence interval.

- Compared to a placebo, *Chang an I hao fang* 肠安I号方 reduced the IBS-SSS score after treatment, but there was no significant difference in the effective rate based on IBS-SSS (Table 5.22).

## *Chang ji tai* 肠吉泰

*Chang ji tai* 肠吉泰 is a self-named formula used in five studies (H12, H30, H31, H32, H33). The formula was based on *Tong xie yao fang* 痛泻要方 and comprised *bai zhu* 白术, *fang feng* 防风, *bai shao* 白芍, *chen pi* 陈皮, and *wu mei* 乌梅; modifications of the formula were seen in the studies.

- Compared to a placebo, *Chang ji tai* 肠吉泰 improved the total effective rate of the IBS-SSS score after treatment (Table 5.22).

- Compared to the conventional medicine pinaverium bromide, *Chang ji tai* 肠吉泰 reduced the IBS-SSS score and stool frequency per day, but there was no significant difference in the effective rate based on the IBS-SSS score (Table 5.22).

## *Tong xie yao fang* 痛泻要方

*Tong xie yao fang* 痛泻要方 is comprised of *bai zhu* 白术, *fang feng* 防风, *bai shao* 白芍, and *chen pi* 陈皮. It was assessed in four studies (H3, H21, H50, H101).

- Compared to pharmacotherapy, *Tong xie yao fang* 痛泻要方 improved the effective rate of the IBS-SSS score after the treatment, but there was no significant difference in the Bristol Stool Form Scale score (Table 5.22).

## Frequently Reported Orally used Herbs in Meta-analyses Showing Favourable Effect

To identify the most promising herbal candidates, the frequency of the herbs used in the studies of the meta-analyses showing favourable effects was calculated. The herb frequency was analysed based on different outcome categories. The global symptoms category consists of meta-analyses of outcomes of AR and the IBS-SSS score, and the category of stool habit consists of stool frequency and stool form; the quality-of-life category includes meta-analyses of the outcomes of IBS-QOL and SF-36 scores, while the psychological category consists of all scales on psychology (SAS, SDS, HADS, HAMA and HRSD). All the included meta-analyses were pooled with estimated results that favoured the CHM groups.

The 10 most common herbs of the meta-analyses favouring the use of CHM are listed in Table 5.23. The outcome category "psychology" only contained two studies, and all the herbs were used once. Among the other outcome categories, it found that the most commonly used herbs were very similar, but the ranking of each herb was

**Table 5.23. Frequently Reported Orally Used Herbs in Meta-Analyses Showing Favourable Effect**

| Herb | Scientific Name | Frequency of Use |
|---|---|---|
| *Global symptoms: 5 meta-analyses, 25 RCTs* | | |
| Bai zhu 白术 | *Atractylodes macrocephala* Koidz. | 24 |
| Bai shao 白芍 | *Paeonia lactiflora* Pall. | 19 |
| Chen pi 陈皮 | *Citrus reticulata* Blanco | 18 |
| Fang feng 防风 | *Saposhnikovia divaricata* (Turcz.) Schischk. | 16 |
| Gan cao 甘草 | *Glycyrrhiza* spp. | 15 |
| Fu ling 茯苓 | *Poria cocos* (Schw.) Wolf | 12 |
| Wu mei/lv e mei 乌梅/绿萼梅 | *Prunus mume* (Sieb.) Sieb. & Zucc. | 6/4 |
| Dang shen 党参 | *Codonopsis pilosula* (Franch.) Nannf. | 10 |
| Yi yi ren 薏苡仁 | *Coix lacryma-jobi* L. var. *ma-yuen* (Roman.) Stapf | 9 |
| Lian zi/he ye 莲子/荷叶 | *Nelumbo nucifera* Gaertn. | 6/2 |
| *Abdominal pain and related symptoms: 2 meta-analyses, 18 RCTs* | | |
| Bai zhu 白术 | *Atractylodes macrocephala* Koidz. | 15 |
| Bai shao 白芍 | *Paeonia lactiflora* Pall. | 13 |
| Fu ling 茯苓 | *Poria cocos* (Schw.) Wolf | 13 |
| Chen pi/qing pi 陈皮/青皮 | *Citrus reticulata* Blanco | 11/1 |
| Gan cao 甘草 | *Glycyrrhiza* spp. | 10 |
| Dang shen 党参 | *Codonopsis pilosula* (Franch.) Nannf. | 9 |
| Fang feng 防风 | *Saposhnikovia divaricata* (Turcz.) Schischk. | 9 |
| Gan jiang/pao jiang/sheng jiang 干姜/炮姜/生姜 | *Zingiber officinale* (Willd.) Rosc. | 3/3/1 |
| Lian zi/he ye 莲子/荷叶 | *Nelumbo nucifera* Gaertn. | 6/1 |
| Qian shi 芡实 | *Euryale ferox* Salisb. | 6 |
| *Stool habit: 8 meta-analyses, 37 RCTs* | | |
| Bai zhu 白术 | *Atractylodes macrocephala* Koidz. | 29 |
| Bai shao/chi shao 白芍/赤芍 | *Paeonia lactiflora* Pall. | 24/1 |
| Fu ling 茯苓 | *Poria cocos* (Schw.) Wolf | 24 |
| Chen pi/qing pi 陈皮/青皮 | *Citrus reticulata* Blanco | 24 |
| Gan cao 甘草 | *Glycyrrhiza* spp. | 19 |

*(Continued)*

**Table 5.23.** *(Continued)*

| Herb | Scientific Name | Frequency of Use |
|---|---|---|
| Fang feng 防风 | *Saposhnikovia divaricata* (Turcz.) Schischk. | 18 |
| Chai hu 柴胡 | *Bupleurum chinense* DC. | 14 |
| Dang shen 党参 | *Codonopsis pilosula* (Franch.) Nannf. | 13 |
| Shan yao 山药 | *Dioscorea opposita* Thunb. | 10 |
| Zhi qiao/Zhishi 枳壳/枳实 | *Citrus aurantium* L. | 8/2 |
| *Quality of life: 8 meta-analyses, 10 RCTs* | | |
| Bai zhu 白术 | *Atractylodes macrocephala* Koidz. | 10 |
| Bai shao 白芍 | *Paeonia lactiflora* Pall. | 9 |
| Chen pi 陈皮 | *Citrus reticulata* Blanco | 8 |
| Fu ling 茯苓 | *Poria cocos* (Schw.) Wolf | 7 |
| Fang feng 防风 | *Saposhnikovia divaricata* (Turcz.) Schischk. | 6 |
| Gan cao 甘草 | *Glycyrrhiza* spp. | 6 |
| Dang shen 党参 | *Codonopsis pilosula* (Franch.) Nannf. | 5 |
| Bai bian dou 白扁豆 | *Dolichos lablab* L. | 4 |
| Huang qi 黄芪 | *Astragalus membranaceus* (Fisch.) Bge. | 4 |
| Wu mei/lv e mei 乌梅/绿萼梅 | *Prunus mume* (Sieb.) Sieb. & Zucc. | 3/1 |
| Yi yi ren 薏苡仁 | *Coix lacryma-jobi* L. var. *ma-yuen* (Roman.) Stapf | 4 |
| *Psychology: 1 meta-analysis, 2 RCTs* | | |
| Fu ling 茯苓 | *Poria cocos* (Schw.) Wolf | 1 |
| Ren shen 人参 | *Panax ginseng* C.A. Mey. | 1 |
| Rou gui 肉桂 | *Cinnamomum cassia* Presl | 1 |
| Shu di huang 熟地黄 | *Rehmannia glutinosa* Libosch. | 1 |
| Suan zao ren 酸枣仁 | *Ziziphus jujube* Mill. Var. *spinosa* (Bunge). Hu ex H. F. Chou | 1 |
| Tian dong 天冬 | *Asparagus cochinchinensis* (Lour.) Merr. | 1 |
| Wu wei zi 五味子 | *Schisandra chinensis* (Turcz.) Baill. | 1 |
| Yan hu suo 延胡索 | *Corydalis yanhusuo* W.T. Wang | 1 |
| Yuan zhi 远志 | *Polygala tenuifolia* Willd. | 1 |

slightly different. The most frequently used herbs were *bai zhu* 白术 among the four outcome categories, followed by *bai shao* 白芍, *chen pi* 陈皮, *fu ling* 茯苓, *fang feng* 防风, and *gan cao* 甘草.

## Controlled Clinical Trials of Oral Chinese Herbal Medicine

One CCT (H102) studied the effects of oral CHM in IBS-D patients using the Rome II criteria with Liver *qi* stagnation and Spleen deficiency syndrome. It allocated participants without randomisation and therefore differed from the RCTs. The study was conducted in China, involving 180 participants in total. The mean age of the participants was 40.5 years, and the duration of IBS was one to eight years. The treatment duration was four weeks without follow-up periods.

The study compared *Xiao yao he ji* 逍遥合剂, consisting of *chai hu* 柴胡, *dang gui* 当归, *bai shao* 白芍, *bai zhu* 白术, *fu ling* 茯苓, *bo he* 薄荷, *sheng jiang* 生姜, and *gan cao* 甘草, to pinaverium bromide. The study reported data on the effective rate based on bloating. However, its data contained errors, thus it was excluded. There was no other outcome measure in the study.

## Non-controlled Studies of Oral Chinese Herbal Medicine

Eight non-controlled studies (H103–H110) were retrieved, involving 2,779 participants. Half of the studies (H106, H108–H110) used the Rome II criteria, and the other half (H103–H105, H107) used the Rome III criteria. Among the five studies that gave information on the CM syndrome, two studies (H106, H108) included multiple syndromes, and the Liver depression and Spleen deficiency syndrome was mentioned the most (twice).

Among the eight studies, two studies (H103, H105) applied self-named formulae, and two studies (H107, H109) prescribed manufactured CMs. Only one study (H109) used CHM in addition to conventional treatment, while the other seven studies did not apply conventional treatments. The treatment duration varied from 14 days to eight weeks.

**Table 5.24. Frequently Reported Orally Used Herbs in Non-controlled Studies**

| Most Common Herb | Scientific Name | Frequency of Use |
| --- | --- | --- |
| Fu ling 茯苓 | *Poria cocos* (Schw.) Wolf | 7 |
| Bai zhu 白术 | *Atractylodes macrocephala* Koidz. | 6 |
| Gan cao 甘草 | *Glycyrrhiza* spp. | 5 |
| Dang shen 党参 | *Codonopsis pilosula* (Franch.) Nannf. | 4 |
| Bai shao 白芍 | *Paeonia lactiflora* Pall. | 4 |
| Chen pi 陈皮 | *Citrus reticulata* Blanco | 4 |
| Huang lian 黄连 | *Coptis chinensis* Franch. | 4 |
| Fang feng 防风 | *Saposhnikovia divaricata* (Turcz.) Schischk. | 3 |

Among the eight studies, one study (H106) included multiple formulae for different syndromes, while the others used only one formula. All formulae were independent. For the frequently reported herbs, *fu ling* 茯苓, *bai zhu* 白术, and *gan cao* 甘草 were the top three herbs. Other frequently reported herbs are presented in Table 5.24.

## Enema with Chinese Herbal Medicine

One RCT (H111) that studied the effects of an enema with CHM in IBS-D patients using the Rome III criteria with the damp-heat syndrome 湿热证 was found. The study was conducted in China involving 40 participants — 17 males and 23 females. The mean age was 43.4 years in the CHM group and 42.7 years in the control group, while the mean duration of IBS was 4.2 years in the CHM group and 3.9 years in the control group. The treatment duration was two weeks without a follow-up period.

The study (H111) compared *Shui liao yi hao fang* 水疗一号方 to otilonium bromide; the formula comprised *huang lian* 黄连, *cang zhu* 苍术, *tu fu ling* 土茯苓, *huai hua* 槐花, *di yu* 地榆, *chi shao* 赤芍, *dan pi* 丹皮, *dan shen* 丹参, and *mu xiang* 木香. It reported data on the score for a stool form based on the *Guiding Principles of Clinical Research on Traditional Chinese Medicine*, rating a lower score as a better effect.[14] The result showed that an enema with CHM was superior at the end of the treatment (MD: −0.89 [−1.08, −0.70]).

## Risk of Bias

The study used computer software for randomisation and was judged as "low" risk for the sequence generation domain. The study did not provide information on allocation concealment, and was judged as an "unclear" risk for allocation concealment. Blinding of the participants and personnel was not achieved, and the study was judged as a "high" risk of bias due to a lack of blinding. There were no dropouts in the study and it was judged as a "low" risk for this domain. No protocol could be located, so the study was judged as an "unclear" risk of bias for selective outcome reporting.

## Oral Chinese Herbal Medicine Plus Enema with Chinese Herbal Medicine

One RCT (H112) studied the effects of oral CHM plus enema CHM in IBS-D patients using the Rome III criteria, with the stagnation of the Liver *qi* attacking the Spleen and Spleen deficiency accompanied by dampness. The study was conducted in China involving 78 participants — 44 males and 34 females. The age range of all the participants was 18–65 years, and the duration of IBS was 1–15.5 years. The treatment duration was four weeks without a follow-up period.

The study used modified *Tong xie yao fang* 痛泻要方加减 for oral CHM and *Chang tai he ji* 肠泰合剂 for the enema, compared to pinaverium bromide. The study reported scores for each subscale of the IBS-QOL; however, the scoring method it presented had errors, so the data could not be analysed.

## Risk of Bias

The study was described as randomised; however, no method of randomisation was described, so it was judged as an "unclear" risk for the sequence generation domain. The study did not provide information on allocation concealment, and was judged as an "unclear" risk for allocation concealment. Blinding of participants and personnel was not achieved, and the study was judged as a "high" risk of bias due to a lack of blinding. There were no dropouts in the study and it was judged as "low" risk for this domain. No protocol could be located, so the study was judged as an "unclear" risk of bias for selective outcome reporting.

## Safety of Chinese Herbal Medicine in Treatment of Irritable Bowel Syndrome with Predominant Diarrhoea

Among all oral CHM studies, 57 studies mentioned checking safety outcomes, including 51 RCTs (H4, H7, H9, H10, H11, H16, H18, H19, H20, H22, H23, H26–H29, H31–H34, H39, H41, H42, H45, H46, H48, H49, H52–H55, H58, H59, H61, H64, H65, H66, H68, H73, H74, H76, H79, H80–H83, H88, H89, H95, H97, H99, H100), one CCT (H102), and five non-controlled studies (H103, H105, H107, H109, H110); however, one RCT (H42) did not provide any details on AEs, so a total of 55 studies involving 6,692 participants reported on the safety outcomes of CHM for IBS-D.

For the RCTs, 50 studies involving 4,214 participants reported safety outcomes. Three studies only reported clinical manifestation of AEs without exact numbers of cases or cases in each group. Among the other 47 studies, the majority reported that no AEs occurred during the study periods. In total, 81 cases of AEs were observed in 15 studies with 1,464 participants. 23 cases of AEs were observed in the CHM groups, while 58 cases were found in the placebo or conventional medicine treatment groups. With CHM treatments, the most common AEs were abdominal pain, nausea and bloating. Other AEs like skin rash, heartburn and bitterness in the mouth were also observed.

The CCT reported no AEs in both groups.

In the non-controlled studies, four studies reported that no AEs were found, while one study reported 35 AEs and 12 adverse reactions, including four patients with decreased haemoglobin level, one with platelets decreasing, one with alanine aminotransferase increasing, one with blood urea nitrogen increasing, one with creatinine increasing, and 37 with abnormal electrocardiography.

The use of CHM for enemas and oral CHM plus enemas did not report on AEs.

# Irritable Bowel Syndrome with Predominant Constipation

A total of 17 studies using CHM to treat IBS-C were found that met our PICO, including 15 RCTs (H113–H126, H129), one CCT (H127), and one non-controlled study (H128).

## Oral Chinese Herbal Medicine

Sixteen studies investigated oral CHM, with 14 RCTs (H113–H126), one CCT (H127), and one non-controlled study (H128). Only one study (H113) used a placebo for the control, while the others used pharmacotherapy.

## Randomised Controlled Trials of Oral Chinese Herbal Medicine

In total, there were 1,148 participants in 14 RCTs (H113–H126) that evaluated CHM for people with IBS-C. All studies were two-arm studies. One study (H113) was conducted in the Australian community, while the others were in Chinese hospitals. Among the 13 RCTs conducted in China, five were conducted in outpatient departments (H118, H119, H122, H124, H126), one (H120) in an inpatients department, and two (H117, H121) were both in outpatients and inpatients departments; the other five studies (H114–H116, H123, H125) only mentioned that they were conducted in hospitals, with no further details.

One study (H126) did not report on gender data, while the other 13 RCTs had more female participants (n = 662) compared to males (n = 406). The lowest mean age in the CHM groups was 34.77 years

(H114), and the highest was 53.16 years (H115). For the control groups, the lowest mean age was 34.93 years (H114), and the highest was 55.04 years (H115). The duration of pre-existing IBS in the treatment groups ranged from a mean of 2.2 years (H116) to 7.2 years (H117) and in the control groups from 2.53 years (H115) to 8.3 years (H117). Four studies (H113, H119, H122, H124) did not report the IBS duration of participants.

The treatment duration of the studies ranged from four weeks to 12 weeks. Only three studies (H113, H117, H118) followed up with the participants after the termination of the treatment. One study (H117) did not present data for the end of the follow-up. The other two studies followed up with the participants for eight weeks (H113) or three months (H118).

Eleven RCTs (H113–H118, H121–H123, H125, H126) utilised the Rome III criteria for participant inclusion and three RCTs (H119, H120, H124) utilised the Rome II criteria. CM syndrome differentiation was used in five studies (H118–H121, H126). Only one study (H120) mentioned the use of a specific syndrome but did not specify what syndrome it was. The other four studies applied specific syndromes, and all of the syndromes were different, including *qi* stagnation and intestinal dryness, *qi* stagnation (or with *yin* deficiency with internal heat), Liver *qi* stagnation and Spleen deficiency, and Spleen deficiency and *qi* stagnation.

The 14 RCTs evaluated 14 different formulae and 51 different herbs. Among these formulae, nine were unnamed or self-named, while the others were traditional formulae (standard and modified), and some were commercial products. All the formulae were different. The largest formula (H121) comprised 14 herbs and the average size was 8 herbs. The commonly used herbs were *zhi shi/zhi qiao* 枳实/枳壳 (7/4 studies), *bai shao* 白芍 (7 studies), *hou pu* 厚朴 (6 studies), *bai zhu* 白术 (6 studies), *gan cao* 甘草 (6 studies), and *bing lang/da fu pi* 槟榔/大腹皮 (5/1 studies) (Table 5.25). The *Wu ling capsule* 乌灵胶囊 (a commercial product) is a single-herb formula tested in one study (H122).

**Table 5.25.** **Frequently Reported Orally Used Herbs in Randomised Controlled Trials for Irritable Bowel Syndrome with Predominant Constipation**

| Most Common Herb | Scientific Name | Frequency of Use |
|---|---|---|
| Zhi shi/zhi qiao 枳实/枳壳 | *Citrus aurantium* L. | 7/4 |
| Bai shao 白芍 | *Paeonia lactiflora* Pall. | 7 |
| Hou pu 厚朴 | *Magnolia officinalis* Rehd. & Wils. | 6 |
| Bai zhu 白术 | *Atractylodes macrocephala* Koidz. | 6 |
| Gan cao 甘草 | *Glycyrrhiza* spp. | 6 |
| Bing lang/da fu pi 槟榔/大腹皮 | *Areca catechu* L. | 5/1 |
| Chai hu 柴胡 | *Bupleurum chinense* DC. | 5 |
| Chen pi/qing pi 陈皮/青皮 | *Citrus reticulata* Blanco | 4/1 |
| Dang shen 党参 | *Codonopsis pilosula* (Franch.) Nannf. | 4 |
| Da huang 大黄 | *Rheum palmatum* L. | 4 |
| Mu xiang 木香 | *Aucklandia lappa* Decne. | 3 |
| Huo ma ren 火麻仁 | *Cannabis sativa* L. | 3 |

Note: The use of some herbs may be restricted in some countries. Readers are advised to comply with relevant regulations.

## Risk of Bias

All studies were described as "randomised"; however, only half of the studies reported an appropriate method for random sequence generation, and the other half did not describe the method of randomisation. Only one study (H113) reported that opaque envelopes were used to conceal allocation. Only one study (H113) was judged as a "low" risk of bias for the blinding of participants, personnel and outcome assessors. A total of 13 out of 14 studies were judged as "high" risk of bias for the blinding of participants and personnel, as the studies were considered unblinded and the outcome assessor was considered an "unclear" risk of bias for these studies. Most of the studies (85.7%) did not have missing data, or the missing data was balanced in numbers with similar reasons across groups. No protocols of any included studies were identified, so there was insufficient

**Table 5.26. Risk of Bias of Randomised Controlled Trials for Irritable Bowel Syndrome with Constipation: Oral Chinese Herbal Medicine**

| Risk of Bias Domain | Low Risk n (%) | Unclear Risk n (%) | High Risk n (%) |
|---|---|---|---|
| Sequence generation | 7 (50) | 7 (50) | 0 (0) |
| Allocation concealment | 1 (7.1) | 13 (92.9) | 0 (0) |
| Blinding of participants | 1 (7.1) | 0 (0) | 13 (92.9) |
| Blinding of personnel | 1 (7.1) | 0 (0) | 13 (92.9) |
| Blinding of outcome assessors | 1 (7.1) | 0 (0) | 13 (92.9) |
| Incomplete outcome data | 12 (85.7) | 1 (7.1) | 1 (7.1) |
| Selective outcome reporting | 0 | 10 (71.4) | 4 (28.6) |

n: Number of studies

information to judge whether the studies reported outcomes as pre-specified, and most of the studies were judged as "unclear" risk of bias for this domain. Four studies (H120, H121, H125, H126) did not report on all planned outcomes and were judged as "high" risk of bias for this domain. The overall methodological quality of the included RCTs was low (Table 5.26), and results should be interpreted with caution because none of the studies were free from bias.

## Outcomes

All categories of the predefined primary outcomes (see Chap. 4) were reported, while several secondary outcomes, including Birminghan, IBS-QOL, SAS, HADS, HAMA and HRSD scores, were not reported in any studies. Single-symptom endpoints, e.g., abdominal pain and related symptoms, and stool form, were the most commonly reported outcomes.

In the following sections, the analysis of results is presented by outcome measures. Within each outcome, there are groups for the type of comparison as follows:

- CHM vs. placebo;
- CHM vs. pharmacotherapy (subgroup by medicine type); and

- CHM + pharmacotherapy vs. pharmacotherapy (subgroup by medicine type).

Some studies included various combinations of dietary and lifestyle management in all groups.

## Adequate Relief

### Chinese herbal medicine vs. placebo

One study (H113) considered AR as the relief of IBS symptoms for the last two weeks; it included 125 participants and compared oral CHM with a placebo for eight weeks. Results showed that treatment effects with CHM were similar to the placebo (RR:1.39 [0.98, 1.95]). The study also reported follow-up data at eight weeks and showed no difference between the CHM group and placebo group (RR:0.90 [0.53, 1.52])

## Irritable Bowel Syndrome Severity Scoring Symptoms

### Chinese herbal medicine vs. placebo

One study (H113) compared oral CHM with a placebo and reported the IBS-SSS score data; however, the study reported data using an incorrect method, so the data could not be analysed.

## Stool Frequency

### Chinese herbal medicine plus pharmacotherapy vs. pharmacotherapy

One study (H124; 148 participants) compared CHM plus mosapride to mosapride, showing that CHM plus mosapride was superior for the score of stool frequency based on *Consensus Opinion of Traditional Chinese Medicine Diagnosis and Treatment Strategy for Irritable Bowel Syndrome*[13] (MD: −0.59 [−1.01, −0.17]).

### Stool Form

Nine studies (H113, H114, H115, H116, H119, H121, H123, H124, H125) reported the score for the stool form using the Bristol scale. One study (H113) only reported the mean for the stool form without information on SD, and another study (H125) only reported the number for each stool type by the Bristol scale, so their data was excluded from the analysis.

### *Chinese herbal medicine vs. pharmacotherapy*

Four studies (H114, H116, H119, H121; 48 participants) reported stool form data by the Bristol stool scale; however, one study scored the stool type according to the Bristol scale's of 1–7 points, with a higher score as a better effect, while the others rated a lower score as a better effect (H116). This study compared CHM to tegaserod, and its results showed no significant difference between the two groups by the Bristol scale (MD: −0.08 [−0.54, 0.38]).

Three studies (H114, H119, H121; 200 participants) rated a lower score as a better effect, and the pooled results from these showed no significant difference between the two groups by the Bristol scale (MD: −0.48 [−1.18, 0.22], $I^2 = 85\%$). When studies were grouped based on different comparators, the results still showed no significant difference, whether they were compared with laxatives (one study (H121), 80 participants, MD: −0.75 [−1.51, 0.01]) or 5-HT4 agonist (2 studies (H114, H119), 120 participants, MD: −0.38 [−1.30, 0.54], $I^2 = 91\%$).

### *Chinese herbal medicine plus pharmacotherapy vs. pharmacotherapy*

Three studies (H115, H123, H124) reported data on stool form by the Bristol scale, comparing CHM plus different pharmacotherapy to pharmacotherapy; the studies rated a lower score as a better effect.

Pooled results showed that CHM as an integrative medicine was superior to pharmacotherapy by the Bristol scale (3 studies (H115,

H123, H124); 299 participants, MD: −1.12 [−1.91, −0.32], $I^2$ = 72%). In the subgroups of different comparators, results that showed significant difference were found when using trimebutine (H115; 91 participants, MD: −0.80 [−1.23, −0.37]) but not with mosapride (H123, H124; 208 participants, MD: −2.52 [−6.18, 1.13], $I^2$ = 85%).

## Abdominal Pain and/or Bloating

Five studies (H113, H118, H120, H125, H126) reported data on abdominal pain and/or bloating. However, one study (H113) that reported THE scores for abdominal pain and related symptoms only presented the mean by VAS, with no SDs presented, so the data was excluded from the analysis. The other four studies all reported the effective rate for abdominal pain and/or bloating; data on abdominal pain and abdominal pain and bloating was pooled for meta-analysis.

### Chinese herbal medicine vs. pharmacotherapy

One study (H120; 120 participants) reported the abdominal pain duration time per day and the frequency per week, so the data could not be pooled with the other studies. The study compared CHM to venlafaxine and tegaserod, and results showed that the effect on the two groups was similar for both abdominal pain outcomes (duration time per day, RR: 1.12 [0.98, 1.28]; frequency per week, RR: 1.12 [0.97, 1.29]).

Two studies (H118, H126; 130 participants) comparing CHM to a 5-HT4 agonist showed that CHM had a similar effect to the 5-HT4 agonist in the effective rate for abdominal pain and bloating (RR: 1.17 [0.99, 1.38], $I^2$ = 39%).

### Chinese herbal medicine + conventional medicine vs. conventional medicine

Another study (H125; 66 participants) comparing CHM plus trimebutine to trimebutine showed no significant difference between the groups in the effective rate for abdominal pain (RR: 1.08 [0.90, 1.30]) or bloating (RR: 1.20 [0.98, 1.47]).

### Recurrence Rate

*Chinese herbal medicine vs. pharmacotherapy*

One study (H118; 38 participants) found the recurrence rate of IBS-C with CHM to be similar to that with tegaserod (RR: 0.46 [0.22, 0.93]).

### 36-item Short-form Survey

Four studies (H113, H117, H120, H123) reported data on the SF-36; however, one study (H113) only presented the mean for physical functioning (PF) and role limitations due to physical health problems (RP), with no SDs presented, so its data was not included in analysis.

*Chinese herbal medicine vs. pharmacotherapy*

Two studies (H117, H120; 220 participants) compared CHM to pharmacotherapy. Results indicated CHM was superior to pharmacotherapy at the end of the treatment for several domains (RP (MD: 15.79 [10.73, 20.86], $I^2 = 0\%$), BP (MD: 5.01 [1.39, 8.62], $I^2 = 65\%$), VT (MD: 9.28 [0.26, 18.29], $I^2 = 95\%$), SF (MD: 7.70 [4.28, 11.12], $I^2 = 0\%$), RE (MD: 19.85 [7.40, 32.29], $I^2 = 88\%$), and MH (MD: 5.11 [3.14, 7.08], $I^2 = 0\%$), except for GH (MD: 7.16 [–1.16, 15.49], $I^2 = 84\%$), and PF (MD: 5.31 [–0.37, 10.99], $I^2 = 81\%$),

*Chinese herbal medicine + pharmacotherapy vs. pharmacotherapy*

One study (H123; 148 participants) compared CHM plus mosapride to mosapride, with results showing that CHM plus mosapride was superior for SF (MD: 6.33 [0.21, 12.45]), RE (MD: 7.57 [0.13, 15.01]), and MH (MD: 5.49 [0.34, 10.64]), but no significant difference for PF (MD: 1.45 [−3.64, 6.54]), RP (MD: −3.67 [−12.29, 4.95]), BP (MD: 7.38 [−1.21, 15.97]), GH (MD: 3.11 [−1.78, 8.00]) or VT (MD: 4.51 [−0.98, 10.00]).

## Self-rating Depression Scale

### Chinese herbal medicine + conventional medicine vs. conventional medicine

One study (H122; 60 participants) compared oral CHM plus polyethylene glycol with polyethylene glycol for eight weeks; results found that oral CHM produced an additional reduction in the SDS score (MD: −8.02 [−10.45, −5.59]).

## Assessment using Grading of Recommendations Assessment, Development and Evaluation

An assessment of the quality of the evidence from the RCTs was made using GRADE. Interventions, comparators and outcomes to be included were selected based on a consensus process, as described in Chap. 4. The comparison of oral CHM versus a placebo was considered critically important. The AR, IBS-SSS score, stool frequency, Bristol stool form and AEs were considered the most important outcomes for assessing the effects of CHM on IBS-C symptoms.

### Oral Chinese herbal medicine vs. placebo

Evidence for oral CHM versus placebo was assessed as "low" for AR (Table 5.27). The results showed that oral CHM might improve AR immediately after the treatment but not at the follow-up.

The study reported on the safety of oral CHM and placebo CHM. There were no serious AEs reported. In the oral CHM group, 33 AEs were reported, including 22 cases of gastrointestinal events (diarrhoea, bloating, cramps, constipation and flatulence), 1 case of lightheadedness, 5 cases of viral infection, 1 case of hypertension, 1 case of body aches, 1 case of vomiting, 1 case of abnormal pathology result, and

**Table 5.27. GRADE: Oral Chinese Herbal Medicine vs. Placebo for Irritable Bowel Syndrome with Constipation**

| Outcome; Mean treatment duration | Estimated Absolute Effect | | Relative effect [95% CI] No. RCTs (Participants) | Certainty of evidence GRADE |
|---|---|---|---|---|
| | Oral CHM | Placebo | | |
| Adequate relief 8w | 61 per 100 | 44 per 100 | RR 1.39 [0.98, 1.95] 1 (125) | ⊕⊕○○ LOW[a] |
| | Difference: 17 more per 100 patients (95% CI: 43 to 85 more per 100 patients) | | | |
| Adequate relief at follow up 8w | 30 | 33 | RR 0.90 [0.53, 1.52] 1 (125) | ⊕⊕○○ LOW[a] |
| | Difference: 3 less per 100 patients (95% CI: 17 to 50 less per 100 patients) | | | |

Abbreviations: CI, confidence interval; FU, follow up; GRADE, Grading of Recommendations Assessment, Development and Evaluation; RR, risk ratio; w, weeks.

[a]High risk of bias from lack of blinding, large CI, small sample size.

References:
AR at 8 weeks: H113.
AR at follow up: H113.

1 case of blood in the urine. In the placebo group, 29 AEs were reported, including 11 cases of gastrointestinal events (diarrhoea, bloating, cramps, constipation and flatulence), 2 cases of lightheadedness, 2 cases of headache, 6 cases of viral infection, 1 case of asthma, 1 case of candida, 3 cases of body aches, 1 case of vomiting, 1 case of abnormal pathology result, and 1 case of fluid retention.

## *Frequently Reported Orally used Herbs in Meta-analyses Showing Favourable Effect*

To identify the most promising herbal candidates, the frequency of herbs used in the studies of meta-analyses showing favourable effects was calculated. The herb frequency was analysed based on different outcome categories. The stool habit category consists of meta-analyses of the outcomes of stool frequency and stool form; however, only

**Table 5.28. Frequently Reported Orally Used Herbs in Meta-Analyses Showing Favourable Effect for Irritable Bowel Syndrome with Predominant Constipation**

| Herbs | Scientific Name | Frequency of Use |
|---|---|---|
| **Stool habit: 1 meta-analysis, 3 RCTs** | | |
| *Bai shao* 白芍 | *Paeonia lactiflora* Pall. | 2 |
| *Bin lang/da fu pi* 槟榔/大腹皮 | *Areca catechu* L. | 1/1 |
| *Chen pi/qing pi* 陈皮/青皮 | *Citrus reticulata* Blanco | 1/1 |
| *Gan cao* 甘草 | *Glycyrrhiza* spp. | 2 |
| *Hou pu* 厚朴 | *Magnolia officinalis* Rehd. & Wils. | 2 |
| *Huo ma ren* 火麻仁 | *Cannabis sativa* L. | 2 |
| *Zhi shi/zhi qiao* 枳实/枳壳 | *Citrus aurantium* L. | 1/1 |
| **Quality of life: 1 meta-analysis, 2 RCTs** | | |
| *Bai zhu* 白术 | *Atractylodes macrocephala* Koidz. | 2 |
| *Bin lang* 槟榔 | *Areca catechu* L. | 2 |
| *Zhi shi* 枳实 | *Citrus aurantium* L. | 2 |

Stool habit: Refer to stool form CHM plus conventional medicine vs. conventional medicine
Quality of life: Refer to SF-36 CHM vs. pharmacotherapy

the stool form had meta-analyses. The categories of quality of life included meta-analyses of all domains of the SF-36.

The most common herbs of the meta-analyses favouring the use of CHM for IBS-C are listed in Table 5.28. It was found that among the two outcome categories, *bin lang/da fu pi* 槟榔/大腹皮 and *zhi shi/zhi qiao* 枳实/枳壳 were used most frequently.

## Controlled Clinical Trials of Oral Chinese Herbal Medicine

One CCT (H127) that studied the effects of oral CHM in IBS-C patients using the Rome III criteria without a specific syndrome was found. The study was conducted in China, involving 65 participants — 27 males and 38 females. The mean age was 43.16 years in the CHM group and 41.67 years in the control group. The duration of IBS was not presented. The treatment duration was four weeks without a follow-up period.

The study compared the manufactured CM product *Si mo tang kou fu ye* 四磨汤口服液 to mosapride, finding that the two groups had similar effects in the effective rate for abdominal pain (RR: 0.90 [0.65, 1.24]) and bloating (RR: 1.06 [0.78, 1.44]).

## Non-controlled Studies of Oral Chinese Herbal Medicine

One non-controlled study (H128; 120 participants) was retrieved using the Rome III criteria without a specific syndrome. The study was conducted in China in an outpatient department with 51 males and 69 females. Their age ranged from 18 to 64 years, and the duration of IBS ranged from 1 to 18 years. The treatment duration was 64 days without a follow-up period.

The study used the self-made formula *Tong bian tang* 通便汤 to treat the participants. It contained *bai shao* 白芍, *bai zhu* 白术, *rou cong rong* 肉苁蓉, *xing ren* 杏仁, *bing lang* 槟榔, *dang gui* 当归, *zhi shi* 枳实, *hou pu* 厚朴, *xiao mai* 小麦, *cu chai hu* 醋柴胡, *gan cao* 甘草, *sheng jiang* 生姜, and *da zao* 大枣.

## Enema Chinese Herbal Medicine

One RCT (H129) that studied the effects of CHM as an enema in IBS-C patients using the Rome II criteria with *qi* stagnation (with dampness-heat) syndrome 气机郁滞（夹湿热）was found. The study was conducted in China involving 64 participants — 22 males and 42 females. The mean age in the CHM group was 38.1 years and 39.5 years in the control group; the mean duration of IBS was 6.9 years in the CHM group and 6.5 years in the control group. The treatment duration was two weeks in the CHM group and four weeks in the control group.

The study compared *Shui liao er hao fang* 水疗 2 号方, including *da huang* 大黄, *zhi shi* 枳实, *mu xiang* 木香, *fu ling* 茯苓, *huang lian* 黄连, *huai hua* 槐花, *di yu* 地榆, *bing pian* 冰片, *chi shao* 赤芍, *dan shen* 丹参, and *dan pi* 丹皮 to tegaserod. The result showed a favourable effect in the CHM group by the Bristol scale, rating a lower score as a better effect (MD: −1.60 [−2.06, −1.14]).

## Risk of Bias

The study used a random table number for randomisation and was judged as "low" risk for the sequence generation domain. The study did not provide information on allocation concealment and was judged as an "unclear" risk for allocation concealment. Blinding of the participants and personnel was not achieved, and the study was judged as a "high" risk of bias due to a lack of blinding. There were no dropouts in the study, and it was judged as a "low" risk for this domain. No protocol could be located, so the study was judged as an "unclear" risk of bias for selective outcome reporting.

## Safety of Chinese Herbal Medicine in Treatment of Irritable Bowel Syndrome with Constipation

Among all oral CHM studies, eight RCTs mentioned checking safety outcomes, with no CCT or non-controlled study reporting AEs. The eight RCTs (H115, H118, H119, H122–H126) involved 680 participants. Three studies (H118, H123, H126) reported that no AEs occurred during the study periods. In total, 97 cases of AEs were observed in the other five studies (H113, H115, H119, H122, H125; 402 participants). Fifty AEs were observed in the CHM group, while 47 cases were found in the conventional medicine treatment group. With CHM treatments, the most common AEs were digestive disorders such as diarrhoea, bloating and flatulence.

The RCT (H129) using CHM as enemas reported that no AEs were observed in both groups.

# Clinical Evidence for Commonly Used Chinese Herbal Medicine Treatments

Several different CHMs were recommended by the CM clinical practice guidelines and textbooks, mostly based on expert consensus (refer to Chapter 2). In this chapter, we have identified clinical trials studying the efficacy and safety of some of these recommended formulae. Therefore, the clinical evidence underpinning these recommended CHM treatments is summarised.

For IBS-D, *Tong xie yao fang* 痛泻要方 was the most frequently studied CHM intervention. A total of 17 RCTs researched *Tong xie yao fang* modified 痛泻要方加减, alone or with other CHM formulae or conventional medicines in participants with IBS-D. They found that *Tong xie yao fang* 痛泻要方 showed an added benefit in reducing global symptoms when used with pharmacotherapy. *Shen ling bai zhu san* 参苓白术散, *Si shen wan* 四神丸 and *Fu zi li zhong tang* 附子理中汤 were commonly used formulae that are found in the guidelines; however, their outcome categories were dispersed and difficult to pool for analysis.

For IBS-C, no formulae used in the studies were the same, so we could not tell which were the most commonly used in clinical studies.

## Summary of Chinese Herbal Medicine Clinical Evidence

In total, 129 clinical studies were identified in this review for the evaluation of IBS. RCTs were the most common study design (118 studies). Among the included studies, CHM was administered orally in all but three studies. There was no fixed treatment course for CHM and the treatment durations varied from 2 to 8 weeks. Except for four studies, all studies were conducted in China. CHM alone or combined with conventional therapy as the intervention and conventional therapy as the control were the most common. CHM was variably administered in the form of decoctions and enemas. Included studies evaluated the effects of CHM on IBS subtypes by examining the outcomes in relation to the IBS-SSS, abdominal pain and related symptoms, stool frequency and stool form, and IBS-related quality of life. The following are summaries of IBS-D and IBS-C clinical studies using CHM.

### IBS-D Summary

The clinical studies evaluated the effects and safety of CHM for IBS-D and IBS-C subtypes, and the majority of the studies were on IBS-D

(112/129 studies, 87%). Information on CM syndrome differentiation was mentioned in 82 IBS-D studies (63.1%). The most common syndrome across the RCTs, CCTs and non-controlled studies was Liver *qi* stagnation with Spleen deficiency. In the IBS-D RCTs, Spleen and/ or Kidney *yang* deficiency was the second most commonly mentioned syndrome. In the two studies that used CHM as enemas, damp-heat was mentioned. The syndromes reported in the clinical studies aligned with those described in contemporary clinical textbooks and guidelines (see Chap. 2).

Oral CHM was the preferred route of administration in the included studies, which also reflects CHM clinical practice. Diversity was seen in the treatments used, with more than 80 different formulae used in the included clinical studies. More than 100 different herbs were used in the included formulae, with the most commonly used herbs being *bai zhu* 白术, *bai shao* 白芍, *fu ling* 茯苓, *chen pi* 陈皮, and *gan cao* 甘草.

For the IBS-D studies, although some formulae were unnamed and some were self-titled, we found by checking the ingredients that *Tong xie yao fang* 痛泻要方 was the core formula across the studies, and the formulae used in many trials were modified based on its composition. It was also used as an enema treatment.

Clinical outcomes were analysed in meta-analyses where possible or presented for individual studies where not possible. Results from meta-analyses of the IBS-D RCTs provided the best estimate of the treatment effect with CHM. Meta-analyses showed benefits with oral CHM, compared to a placebo and pharmacotherapy, in improving the TER of the IBS-SSS, total IBS-SSS score, and SF-36 domains. Oral CHM was more effective than pharmacotherapy in improving the subscales of IBS quality of life in dysphoria and interference with activity at the end of the treatment and follow-up. Compared to pharmacotherapy, oral CHM showed benefits in improving abdominal pain, including bloating or discomfort, and improving stool frequency and form.

Benefits were also seen when oral CHM and conventional therapies such as probiotics and pharmacotherapy were used together; improvements were observed in the IBS-SSS score, effective rate, quality of life scales, abdominal pain, abdominal bloating, and stool frequency and form.

One RCT using an enema for IBS-C showed a favourable effect when using CHM for the Bristol scale. Meta-analysis was not possible when oral CHM and enemas were used together.

Many studies reported on the safety of CHMs. AEs with CHMs were lower than with pharmacotherapy. AEs in the CHM groups included abdominal pain and nausea, which were also seen in the control groups using pharmacotherapy.

## IBS-C Summary

Seventeen IBS-C studies were identified. Six RCTs (23.5%) applied specific syndromes as one of the study inclusion criteria; the different syndromes used were *qi* stagnation and intestinal dryness, *qi* stagnation (or with *yin* deficiency with internal heat), Liver stagnation and Spleen deficiency, and Spleen deficiency and *qi* stagnation. The damp-heat syndrome was mentioned in one RCT that used CHM as an enema for IBS-C. The syndromes reported in the clinical studies aligned with those described in contemporary clinical textbooks and guidelines (see Chap. 2).

For IBS-C, the formulae were very different, so it was difficult to identify one core formula. All studies evaluated different formulae. Among these formulae, nine were unnamed or self-named, while others were traditional formulae (standard and modified) as well as commercial products.

Meta-analyses showed benefits with oral CHM when compared to pharmacotherapy in improving all SF-36 domains and in three domains (SF, RE, MH) when CHM was used in combination with conventional medicine. When CHM was added to conventional therapy, benefits were seen in the reduction of the SDS score and improved stool frequency. One RCT using an enema for IBS-C showed a favourable effect of using CHM for the Bristol scale.

There are several limitations of this review. None of the studies were free from bias. Although called RCTs, the included studies lacked details of randomisation and allocation concealment, with no blinding of treatment groups. The meta-analysis largely focused on the overall effect of CHM on different outcomes, while CHM treatment details, such as formula ingredients, herb dosage, and treatment duration, varied from study to study. Not surprisingly, therefore, substantial heterogeneity was detected.

Further, different measurements of the Bristol stool form score led to studies not being able to be grouped for meta-analysis, resulting in a small sample size and lacking the value of the measurement.

Finally, only a few studies included follow-up data, so the long-term effect of CHM on IBS-D and IBS-C is unknown.

# References

1. Liu JP, Yang M, Liu Y, *et al.* (2006) Herbal medicines for treatment of irritable bowel syndrome. *Cochrane Database of Syst Rev.* **(1):** CD004116.
2. 魏秋月. (2016) 中药治疗腹泻型肠易激综合征疗效的 Meta 分析. 辽宁中医药大学, 中国沈阳.
3. Shi J, Tong Y, Shen JG, Li HX. (2008) Effectiveness and safety of herbal medicines in the treatment of irritable bowel syndrome: A systematic review. *World J Gastroenterol.* **14(3):** 454–462.
4. Bian Z, Wu T, Liu L, *et al.* (2006) Effectiveness of the Chinese herbal formula TongXieYaoFang for irritable bowel syndrome: A systematic review. *J Altern Complement Med.* **2(4):** 401–407.
5. 侯飞飞, 郭晓钟, 吴春燕, *et al.* (2016) 中医疏肝健脾法治疗腹泻型肠易激综合征临床疗效荟萃分析. *辽宁中医药大学学报.* **18(5):** 183–186.
6. 黄绍刚, 张海燕. (2011) 疏肝健脾法治疗腹泻型肠易激综合征 (IBS-D) 随机对照试验的 Meta 分析. *中国中医基础医学杂志.* **17(1):** 80–81.
7. 张莎, 王文, 李哲, *et al.* (2016) 从肝脾辨治腹泻型肠易激综合征的 Meta 分析. *中国医导报.* **22(20):** 69–73.
8. Xiao Y, Liu Y, Huang S, *et al.* (2015) The efficacy of Shugan Jianpi Zhixie therapy for diarrhea-predominant irritable bowel syndrome: A meta-analysis of randomized, double-blind, placebo-controlled trials. *PLoS One.* **10(4):** e0122397.
9. Zhu JJ, Liu S, Su XL, *et al.* (2016) Efficacy of Chinese herbal medicine for diarrhea-predominant irritable bowel syndrome: A meta-analysis of

randomized, double-blind, placebo-controlled trials. *Evid Based Complement Alternat Med.* **2016:** 4071260.

10. Li Q, Liu F, Hou Z, Luo D. (2013) Treatment of constipation-predominant irritable bowel syndrome by focusing on the liver in terms of traditional Chinese medicine: A meta-analysis. *J Tradit Chin Med.* **33(5):** 562–571.

11. Li DY, Dai YK, Zhang YZ, *et al.* (2017) Systematic review and meta-analysis of traditional Chinese medicine in the treatment of constipation-predominant irritable bowel syndrome. *PLoS One.* **12(12):** e0189491.

12. Li C-Y, Tahir NAM, Li S-C. (2015) A systematic review of integrated traditional Chinese and Western medicine for managing irritable bowel syndrome. *Am J Chinese Med.* **43(3):** 385–406.

13. 中华中医药学会脾胃病分会. (2010) 肠易激综合征中医诊疗共识意见. *中华中医药杂志.* **25(7):** 1062–1065.

14. 郑筱萸. (2002) 中药新药临床研究指导原则. 中国医药科技出版社, 中国北京.

15. 中国中西医结合学会消化系统委员会. (2010) 胃肠疾病中医症状评分表. *中国中西医结合消化杂志.* **19(1):** 66–69.

16. 危北海, 陈治水, 张万岱. (2004) 胃肠疾病中医证候评分表. *世界华人消化杂志.* **12(11):** 2701–2703.

17. 李乾构. 周学文, 单兆伟. (2006) *中医消化病诊疗指南.* 中国中医药出版社, 中国北京.

# References for Included Chinese Herbal Medicine Clinical Studies

| Study No. | Reference |
| --- | --- |
| H1 | 熊潭玮. (2016) 疏肝健脾方加不同风药治疗腹泻型肠易激综合征临床观察. *华夏医学.* **29(4):** 28–32. |
| H2 | 吴皓萌. (2016) 疏肝健脾法干预腹泻型肠易激综合征的临床和实验研究. 广州中医药大学, 中国广州. |
| H3 | 张声生, 许文君, 陈贞, *et al.* (2010) 疏肝健脾法与健脾化湿法治疗腹泻型肠易激综合征对比疗效观察. *中华中医药杂志.* **25(1):** 127130. |
| H4 | 赵庆卫, 吕道仙. (2015) 痛泻宁颗粒联合金双歧治疗腹泻型肠易激综合征随机对照研究. *中国医学创新.* **12(26):** 68–71. |

| Study No. | Reference |
|---|---|
| H5 | 梁枫. (2006) 固肠止泻汤治疗腹泻型肠易激综合征 68 例. *江苏中医药*. **27(12):** 29–30. |
| H6 | 骆天炯. (2003) 健脾疏肝法对肠易激综合征血浆及粘膜β内啡肽的调节作用. *中国中西医结合杂志*. **23(8):** 616–618. |
| H7 | 蔡键锋. (2005) 病症结合治疗腹泻型肠易激综合征有效性的临床观察. 湖北中医药大学硕士学位论文, 中国武汉. |
| H8 | Ko S-J, Han G, Kim S-K, *et al.* (2013) Effect of Korean herbal medicine combined with a probiotic mixture on diarrhea-dominant irritable bowel syndrome: A double–blind, randomized, placebo-controlled trial. *ECAM.* **2013:** 824605. |
| H9 | 张超贤, 郭李柯, 秦咏梅. (2016) 针刺联合参苓健脾胃颗粒治疗肠易激综合征腹泻型的近远期疗效观察. *中华中医药学刊*. **34(4):** 854–859. |
| H10 | 李玲.（2005）参苓白术散配合耳穴按压治疗腹泻型肠易激综合征（脾虚湿阻证）的临床研究. 湖南中医药大学硕士学位论文, 中国长沙. |
| H11 | 刘启泉. (2010) 隔山逍遥方配合针刺疗法对肠易激综合征患者生活质量影响的临床观察. *浙江中医药大学学报*. **34(4):** 510–511, 513. |
| H12 | 李熠萌, 林江, 蔡淦, 陈明显. (2014) 肠吉泰联合经皮穴位电刺激法治疗腹泻型肠易激综合征的随机、双盲、安慰剂对照研究. *中国中西医结合消化杂志*. **22(1):** 1–4. |
| H13 | Alam MS, Roy PK, Miah AR, *et al.* (2013) Efficacy of Peppermint oil in diarrhea predominant IBS — a double blind randomized placebo — controlled study. *Mymensingh Med. J* **22(2):** 27–30. |
| H14 | Aniwan S, Gonlachanvit S. (2014) Effects of chili treatment on gastrointestinal and rectal sensation in diarrhea-predominant irritable bowel syndrome: A randomized, double–blinded, crossover study. *J Neurogastroenterol.* **20(3):** 400–406. |
| H15 | 文廷玉. (2016) 附子理中汤合四神丸加减治疗脾肾阳虚型腹泻型肠易激综合征. *中国实验方剂学杂志*. **22(9):** 177–180. |
| H16 | 钱潇, 章静, 张娅丽. (2016) 痛泻要方加减治疗腹泻型肠易激综合征疗效及安全性观察. *浙江中西医结合杂志*. **26(10):** 941–943. |
| H17 | 刘倩, 田洁, 张海超, *et al.* (2016) 自拟运脾清肠方治疗腹泻型肠易激综合征 60 例. *中国中西医结合消化杂志*. **24(5):** 393–396. |
| H18 | 黎颖婷. (2012) 基于肝脾辨证中医药治疗腹泻型肠易激综合征的临床研究. 广州中医药大学, 中国广州. |

(*Continued*)

**(Continued)**

| Study No. | Reference |
| --- | --- |
| H19 | 刘嘉梦. (2016) 肠激灵治疗腹泻型肠易激综合征对生存质量影响的观察. 广州中医药大学硕士学位论文, 中国广州. |
| H20 | 闫丹丹. (2015) 合欢苓术方治疗肝气郁滞心神失养型 IBS–D 的临床研究. 河北医科大学硕士学位论文, 中国石家庄. |
| H21 | 陶琳, 张声生, 肖旸, *et al.* (2012) 健脾疏肝法对腹泻型肠易激综合征患者生活质量的影响. *北京中医药.* **31(6):** 437–440. |
| H22 | 成亚亚. (2015) 柴芍调肝方治疗肝郁脾虚型肠易激综合征临床研究. 河北医科大学硕士学位论文, 中国石家庄. |
| H23 | 李文花. (2013) 辨证分型治疗腹泻型肠易激综合征随机平行对照研究. *实用中医内科杂志.* **27(7):** 41–43. |
| H24 | 张声生, 汪红兵, 李振华, *et al.* (2010) 中医药辨证治疗腹泻型肠易激综合征多中心随机对照研究. *中国中西医结合杂志.* **30(1):** 9–12. |
| H25 | 林李淼, 陈浩, 陈碧红, *et al.* (2008) 乌灵胶囊治疗伴有抑郁症状的腹泻型肠易激综合征的对照研究. *安徽医药.* **12(5):** 445–446. |
| H26 | 夏东俊. (2014) 温中健脾方联合马来酸曲美布汀治疗腹泻型肠易激综合征脾阳虚证的临床研究. 湖北中医药大学硕士学位论文. |
| H27 | 卞立群. (2011) 肠安 Ⅰ 号方治疗 IBS–D 的临床疗效评价暨临床疗效评价指标的比较研究. 中国中医科学院博士学位论文, 中国北京. |
| H28 | Leung WK, Wu, JCY, Liang SM, *et al.* (2006) Treatment of diarrhea-predominant irritable bowel syndrome with traditional Chinese herbal medicine: A randomized placebo-controlled trial. *Am J Gastroenterol.* **101(7):** 1574–1580. |
| H29 | Tang XD, Lu B, Li ZH, *et al.* (2016) Therapeutic effect of Chang'an I recipe (I) on irritable bowel syndrome with diarrhea: A multicenter randomized double–blind placebo-controlled clinical trial. *Chin J Integr Med.* **24(9):** 645–652. |
| H30 | 蔡淦, 雷云霞, 郑顺化, 李熠萌. (2006) 肠吉泰治疗腹泻型肠易激综合征 60 例疗效观察. *江西中医药.* **37(5):** 20–21. |
| H31 | 李熠萌, 张亚楠, 蔡淦, 林江. (2010) 肠吉泰治疗腹泻型肠易激综合征的随机双盲安慰剂平行对照试验. *上海中医药杂志.* **44(12):** 33–36. |
| H32 | 雷云霞, 刘新, 蔡淦, 张正利. (2011) 肠吉泰对腹泻型肠易激综合征患者生活质量影响的临床研究. *新疆医学.* **41(11):** 8–12. |
| H33 | 沈芸, 蔡淦, 孙旭, 赵昊龙. (2003) 中药复方肠吉泰治疗腹泻型肠易激综合征的临床随机对照观察. *中国中西医结合杂志.* **23(11):** 823–825. |

**(*Continued*)**

| Study No. | Reference |
|---|---|
| H34 | 陈明显, 陈军贤, 夏亮, *et al.* (2014) 抑肝扶脾汤治疗腹泻型肠易激综合征的随机对照临床研究. *中国中西医结合杂志*. **34(6):** 656–660. |
| H35 | 杨静, 张声生. (2009) 疏肝健脾化湿法治疗腹泻型肠易激综合征临床观察. *中国中西医结合消化杂志*. **17(1):** 12–14. |
| H36 | 来要良, 杨晋翔, 黄海啸. (2012) 固本调肠汤治疗腹泻型肠易激综合征疗效观察. *中国中西医结合消化杂志*. **20(4):** 153–155. |
| H37 | 李小兰, 苏振政, 顾向东. (2014) 肠益清治疗肠易激综合征脾虚湿盛证的疗效观察. *中国中西医结合消化杂志*. **22(8):** 475–477. |
| H38 | 郭晨希. (2016) 健脾清化法联合微生态制剂治疗腹泻型肠易激综合征脾虚湿热证的临床观察. 南京中医药大学硕士学位论文, 中国南京. |
| H39 | 蔡利军, 吕宾, 孟立娜, *et al.* (2013) 疏肝健脾温肾法治疗腹泻型肠易激综合征疗效观察. *中华中医药学刊*. **31(5):** 1097–1099. |
| H40 | 李医芳. (2011) 温肾健脾法治疗腹泻型肠易激综合征的临床观察. 北京中医药大学硕士学位论文, 中国北京. |
| H41 | 齐增产. (2016) 益气固肠方治疗腹泻型肠易激综合征的临床研究及对结肠粘膜电镜下超微结构的影响. 河北医科大学硕士学位论文, 中国石家庄. |
| H42 | 张莹. (2015) 温肾健脾方治疗腹泻型肠易激综合征的临床疗效观察. 北京中医药大学硕士学位论文, 中国北京. |
| H43 | 李从燕. (2015) 健脾化湿方治疗脾虚湿阻证腹泻型肠易激综合征的临床研究. 安徽中医药大学硕士论文, 中国合肥. |
| H44 | 杨志. (2016) 九味镇心颗粒联合匹维溴铵治疗肠易激综合征的效果分析. *中国中西医结合消化杂志*. **24(5):** 379–382. |
| H45 | 王兵. (2014) 缓肝理脾汤治疗腹泻型肠易激综合征临床观察. *中国中医急症*. **23(10):** 1943–1944. |
| H46 | 马冬颖, 彭莉莉. (2016) 四逆散合痛泻要方加味治疗腹泻型肠易激综合征疗效观察. *山西中医*. **32(1):** 16–17. |
| H47 | 池美华, 王忠建, 姚憬, 黄金海. (2012) 葛连藿苏汤治疗腹泻型肠易激综合征 35 例. *浙江中西医结合杂志*. **22(6):** 483–484. |
| H48 | 丁倩. (2015) 补脾清肠法对肠易激综合症小肠细菌过度生长影响的临床疗效观察. 南京中医药大学硕士学位论文, 中国南京. |
| H49 | 孙光裕, 陈壁亮. (2003) 匹维溴铵联合固肠止泻丸治疗腹泻为主型肠易激综合征. *广东医学*. **24(12):** 1365–1366. |
| H50 | 徐建军. (2012) 痛泻要方加味治疗腹泻型肠易激综合征疗效观察. *浙江中西医结合杂志*. **22(10):** 775–776. |

(*Continued*)

**(Continued)**

| Study No. | Reference |
|---|---|
| H51 | 詹程胹, 潘锋, 张涛. (2011) 基于血浆及结肠黏膜 Ghrelin 变化探讨半夏泻心汤干预腹泻型肠易激综合征临床研究. *中华中医药学刊*. **29(11):** 2588–2591. |
| H52 | 潘瑞东. (2014) 五苓散合四逆散加减治疗肠易激综合征腹泻型（脾虚肝郁证）的临床研究. 成都中医药大学硕士学位论文, 中国成都. |
| H53 | 陈默. (2016) 八神汤治疗腹泻型肠易激综合征脾肾阳虚型的疗效观察. 福建中医药大学硕士学位论文, 中国福州. |
| H54 | 董倩. (2011) 加味黄芪建中汤加减治疗腹泻型肠易激综合征（脾气虚型）的临床观察. 成都中医药大学硕士学位论文, 中国成都. |
| H55 | 韩文冬. (2012) 固本安肠汤治疗腹泻型肠易激综合征的临床研究. 陕西中医学员硕士学位论文, 中国咸阳. |
| H56 | 陈春音. (2016) 中西医结合治疗腹泻型肠易激综合征 54 例. *光明中医*. **31(22):** 3340–3341. |
| H57 | 陈建林, 陈锦锋, 邓健敏, 韩宇斌. (2016) 加味痛泻要方对肝郁脾虚型肠易激综合征患者小肠黏膜 5– 羟色胺含量及其受体 mRNA 表达的影响. *中国中西医结合消化杂志*. **24(6):** 442–445. |
| H58 | 甄杰武. (2009) 健脾化湿法治疗腹泻型肠易激综合征的临床研究. 广州中医药大学硕士学位论文, 中国广州. |
| H59 | 陈一斌, 吴耀南, 王芸素, 曹健. (2015) 调肠方治疗腹泻型肠易激综合征肾阳虚证综合疗效评价. *光明中医*. **30(5):** 966–968. |
| H60 | 刘晓辉, 刘启泉. (2006) 合欢逍遥颗粒治疗腹泻型肠易激综合征的临床观察. *辽宁中医药大学学报*. **8(4):** 91. |
| H61 | 谢彬. (2010) 平调肝脾法治疗腹泻型肠易激综合征肝郁脾虚型的临床研究. 南京中医药大学硕士学位论文, 中国南京. |
| H62 | 陈奕霞, 王海燕, 邓素萍. (2014) 四逆散合痛泻要方加味对肠易激综合征患者血清 5– 羟色胺表达水平的影响研究. *检验医学与临床*. **11(11):** 1462–1463, 1467. |
| H63 | 陆玲英. (2009) 逍遥散加味治疗腹泻型肠易激综合征 36 例. *山东中医杂志*. **28(4):** 228–229. |
| H64 | 宋玉琴. (2015) 抑木扶土汤治疗腹泻型肠易激综合征 (肝郁脾虚证) 的临床观察. 云南中医学院硕士学位论文, 中国昆明. |
| H65 | 王聪. (2012) 加减升阳益胃汤合马来酸曲美布汀治疗腹泻型肠易激综合征临床观察. 湖北中医药大学硕士学位论文, 中国武汉. |
| H66 | 张震坤, 王宁宁, 李倩雯. (2014) 参苓白术散加减对肠易激综合征患者脑肠肽的影响. *光明中医*. **29(8):** 1633–1635. |

**(*Continued*)**

| Study No. | Reference |
|---|---|
| H67 | 郭爱华. (2014) 参苓白术散加味治疗肠易激综合征(腹泻型)脾胃虚弱证的临床研究. 陕西中医学院硕士学位论文, 中国咸阳. |
| H68 | 段晓东. (2012) 健脾安肠汤治疗腹泻型肠易激综合征的临床研究. 山东中医药大学硕士学位论文, 中国济南. |
| H69 | 张声生, 汪红兵, 陶琳, *et al.* (2004) 健脾化湿法治疗腹泻型肠易激综合征及其对胃肠激素影响的研究. *中国医药学报*. **19(8):** 479–481. |
| H70 | 张艳霞. (2015) 四逆当归方对腹泻型肠易激综合征患者 vip, Ss, Mot 含量的影响. *辽宁中医杂志*. **42(11):** 2146–2148. |
| H71 | 楚梦颖. (2013) 中药联合马来酸曲美布汀治疗肠易激综合征. *长春中医药大学学报*. **29(1):** 132–133. |
| H72 | 张玉柱. (2006) 自拟疏肝止泻汤治疗腹泻型肠易激综合征 50 例临床观察. *北京中医*. **25(7):** 419–421. |
| H73 | 郑娟霞. (2014) 缓急止痛颗粒治疗腹泻型肠易激综合征的临床研究. 山西省中医药研究院硕士学位论文, 中国太原. |
| H74 | 包永欣. (2015) 肝脾肾同调对腹泻型肠易激综合征患者腹痛视觉模拟评分及排便情况的影响. *中华中医药学刊*. **33(3):** 650–652. |
| H75 | 王海芬, 韩宝娟, 赵慧敏, *et al.* (2014) 自拟心肠易激宁液治疗抑郁状态腹泻型肠易激综合征患者的临床疗效. *临床合理用药杂志*. **7(17):** 55–56. |
| H76 | 陆彩霞, 焦建华. (2010) 益肠汤治疗腹泻型肠易激综合征的疗效观察. *现代中西医结合杂志*. **19(31):** 3407–3408. |
| H77 | 岳妍, 王文仲, 杨强, *et al.* (2004) 蒺藜汤治疗腹泻型肠易激综合征. *中国中医药信息杂志*. **11(5):** 447. |
| H78 | 邱允忠. (2010) 辛开苦降法治疗腹泻型肠易激综合症的疗效观察. *实用临床医药杂志*. **14(23):** 104, 111. |
| H79 | 余超. (2013) 调和肝脾法治疗腹泻型肠易激综合征临床疗效观察. 南京中医药大学, 中国南京. |
| H80 | 李力强, 张贵锋, 曾艺文, *et al.* (2016) 左金丸合四逆散辨证治疗腹泻型肠易激综合征 72 例临床观察. *中医杂志*. **57:** 1214–1217. |
| H81 | Wang G, Li TQ, Wang L, *et al.* (2006) Tong-xie-ning, a Chinese herbal formula, in treatment of diarrhea-predominant irritable bowel syndrome: A prospective, randomized, double-blind, placebo-controlled trial. *Chin Med J.* **119(24):** 2114–2119. |
| H82 | 吴宇. (2016) 加味痛泻要方联合培菲康治疗腹泻型肠易激综合征疗效观察. *现代中西医结合杂志*. **25(11):** 1198–1200. |

*(Continued)*

**(*Continued*)**

| Study No. | Reference |
|---|---|
| H83 | 王新磊. (2014) 加味黄芪建中汤治疗伴轻中度焦虑抑郁 IBS–D（脾阳虚证）临床观察. 成都中医药大学, 中国成都. |
| H84 | 刘添文, 陈新林, 缪旺冬, 钟亮环. (2016) 半夏泻心汤治疗腹泻型肠易激综合征临床观察. *新中医*. **48(8):** 76–79. |
| H85 | 田艳朋, 袁旭潮, 王康永, *et al.* (2016) 腹泻 II 号方治疗腹泻型肠易激综合征 23 例. *江西中医药*. **47(8):** 56–57, 62. |
| H86 | 李恺. (2015) 痛泻药方加减对肠易激综合征肝郁脾虚型腹泻患者的临床研究. *检验医学与临床*. **12(12):** 1707–1709. |
| H87 | 张艳霞. (2016) 加味当芍药散治疗腹泻型肠易激综合征 60 例. *环球中医药*. **9(1):** 100–102. |
| H88 | 潘相学, 谢建群. (2006) 疏肝饮治疗肠易激综合征的临床疗效观察. *上海中医药大学学报*. **20(4):** 48–50. |
| H89 | 张琼, 陈定玉. (2014) 疏补温肾固肠方治疗腹泻型肠易激综合征的疗效观察. *中国药房*. **25(35):** 3338–3340. |
| H90 | 辛红. (2015) 抑木扶土方治疗腹泻型肠易激综合征肝气乘脾证临床观察. *上海中医药杂志*. **49(4):** 47–49. |
| H91 | 顾勇刚, 乔春萍, 陆红, *et al.* (2016) 二姜四神汤治疗腹泻型肠易激综合征临床观察. *四川中医*. **34(7):** 85–88. |
| H92 | 孔梅, 邢常永, 王莺. (2010) 痛泻要方颗粒剂干预腹泻型肠易激综合征结肠黏膜 VIP, SP 表达的临床研究. *中药材*. **33(10):** 1668–1671. |
| H93 | 许德坚. (2009) 肠吉饮治疗腹泻型肠易激综合征 30 例. *江西中医药*. **10(40):** 28–29. |
| H94 | 彭万枫. (2016) 二神丸联合参苓白术散对肠易激综合征 (腹泻型) 脾胃虚弱证的临床干预作用. *新疆中医药*. **34(1):** 7–9. |
| H95 | 刘倩. (2015) 升阳益胃汤加减治疗腹泻型肠易激综合征临床疗效观察. 河北医科大学, 中国石家庄. |
| H96 | 聂玮, 张立平, 孟捷, *et al.* (2014) 疏肝健脾法治疗腹泻型肠易激综合征的研究. *现代中西医结合杂志*. **23(31):** 3421–3423, 3427. |
| H97 | 曹洋, 朱宏, 王永庆. (2016) 气滞胃痛颗粒治疗腹泻型肠易激综合征的疗效. *江苏医药*. **42(10):** 1120–1122. |
| H98 | 卢亮. (2014) 抑肝扶脾养心安神法治疗腹泻型肠易激综合征肝郁脾虚型的临床研究. 南京中医药大学, 中国南京. |
| H99 | 陈峰松, 索红军, 范辉. (2010) 疏肝解郁汤治疗腹泻型肠易激综合征 30 例. *世界华人消化杂志*. **18(25):** 2715–2718. |

**(*Continued*)**

| Study No. | Reference |
| --- | --- |
| H100 | 张芸. (2011) 中西医结合治疗腹泻型肠易激综合征伴焦虑状态疗效观察. *光明中医*. **27(7):** 1422–1424. |
| H101 | Pan F, Zhang T, Zhang Y-H, *et al.* (2009) Effect of Tongxie Yaofang Granule in treating diarrhea–predominate irritable bowel syndrome. *Chin Med J.* **15(3):** 216–219. |
| H102 | 宫毅, 杨阳. (2007) 逍遥合剂治疗肠易激综合征肝郁脾虚证的临床观察. *中国肛肠病杂志.* **27(7):** 35–36. |
| H103 | 张强. (2016) 柴术愈肠饮治疗肠易激综合征肝郁脾虚夹湿证的临床观察. |
| H104 | 叶涛, 陶夏平. (2013) 乌梅丸用于寒热错杂型腹泻型肠易激综合征的疗效评价. *国际中医中药杂志.* **35(8):** 689–691. |
| H105 | 张艳国, 佟秀芳, 郑素梅, *et al.* (2011) 通络安肠饮治疗情志不遂所致腹泻型肠易激综合症的疗效观察. *中国美容医学.* **20(6):** 367. |
| H106 | 高志远, 张正利. (2008) 辨证治疗腹泻型肠易激综合征 82 例. *山东中医杂志.* **27(11):** 736–738. |
| H107 | 邱春华. (2016) 参倍固肠胶囊治疗腹泻型肠易激综合征开放、多中心、Ⅳ期临床试验. *中国中药杂志.* **41(10):** 1947–1951. |
| H108 | 马玉萍, 苏进义, 丁乾, *et al.* (2011) 升阳益胃汤加减治疗腹泻型肠易激综合征 240 例. *辽宁中医杂志.* **38(4):** 657–659. |
| H109 | 王莹, 万霞. (2013) 中西医结合治疗肠易激惹综合征疗效观察. *中国伤残医学.* **21(6):** 283–284. |
| H110 | 黄沁, 许尊贤, 魏睦新. (2008) 痛泻要方加味治疗腹泻型肠易激综合征 50 例. *江苏中医药.* **40(1):** 47–48. |
| H111 | 朱永苹, 林寿宁, 杨秀静, *et al.* (2013) 水疗一号方对腹泻型肠易激综合征患者血清中乙酰胆碱和血管活性肠肽的影响. *辽宁中医杂志.* **40(8):** 1658–1660. |
| H112 | 梁振平, 李平. (2012) 痛泻要方加味联合微生态制剂经结肠途径治疗腹泻型肠易激综合征. *中国实验方剂学杂志.* **18(5):** 217–219. |
| H113 | Bensoussan A, Kellow JE, Bourchier SJ, *et al.* (2015) Efficacy of a Chinese herbal medicine in providing adequate relief of constipation–predominant irritable bowel syndrome: A randomized controlled trial. *Clin. Gastroenterol. Hepatol.* **13(11):** 1946–1954. |
| H114 | 龙文醒, 钟毅. (2013) 肠激宁治疗功能性消化不良重叠便秘型肠易激综合征 30 例疗效观察. *云南中医中药杂志.* **34(5):** 44–45. |
| H115 | 姜岩. (2016) 自拟运肠通腑煎剂联合马来酸曲美布汀治疗便秘型肠易激综合征患者 46 例. *环球中医药.* **9(9):** 1127–1129. |

(*Continued*)

**(*Continued*)**

| Study No. | Reference |
|---|---|
| H116 | 高影. (2008) 枳术汤加减治疗便秘型肠易激综合征的临床观察. *中国实用医药*. **3(33):** 9–10. |
| H117 | 王艳艳, 朱叶姗, 石志敏. (2011) 中医疗法结合护理干预对改善便秘型肠易激综合征患者生活质量作用的研究. *贵阳中医学院学报*. **33(4):** 17–19. |
| H118 | 苏月娴. (2014) 枳实消痞丸配合饮食治疗便秘型肠易激综合征（脾虚气滞证）的临床观察. |
| H119 | 汪运鹏. (2007) 通幽清治疗便秘型肠易激综合征疗效观察. |
| H120 | 张家炎, 黎达. (2009) 疏肝健脾法治疗便秘型肠易激综合征的临床疗效分析. *甘肃中医*. **22(7):** 23–24. |
| H121 | 梁雪, 黄祖美, 王鹏. (2016) 调气清热方治疗气滞肠燥证便秘型肠易激综合征临床观察. *广西中医药*. **39(2):** 13–17. |
| H122 | 林李淼, 陈浩, 陈碧红, *et al.* (2008) 乌灵胶囊治疗伴有抑郁症状的便秘型肠易激综合征的对照研究. *现代中西医结合杂志*. **17(17):** 2597–8, 601. |
| H123 | 李志涵. (2015) 木香顺气丸联合莫沙必利治疗便秘型肠易激综合征的疗效观察. *现代药物与临床*. **30(8):** 999–1003. |
| H124 | 邬美萍. (2005) 中西医结合治疗便秘型肠易激综合征 30 例临床观察. *中国中医药科技*. **12(6):** 400. |
| H125 | 俞峻. (2010) 马来酸曲美布汀联合六味安消胶囊治疗便秘型肠易激综合征. *中国临床医生*. **38(1):** 55–56. |
| H126 | 王飞达. (2015) 三脏调和润肠汤治疗便秘型易激综合征的临床研究. 浙江中医药大学硕士学位论文, 中国杭州. |
| H127 | 曹曙光, 王建嶂, 蔡振寨, *et al.* (2010) 四磨汤治疗便秘型肠易激综合征患者肠道气体的临床观察. *中国中西医结合杂志*. **30(1):** 94–96. |
| H128 | 赵彬, 孙玉芳. (2012) 通便汤为主治疗便秘型肠易激综合征 120 例. *河南中医*. **32(7):** 867–868. |
| H129 | 吴晓君. (2007) 水疗 2 号方治疗便秘型肠易激综合征疗效观察. *广西中医学报*. **10(1):** 16–17. |

# 6

# Pharmacological Actions of Frequently Used Herbs

## OVERVIEW

The therapeutic effects of Chinese herbal formulae and herbs for irritable bowel syndrome (IBS) are largely attributed to their active compounds. This section reviews the experimental evidence to explore the possible biological activities and mechanisms of the 10 most frequently used Chinese herbs from the randomised clinical trials identified in Chap. 5.

## Introduction

This chapter reviews experimental evidence from *in vitro* experimental cells and *in vivo* animal models for the 10 most frequently used herbs identified in Chap. 5 for irritable bowel syndrome (IBS) subtypes with prominent diarrhoea (IBS-D) and with prominent constipation (IBS-C), to possibly explain the findings from the randomised controlled clinical trials (RCTs) for IBS. Some herbs are used in both subtypes, including *bai zhu* 白术, *bai shao/chi shao* 白芍/赤芍, *gan cao* 甘草, and *chai hu* 柴胡, while *fu ling* 茯苓, *chen pi/qin pi* 陈皮/青皮 and *fang feng* 防风 are used in IBS-D and *zhi shi/zhi qiao* 枳实/枳壳, *hou po* 厚朴, and *bing lang/da fu pi* 槟榔/大腹皮 are used in IBS-C. Common formulae are also reviewed: *Tong xie yao fang* 痛泻要方 and *Si ni san* 四逆散.

In relation to the pathological processes and mechanisms of IBS described in Chap. 1, although the pathogenesis of IBS has many mechanisms, low-grade mucosal inflammation, gastrointestinal motility impairment, and visceral hypersensitivity are the key factors among its multifactorial pathogenesis. To identify experimental studies by their pharmacological actions of relevance to IBS, the pharmacological activities of each herb and/or compound will be focused on in relation to their therapeutic effects of anti-gastrointestinal inflammation, improvement in gastrointestinal motility, promotion of intestinal laxity and restoration of intestinal permeability, if available.

## Methods

The constituent compounds were identified by searching herbal medicine encyclopedias,[1] materia medica,[2] high-quality reviews of Chinese herbal medicine (CHM), and PubMed. To identify pre-clinical studies, literature searches in PubMed and Pubmed Central were undertaken. Search terms included the names of the plant in Chinese *pinyin* and their scientific names, and the names of the compounds contained within. These were combined with the terms "irritable bowel syndrome", "constipation", "diarrhoea", "gastrointestinal disorder", "gastrointestinal motility", and "visceral hypersensitivity".

## Experimental Studies of *bai zhu* 白术

The rhizome of *bai zhu* 白术 (*Atractylodes macrocephala* Koidz) has long been used as a tonic agent for the treatment of gastrointestinal hypofunction in East Asia, especially in China. At least 79 chemical compounds have been identified from *A. macrocephala*, including sesquiterpenoids, triterpenoids, polyacetylenes, coumarins, phenylpropanoids, flavonoids and flavonoid glycosides, steroids, benzoquinones, polysaccharides, and others. Among them, sesquiterpenoids, polyacetylenes and polysaccharides are the most abundant and major bioactive constituents that contribute most of the pharmacological activities of *A. macrocephala*.[2,3]

Pharmacological effects in relation to IBS, such as improving the gastrointestinal function and immunomodulatory activity, which make *A. macrocephala* outstanding in the treatment of IBS, are reviewed below.

## Anti-gastrointestinal Inflammation

Recently, researchers have focused their attention on the pivotal role of low-grade mucosal inflammation in IBS, with evidence showing that in some IBS patients have an increased number of inflammatory cells in the colonic and ileal mucosa.[4]

It has been reported that sesquiterpenoids, especially atractyle-nolides, demonstrated significant anti-inflammatory activity on the peritoneal capillary permeability induced by acetic acid in mice.[5] Polyacetylenes, particularly 14-acetoxy-12-senecioyloxytetradeca-2E, 8E,10E-trien-4,6-diyn-1-ol 41 derived from *A. macrocephala*, could be comparable to L-N6 -(1-iminoethyl)-lysine, a selective inhibitor of inducible nitric oxide synthase,[6] while some phenylpro-panoids, including Z-methyl caffeate, ferulic acid, 2-hydroxy ferulic acid and Z-5-hydroxy ferulic acid, have also been shown to have remarkable anti-inflammatory activity.[7] Moreover, the protection of gastric mucosa from low-grade inflammation through its anti-oxidant effects and increased vascular endothelial growth factor (VEGF) expression has been shown in a study with a *Zhizhu* decoction composed of *A. macrocephala* and *A. fructus* in an ethanol-induced ulcer rat model.[8]

## Intestinal Protective Effect

In intestinal epithelial cell 6 (IEC-6) cells, a methanol extract of *A. macrocephala* significantly improved cellular polyamine content, membrane hyperpolarisation, and cytoplasmic $Ca^{2+}$ level, and stimulated the migration of intestinal epithelial cells to promote the healing of intestinal injuries. These effects might involve the polyam-ine-Kv1.1 channel signalling pathway.[9] In a rat model, oral administration of atractylenolide I, atractylenolide III, and 4,15-epoxy-8$\beta$hydroxyasterolide from *A. macrocephala* notably reduced muscle contractility, suggesting that atractylenolides might have gastrointestinal protective activity.[10]

## Anti-gut Hypersensitivity/Anti-gut Allergic Responses

Treatment with *A. macrocephala* in lymphocyte *in vitro* and using *A. macrocephala* in an ovalbumin (OVA)-mediated allergic diarrhoea mouse model have demonstrated that *A. macrocephala* can modulate gut hypersensitivity via its anti-allergic effects by stimulating lymphocyte proliferation, antibody production, cytokine secretion, and gamma interferon (IFN-gamma) production, and suppressing Th2-type immune response-mediated allergic diarrhoea.[11]

# Experimental Studies of *bai shao/chi shao* 白芍/赤芍

*Bai shao/chi shao* 白芍/赤芍 (white peony/red peony) is mainly derived from the dried root without the bark of *P. lactiflora* Pall. The characteristic constituents of *P. lactiflora* Pall contain monoterpenoids, triterpenoids, flavonoids, phenols and tannins.[2] It consists of more than 15 components, with the main bioavailable compounds being paeoniflorin (PF), pentagalloylglucose, gallic acid, albiflorin and benzoic acid. Most of these are monoterpene glucosides, and among them, PF, a chief active ingredient in the root of *P. lactiflora* Pall, is the most abundant (>90%), accounting for the pharmacological activities.[12,13] Pharmacological effects in relation to IBS are reviewed below.

## Anti-visceral Hyperalgesic Effect

It was reported that *P. lactiflora* can effectively relieve muscle cramps of various types, particularly when combined with licorice (*gan cao*). PF and glycyrrhizin (a major active glycoside in licorice) were individually too low in level to inhibit muscle contraction but were very active when applied simultaneously on isolated sciatic nerve-sartorius muscle preparations in frogs or on isolated or *in situ* phrenic nerve-diaphragm muscle preparations in mice.[14] Furthermore, PF has been demonstrated to relieve pain, especially visceral pain,[15] in neonatal maternal separation-induced visceral hyperalgesic rats in a dose-dependent manner by kappa-opioid receptors and alpha(2)-adrenoceptors in the central nervous system. This analgesic effect of *P. lactiflora* could be mediated through nor-binaltorphimine (nor-BNI), dl-alpha-methyltyrosine (alpha-AMPT) and yohimbine,[15] as well as through the adenosine A1 receptor by inhibiting the extracellular signal-regulated protein kinase (ERK) pathway.[16]

## Improvement of Intestinal Motility

Using an atropine-diphenoxylate-induced slow transit constipation (STC) rat model, the total glucosides from *P. lactiflora* Pall could alleviate STC with improvements in faecal volume, moisture content, and intestinal transit rate by enhancing the function of interstitial cells of Cajal (ICC) and reducing the production of inhibitory neurotransmitters such as nitric oxide (NO), nitric oxide synthase (NOS), vasoactive intestinal peptide (VIP), and the P substance (SP).[17]

## Anti-gut Hypersensitivity/Anti-gut Allergic Responses

On mucosal-type murine bone marrow-derived mast cells (mBM-MCs), treatment with pentagalloylglucose (PGG) could reduce immunoglobulin E (IgE)-mediated mast cell activation, which plays a key role in the pathogenesis of allergic disorders. Moreover, in a food-allergy mouse model, PGG prevented the development of allergic diarrhoea by inhibiting upregulated Fc epsilon RI surface expression on mast cells.[18]

# Experimental Studies of *gan cao* 甘草

The three original plants of *gan cao* 甘草 (licorice) in Chinese medicine (CM) are *Glycyrrhiza uralensis* Fisch., *Glycyrrhiza inflata* Bat. and *Glycyrrhiza glabra* L.[2] Among at least 400 isolated compounds, the main bioactive constituents of licorice are triterpene saponins (more than 20) and various types of flavonoids (more than 300).[19–21] Pharmacological effects in relation to IBS are reviewed below.

## Improvement of Intestinal Motility

Isoliquiritigenin, a flavonoid isolated from the roots of licorice, plays a dual role in regulating gastrointestinal motility, both spasmogenic and spasmolytic. *In vitro,* isoliquiritigenin demonstrated an atropine-sensitive concentration-dependent spasmogenic effect in isolated rat stomach fundus and a spasmolytic effect in isolated rabbit jejunums, guinea pig ileums, and atropinised rat stomach fundus.[22] *In vivo,* isoliquiritigenin also showed a dual-dose-related effect on charcoal meal travel with an inhibitory effect at low doses and a prokinetic effect at high doses. The spasmogenic effect may be mediated by the activation of muscarinic receptors, while the spasmolytic effect is predominantly involved in the blockage of the calcium channels.[22]

Recently, AD-lico/Healthy Gut™, a commercial formulation of *Glycyrrhiza inflata* extract under clinical development for gastrointestinal diseases, including inflammatory bowel disease, demonstrated gastroprotective and gastric motility benefits. Treatment with AD-lico/ Healthy Gut™ significantly improved mucosal damage from *Helicobacter pylori* pathogen in a dose-dependent manner accompanied by a decreased expression of the inflammatory markers iNOS and COX-2 in the cells. Also, AD-lico/Healthy Gut™ could accelerate gastric emptying (GE) in normal rats and provide relief in gastric relaxation in a delayed-GE animal model.[23]

This effect in improving gastrointestinal motility disorders has been explained as linked to 5-HT3A receptor antagonism. The flavonoids — liquiritigenin, glabridin and licochalcone A — from licorice were identified as the most effective inhibitors on heterologously expressed human5-HT3A receptors using the two-electrode voltage-clamp technique.[24] In addition, herbal mixtures of licorice, together with *Liriope platyphylla* and *Cinnamomum cassia,* have shown a potent laxative effect in loperamide (Lop)-induced constipated Sprague-Dawley rats.[25]

# Experimental Studies of *chai hu* 柴胡

*Chai hu* 柴胡 (*Radix Bupleuri*) is derived from the dried roots of *Bupleurum chinense* DC. and *Bupleurum scorzonerifolium* Willd.[2] More than 281 components have been isolated from *Radix Bupleuri*, including 15 flavonoids, 66 triterpenoid saponins, 430 lignins, 12 phenyl propanol derivatives, and 158 volatile oils. Among these, triterpenoid saponins are the major bioactive compounds. Saikosaponins a and d are used as chemical standards for a quality evaluation of *Radix Bupleuri*.[26,27]

Crude extracts and pure compounds isolated from *Radix Bupleuri* exhibit extensive pharmacological properties. Pharmacological effects in relation to IBS are reviewed below.

## Anti- gastrointestinal Inflammation

Numerous studies *in vitro* and *in vivo* have suggested that triterpenoid saponins have potential in the inhibition of intestinal inflammation by suppressing intestinal inflammation through NF-$\kappa$B, MAPKs and TLR4 pathways, enhancing intestinal epithelial barrier repair, and maintaining the diversity of the intestinal microbiota to achieve the treatment of a wide range of intestinal-inflammation-related digestive diseases.[28]

## Anti-gut Hypersensitivity/Anti-gut Allergic Responses

In a rat basophilic leukemia-2H3 cell line, saikosaponins d, one of the most important active saikosaponins in *Radix Bupleuri,* demonstrated anti-allergic activity against allergic reactions caused by $\beta$-conglycinin by suppressing $\beta$-conglycinin-induced rat basophilic leukemia-2H3 cell degranulation and inhibiting intracellular calcium mobilisation and tyrosine phosphorylation.[29]

There is a limited number of studies evaluating the effects of *Radix Bupleuri* alone on IBS; however, in combination with other herbs in formulae, it offers great treatment potential for IBS (see Experimental Studies on Herbal Formulae).

# Experimental Studies of *fu ling* 茯苓

*Fu ling* 茯苓 (*Poria cocos*) is a well-known medicinal fungus used in traditional CM for its diuretic, sedative and tonic effects. The major phytochemical compounds present in *Poria cocos* are triterpenoids (lanostane and 3,4-secolanostane skeletons) and polysaccharides (beta-pachyman).[2] Other minor compounds are hyperin, ergosterol, amino acids, choline, histidine and potassium salt (see reviews)[30,31].

## Anti-visceral Hyperalgesic Effect

A study reported that three triterpenoids from *Poria cocos* (dehydroeburicoic acid, 3$\beta$-hydroxylanosta-7,9 and 24-trien-21-oic acid) suppressed 5-hydroxytryptamine-induced inward current (I5-HT) in a dose-dependent and reversible manner in Xenopus oocytes, indicating that the three triterpenoids could inhibit the expression of 5-hydroxytryptamine 3A (5-HT3A) receptors, which are involved in visceral pain in IBS.[32]

## Intestinal Protective Effect/Gastrointestinal Protective Effect

More recently, carboxymethylated pachyman (CMP), a polysaccharide isolated from *Poria cocos,* has been reported to exert an intestinal protective effect in a CT26 colon carcinoma xenograft mice model. The results showed that CMP could attenuate 5-fluorouracil (5-FU)-induced intestinal mucositis and reverse 5-FU-induced intestinal microflora disorders via downregulating the expression of ROS, NF-$\kappa$B, p-p38 and Bax, and upregulating the expression of CAT, GSH-Px , GSH, Nrf2 and Bcl-2.[33]

There is scarce data available for evaluating *Poria cocos* alone for IBS, but with other herbs in the formulae, it offers great treatment potential for IBS (see Experimental Studies on Herbal Formulae).

# Experimental Studies of *chen pi/qin pi* 陈皮/青皮

*Chen pi/qin pi* 陈皮/青皮 (*Citrus aurantium* L. (Rutaceae)), the dried pericarp derived from mature *Citrus reticulata* Blanco, has been used to treat various diseases for thousands of years in China. So far, at least 140 chemical components have been isolated and identified from *Citrus aurantium*, including alkaloids, flavonoids and essential oils.[2] Among these, volatile oils (mainly including limonene, β-myrcene, α-pinene and β-pinene) and flavonoids (mainly including flavone C-glycosides, flavone O-glycosides, flavonoid glycosides, and polymethoxy flavones) are the main bioactive compounds (see review).[34]

## Improvement of Intestinal Motility

A crude extract of *C. aurantium* has been shown to have a bidirectional action of promoting gastrointestinal motility in mice and inhibiting intestinal smooth muscle contraction in rats through stimulating the secretion of the digestive organs or acting directly on the intestinal smooth muscle.[35,36] Pure compounds have further validated this dual effect. Hesperidin and synephrine could promote gastrointestinal motility by different mechanisms. The former was mediated by increasing the levels of gastrin and decreasing the levels of acetylcholine (ACh), SP, motilin (MTL) and VIP. The latter was mediated by increasing the expression of MTL and ACh and decreasing the expression of SP and VIP.[37] Another flavonoid, polymethoxy flavones (PMFs) from *C. aurantium*, also has the effect of promoting gastrointestinal motility by increasing GE and small bowel peristalsis activity,[37,38] indicating the role of *C. aurantium* in the treatment of gastrointestinal disorders.

## Intestinal Protective Effect/Gastrointestinal Protective Effect

It has been reported that hesperidin, belonging to the flavanone O-glycosides, could significantly improve gastric ulcer conditions in rats in relation to the pH, the volume of gastric content, total acidity, and ulcer index.[39] This improvement was further confirmed, in that hesperidin protected rats from all ethanol-induced gastric damage and had an anti-gastric ulcer effect through regulating MDA, $H_2O_2$, TNF-α, GPX and SOD.[40]

# Experimental Studies of *fang feng* 防风

*Fang feng* 防风 (*Saposhnikoviae Radix*) is the dried root of *Saposhnikovia divaricata* (Turcz.) Schischk. (Umbelliferae).[2] A total of 45 compounds have been identified, including 13 chromones, 28 coumarins and 4 others. In relation to IBS, crude extracts and bioactive constituents of *S. divaricata* exert pharmacological effects on anti-inflammatory, anti-gut hypersensitivity/anti-gut allergic responses, and anti-visceral hyperalgesic effects, as presented below.

## Anti-inflammatory Activity

In LPS-induced RAW 264.7 cells, *S. divaricata* demonstrated anti-inflammatory activity by inhibiting the production of NO, prostaglandin E2 (PGE2), tumour necrosis factor-$\alpha$ (TNF-$\alpha$), and interleukin-6 (IL-6).[41] This anti-inflammatory activity was further confirmed with a pyrano-coumarin constituent of *S. divaricata*, anomalin, which also exhibited potent anti-inflammatory activity in a dose-dependent manner.[42]

## Anti-gut Hypersensitivity/Anti-gut Allergic Responses

During the degranulation process, activated mast cells release various biological molecules (such as histamine, $\beta$-hexosaminidase, leukotriene), which are responsible for allergic symptoms. Recently, three main components of *S. divaricate*, prim-O-glucosylcimifugin (PGC), cimifugin (CF) and 4'-O-$\beta$-D-glucosyl-5-Omethylvisamminol (MV), have been identified based on retention time and mass spectrometry fragment information to possess anti-allergic potential by inhibiting the degranulation process in mast cells with decreased C48/80-induced histamine release in LAD2 cells in a dose-dependent manner.[43]

## Anti-visceral Hyperalgesic Effects

In addition to the above activities, a methanol extract of *S. divaricata* showed an analgesic property in mice by the acetic acid-induced writhing method and a prolongation effect on pentobarbital-induced hypnosis in mice. This analgesic effect was a combination of several types of compounds, including chromones, coumarins, furanocoumarins, polyacetylenes and monoacylglycerides. Among these, chromones such as divaricatol, ledebouriellol and hamaudol were observed to be the most potent analgesia with significant writhing inhibition.[44]

# Experimental Studies of *zhi shi/zhi qiao* 枳实/枳壳

*Zhi shi/zhi qiao* 枳实/枳壳 comes from *Citrus sinensis* O (sweet orange)/*Citrus aurantium* L (bitter orange).[2] Several types of chemical compounds have been identified in the fruit, peel, leaves, juice and roots of *C. sinensis*, including flavonoids, steroids, hydroxyamides, alkanes, fatty acids, coumarins, peptides, carbohydrates, carbamates, alkylamines, carotenoids, and volatiles.[2]

## Anti-intestinal Inflammation

In a mouse model with dextran sodium sulfate (DSS)-induced ulcerative colitis, a hydroalcoholic extract of *C. aurantium* consisting of 4 alkaloids, 7 coumarins, 18 flavonoids, 2 lignans, 2 phenolics, and 10 terpenoids significantly prevented body weight loss and colon shortening, accompanied by reduced DSS-related mucosal inflammatory lesions in the colon through decreasing the expression levels of IL-6, interferon-$\gamma$, TNF-$\alpha$, and monocyte chemotactic protein-1.[45]

## Intestinal Laxative Effect

In isolated rat colonic crypts, the flavanone naringenin (NAR, aglycone), a main active flavonol compound extracted from citrus fruit (oranges and grapefruits), could stimulate Cl⁻ secretion in a concentration-dependent manner in the colonic epithelium via a signalling pathway involving cyclic adenosinemonophosphate (cAMP) and protein kinase A (PKA).[46] Indeed, this effect of cAMP-dependent Cl⁻ secretion obtained *in vitro* was validated in an *in vivo* Lop-induced constipation rat model. In this rat constipation model, naringenin could restore the levels of faecal output, water content, and mucus secretion, compared to a control group, indicating that naringenin is a potent stimulator of chloride secretion in colonic epithelia with a great improvement in the symptoms of constipation.[46]

Recently, the precise effects of naringenin on laxative effects were further evaluated in mice with Lop-induced constipation. Naringenin enhanced stool excretion and increased the intestinal charcoal transit ratio to relieve Lop-induced constipation in mice by regulating the expression of gastrointestinal metabolic components and increasing the expression of enteric nerve-related factors, which play a key role in water reabsorption across colonic surface cells.[47]

# Experimental Studies of *hou po* 厚朴

*Hou po* 厚朴 is the dried bark of *Magnolia officinalis* Rehd. et Wils (MO) and *Magnolia officinalis* var. *biloba* (MOV). More than 250 chemical constituents have been isolated from the root, bark, leaf, flower and fruit of *M. officinalis*. The main constituents are phenols, including lignans, phenylethanoid glycosides, phenolic glycosides, alkaloids, steroids, essential oils and others.[2] The two principal phenolic compounds, the neolignan derivatives magnolol (5,5'-diallyl-2,2'-dihydroxybiphenyl) and honokiol (5,3'-diallyl-2,4'-dihydroxybiphenyl), are generally considered the main bioactive and characteristic ingredients in the bark (see review in Ref. 48).

## Improvement of Gastrointestinal Motility

The total phenols of *M. officinalis* have beneficial effects on atropine-induced gastrointestinal tract dysmotility rats with an improved atropine-induced gastric residual rate increase, normalised gastrointestinal hormones, and an increased number of interstitial cells of Cajal (ICC). The mechanism may be the activation of the c-kit/stem cell factor (SCF) pathway in ICCs.[49] Moreover, in ICC, an ethanol extract of *M. officinalis* could depolarise the pacemaker potential in a dose-dependent manner via the whole-cell patch-clamp technique. In normal mice, *M. Officinalis* could increase GE and intestinal transit rates, while in Lop- and cisplatin-induced GE delay models, *M. officinalis* could reverse gastrointestinal motility dysfunction. The mechanism might be through M2 and M3 receptors via internal and external $Ca^{2+}$ regulation through G protein pathways.[50]

Magnolol and honokiol, two major bioactive constituents of the bark of *M. officinalis*, have been reported to relieve spasms of smooth muscle and inhibit contractility in the isolated ACh- or 5-hydroxytryptamine (5-HT)-treated gastric fundus strips of rats and isolated ACh- or $CaCl_2$-treated ileum segments of guinea pigs. This inhibitory effect on the contractility of the smooth muscles is associated with a calcium antagonistic effect.[51] Magnolol and honokiol were also demonstrated to improve the GE of a semi-solid meal and intestinal propulsive activity in mice,[51] suggesting that magnolol and honokiol may be the main active ingredients of *M. officinalis* for promoting gastrointestinal motility.

The effect of magnolol was further confirmed by another two studies, one of which showed contractile activity using rat-isolated gastrointestinal strips with different regulation of gastrointestinal motility according to the region of gastrointestinal tracts and orientation of smooth muscles, which may be mediated by the activation of ACh and 5-HT receptors.[52] The other study indicated that inhibition of the contractions of distal colonic segments in rats by magnolol was due to inhibiting L-type $Ca^{2+}$ channels.[53]

## Anti-visceral Hyperalgesic Effect

Honokiol and magnolol have been shown to possess anti-nociceptive effects. Both could block glutamate-, SP- and PGE2-induced inflammatory pain in mice.[54] This effect has been further explored in that an anti-nociceptive effect of honokiol in carrageenan-induced acute and chronic inflammatory pain models was mediated through inhibiting mechanical hyperalgesia, mechanical allodynia, and thermal hyperalgesia by targeting NF-$\kappa$B and Nrf2 signalling.[55]

# Experimental Studies of *bing lang/da fu pi* 槟榔/大腹皮

*Bing lang/da fu pi* 槟榔/大腹皮 (*Areca catechu* L) compounds identified from *A. catechu* include alkaloids, flavonoids, tannins, triterpenes, fatty acids, and others.[2] Among these, pyridine-type alkaloids and condensed tannins are generally considered the characteristic constituents. Arecoline, belonging to the alkaloids, is commonly used as an indicator to standardise and characterise the quality of the areca nut (see review).[56]

## Improvement of Gastrointestinal Motility

Crude water extracts of the pericarp of *A. catechu* could markedly enhance gastrointestinal motility in rabbits and mice through stimulating the M receptor and the verapamil-sensitive $Ca^{2+}$ channel.[57–59] Similarly, ethyl acetate extracts of *A. catechu* also affected gastrointestinal motility in mice.[60] These mechanisms have also been considered to be relevant with increasing the content of SP and MTL and decreasing the content of VIP.[61]

Moreover, an active component, arecoline, which belongs to the alkaloids category of *A. catechu,* has been reported to notably improve the contraction of gastric smooth muscle and muscle strips of the duodenum, ileum and colon.[62] Another fraction, named F57, was identified from *A. catechu* using various chromatographic techniques (HPLC, membrane filtration and exclusion chromatography (Sephadex G-25)) and could significantly promote gastric smooth muscle contraction in rats.[63]

Additionally, increasing the colonic muscle strip motility by *A. catechu* was also noted. The dose-dependent stimulation of *A. catechu* on the contraction of proximal and distal colonic smooth muscle strips of rats was also observed. *A. catechu* could mix, stir, promote and even excrete colonic contents through a mechanism possibly relevant to a stimulation of the cholinergic M receptor, which caused increased influx of extracellular and intracellular $Ca^{2+}$, in turn contracting the colonic smooth muscle.[64] Besides increasing gastrointestinal motility, *A. catechu* also could improve gastrointestinal function in rats with functional dyspepsia.[65]

## Anti-visceral Hyperalgesic Effect

*A. catechu* has also shown significant analgesic activity. Using hot-plate and formalin tests in mice, oral administration with a hydroalcoholic extract of *A. catechu* could inhibit nitroglycerine infusion-induced inflammatory responses and induce analgesic and anti-inflammatory effects with a maximum increase in hot-plate reaction time and decrease in the duration of licking/biting behaviours in formalin tests.[66]

Furthermore, UP446, a standardised bioflavonoid composition consisting of catechin from *A. catechu* and baicalin from *Scutellaria baicalensis*, demonstrated analgesic effects on carrageenan-induced mechanical hyperalgesia, formalin-induced hind-paw licking (acute inflammatory pain), and acetic acid-induced visceral pain. This pain inhibition could be comparable to that of ibuprofen, a pharmaceutical drug used as a non-steroidal anti-inflammatory drug (NSAID).[67]

## Anti-gut Hypersensitivity/Anti-gut Allergic Responses

Besides the above-mentioned effects, the rich amount of polyphenols in *A. catechu* makes it possible to modulate the functionality of mast cells and T cells against allergy. Water extracts of *A. catechu* could inhibit mast cell-mediated allergic reactions *in vitro* and *in vivo*. *A. catechu* not only showed suppression of DNP-BSA- and compound 48/80-induced degranulation in RBL-2H3 mast cells but also showed the inhibition of compound 48/80-induced systemic anaphylaxis in mice.[68]

Recently, it was found that this anti-allergic response might be attributed to polyphenols. In mice challenged with OVA by gavage to induce food-allergic responses, an oral intake of *A. catechu*-derived polyphenols could reduce OVA-induced allergic responses (including diarrhoea and infiltration and degranulation of mast cells in the duodenum) through the suppression of Th2 immunity and the induction of myeloid-derived suppressor cells (MDSC) in the duodenum of food-allergic mice.[69]

## Experimental Studies of Herbal Formulae

### *Tong xie yao fang* 痛泻要方

*Tong xie yao fang* 痛泻要方 (TXYF), the core formula for the treatment of IBS-D, containing *bai zhu* 白术, *bai shao* 白芍, *fu ling* 茯苓, *chen pi* 陈皮, and *gan cao* 甘草, has been extensively investigated for its effect on relieving IBS-associated symptoms *in vitro* and *in vivo*.

TXYF on IBS-model rats with rectum expansion to produce chronic visceral hypersensitivity has shown significant analgesic effects, reduction of the increased colonic smooth muscle tension, and contract frequency in IBS-model rats through the regulation of 5-HT and SP.[70,71]

Further investigation of TXYF intragastrically fed at different doses to rats with post-infectious irritable bowel syndrome (PI-IBS) showed that it notably reversed PI-IBS-induced increases in the intestinal mucosal mast-cell activation ratio, levels of serum TNF-$\alpha$ and histamine, and rat abdominal withdrawal reflex and faecal water content, which indicates intestinal sensitivity, suggesting that TXYF improves PI-IBS by attenuating behavioural hyperalgesia and anti-diarrhoea.[72] By a novel method of faecal transplantation, TXYF was also shown to relieve IBS-D by modulating gut microbiota and regulating colonic 5-HT levels.[73]

### *Si ni san* 四逆散

*Si ni san* 四逆散 decoction, composed of *Bupleurum chinensis Chaihu* 柴胡, *P. lactiflora* Pall *Baishao*白芍, *Citrus aurantium* L. *Zhishi*枳实, and *Glycyrrhiza* spp. *Gancao* 甘草 has been beneficial in the treatment of IBS in mice with atropine-induced gastrointestinal motility dysfunction through synergy between multiple components, multiple targets, and multiple pathways. In particular, *Bupleurum* polysaccharide, *Citrus aurantium* flavonoid, *Citrus* *aurantium* essential oil, and *Cyperus rotundus* flavonoids could significantly modulate glycerophosphocholine, tryptophan, 25-Hydroxycholecalciferol, and 5, 6-Indolequinone-2-carboxylic acid, which are associated with gastrointestinal movement in the body to promote gastrointestinal motility.[74]

## Summary of Pharmacological Actions of the Common Herbs

Each of these ten herbs, frequently reported in the formulae in the RCTs, has received great research attention in experimental models of relevance to IBS.

Improvement in gastrointestinal motility to maintain normal bowel movement was observed in most of the herbs, including *bai shao/chi shao* 白芍/赤芍, *gan cao* 甘草, *chen pi/qin pi* 陈皮/青皮, *hou po* 厚朴, and *bing lang/da fu pi* 槟榔/大腹皮 via stimulation of the cholinergic M receptor to regulate the influx of extracellular and intracellular Ca2+ and activate ACh and 5-HT receptors.

An anti-visceral hyperalgesic effect against visceral pain in acetic acid-induced visceral pain models was observed in most extracts and/or compounds including *bai shao/chi shao* 白芍/赤芍, *fu ling* 茯苓, *fang feng* 防风, *hou po* 厚朴, and *bing lang/da fu pi* 槟榔/大腹皮 through inhibiting 5-HT3A receptors, which are involved in visceral pain in IBS, and adenosine A1 receptor kappa-opioid receptors, as well as alpha(2)-adrenoceptors in the central nervous system.

Anti-gut hypersensitivity/anti-gut allergic responses to avert bowel hypersensitivity were observed in extracts and/or compounds derived from *bai zhu* 白术, *bai shao/chi shao* 白芍/赤芍, *chai hu* 柴胡, *fang feng* 防风, and *bing lang/da fu pi* 槟榔/大腹皮 via suppression of immunoglobulin E (IgE)-mediated mast cell infiltration, activation and degranulation, as well as intracellular calcium mobilisation.

An intestinal protective effect/gastrointestinal protective effect that protected the gastrointestinal tract from injuries and microflora disorders was observed in *bai zhu* 白术, *fu ling* 茯苓, and *chen pi/qin pi* 陈皮/青皮.

An intestinal laxative effect *in vitro* and *in vivo* in mice with Lop-induced constipation was only found in *zhi shi/zhi qiao* 枳实/枳壳 through cAMP-dependent Cl⁻ secretion.

A general anti-inflammation effect for the whole body that is also beneficial in the inhibition of intestinal inflammation has been reported in relation to the general pharmacological properties of all extracts of these herbs or their bioactive compounds. In particular, anti-gastrointestinal inflammation against low-grade mucosal inflammation in IBS was observed in *in vitro* and *in vivo* models in *bai zhu* 白术, *chai hu* 柴胡, and *zhi shi/zhi qiao* 枳实/枳壳 through inhibiting the plurality of inflammation pathways.

In addition, the herbal formulae reviewed in this chapter, namely *Tong xie yao fang* 痛泻要方 and *Si ni san* 四逆散, containing most of the 10 most frequently used herbs, have been observed to significantly relieve IBS-associated symptoms *in vitro* and *in vivo*. However, the number of available studies is limited, and there is a lack of direct evidence links to IBS. Further research is recommended with either the main compounds alone or combined in relevant specific symptom animal models to clarify the capacity of the compound and their synergistic effects with other herbs based on the compatibility theory of traditional CM and disclose the underlying mechanisms.

*In vitro* and *in vivo* studies of IBS-relevant activities, along with more general anti-inflammatory, anti-oxidant, anti-allergic and anti-hyperalgesic activities, would provide potential explanations of the clinical benefits of the herbs contained in the formulae used in the clinical of IBS that act through multi-component, multi-target, multiple pathways to play a role in treating IBS-relevant symptoms, fully reflecting the synergistic characteristics of traditional CM.

# References

1. Zhou J, Xie G, Yan X. (2011) *Encyclopedia of Traditional Chinese Medicine: Molecular Structures, Pharmacological Activities, Natural Sources and Applications.* Springer, Berlin, Germany.
2. Bensky D, Clavey S, Stoger E. (2004) *Chinese Herbal Medicine Materia Medica,* 3rd ed. Eastland Press, Inc., Seattle, US.

3. Zhu B, Zhang QL, Hua JW, *et al.* (2018) The traditional uses, phyto-chemistry, and pharmacology of Atractylodes macrocephala Koidz.: A review. *J Ethnopharmacol.* **226:** 143–167.

4. Barbara G, De Giorgio R, Stanghellini V, *et al.* (2002) A role for inflammation in irritable bowel syndrome? *Gut.* **51(Suppl 1):** i41–i44.

5. Dong H, He L, Huang M, Dong Y. (2008) Anti-inflammatory components isolated from Atractylodes macrocephala Koidz. *Nat Prod Res.* **22(16):** 1418–1427.

6. Yao CM, Yang XW. (2014) Bioactivity-guided isolation of polyacetylenes with inhibitory activity against NO production in LPS-activated RAW264.7 macrophages from the rhizomes of Atractylodes macrocephala. *J Ethnopharmacol.* **151(2):** 791–799.

7. Hoang le S, Tran MH, Lee JS, *et al.* (2016) Inflammatory inhibitory activity of sesquiterpenoids from Atractylodes macrocephala rhizomes. *Chem Pharm Bull (Tokyo).* **64(5):** 507–511.

8. He W, Zhang Y, Wang X, *et al.* (2013) Zhizhu decoction promotes gastric emptying and protects the gastric mucosa. *J Med Food.* **16(4):** 306–311.

9. Song HP, Li RL, Chen X, *et al.* (2014) Atractylodes macrocephala Koidz promotes intestinal epithelial restitution via the polyamine — voltage-gated K+ channel pathway. *J Ethnopharmacol.* **152(1):** 163–172.

10. Zhang YQ, Xu S, Lin YC. (1999) Gastrointestinal Inhibitory effects of sesquiterpene lactones from *Atractylodes macrocephala. J Chin Med Mater.* **22:** 636–640.

11. Kim SH, Jung HN, Lee KY, *et al.* (2005) Suppression of Th2-type immune response-mediated allergic diarrhea following oral administration of traditional Korean medicine: Atractylodes macrocephala Koidz. *Immunopharmacol Immunotoxicol.* **27(2):** 331–343.

12. He DY, Dai SM. (2011) Anti-inflammatory and immunomodulatory effects of paeonia lactiflora pall., a traditional Chinese herbal medicine. *Front Pharmacol.* **2:** 10.

13. Parker S, May B, Zhang C, *et al.* (2016) A pharmacological review of bioactive constituents of Paeonia lactiflora Pallas and Paeonia veitchii Lynch. *Phytother Res.* **30(9):** 1445–1473.

14. Kimura M, Kimura I, Takahashi K, *et al.* (1984) Blocking effects of blended paeoniflorin or its related compounds with glycyrrhizin on neuromuscular junctions in frog and mouse. *Jpn J Pharmacol.* **36(3):** 275–282.

15. Zhang XJ, Li Z, Leung WM, *et al.* (2008) The analgesic effect of paeoniflorin on neonatal maternal separation-induced visceral hyperalgesia in rats. *J Pain.* **9(6):** 497–505.

16. Zhang XJ, Chen HL, Li Z, *et al.* (2009) Analgesic effect of paeoniflorin in rats with neonatal maternal separation-induced visceral hyperalgesia is mediated through adenosine A(1) receptor by inhibiting the extracellular signal-regulated protein kinase (ERK) pathway. *Pharmacol Biochem Behav.* **94(1):** 88–97.

17. Zhu JJ, Liu S, Su XL, *et al.* (2016) Efficacy of Chinese herbal medicine for diarrhea-predominant irritable bowel syndrome: A meta-analysis of randomized, double-blind, placebo-controlled trials. *Evid Based Complement Alternat Med.* **2016:** 4071260.

18. Kageyama-Yahara N, Suehiro Y, Maeda F, *et al.* (2010) Pentagalloylglucose down-regulates mast cell surface FcepsilonRI expression *in vitro* and *in vivo*. *FEBS Lett.* **584(1):** 111–118.

19. Asl MN, Hosseinzadeh H. (2008) Review of pharmacological effects of Glycyrrhiza sp. and its bioactive compounds. *Phytother Res.* **22(6):** 709–724.

20. Ji S, Li Z, Song W, *et al.* (2016) Bioactive constituents of Glycyrrhiza uralensis (licorice): Discovery of the effective components of a traditional herbal medicine. *J Nat Prod.* **79(2):** 281–292.

21. Zhang Q, Ye M. (2009) Chemical analysis of the Chinese herbal medicine Gan-Cao (licorice). *J Chromatogr A.* **1216(11):** 1954–1969.

22. Chen G, Zhu L, Liu Y, *et al.* (2009) Isoliquiritigenin, a flavonoid from licorice, plays a dual role in regulating gastrointestinal motility *in vitro* and *in vivo*. *Phytother Res.* **23(4):** 498–506.

23. Sadra A, Kweon HS, Huh SO, Cho J. (2017) Gastroprotective and gastric motility benefits of AD-lico/healthy gut Glycyrrhiza inflata extract. *Anim Cells Syst (Seoul).* **21(4):** 255–262.

24. Herbrechter R, Ziemba PM, Hoffmann KM, *et al.* (2015) Identification of Glycyrrhiza as the *rikkunshito* constituent with the highest antagonistic potential on heterologously expressed 5-HT3A receptors due to the action of flavonoids. *Front Pharmacol.* **6:** 130.

25. Kim JE, Yun WB, Lee ML, *et al.* (2019) Synergic laxative effects of an herbal mixture of Liriope platyphylla, Glycyrrhiza uralensis, and Cinnamomum cassia in loperamide-induced constipation of sprague dawley rats. *J Med Food.* **22(3):** 294–304.

26. Sun P, Li Y, Wei S, *et al.* (2019) Pharmacological effects and chemical constituents of Bupleurum. *Mini Rev Med Chem.* **19(1):** 34–55.

27. Yang F, Dong X, Yin X, *et al.* (2017) Radix Bupleuri: A review of traditional uses, botany, phytochemistry, pharmacology, and toxicology. *Biomed Res Int.* **2017:** 7597596.

28. Dong J, Liang W, Wang T, *et al.* (2019) Saponins regulate intestinal inflammation in colon cancer and IBD. *Pharmacol Res.* **144:** 66–72.

29. Hao Y, Piao X, Piao X. (2012) Saikosaponin-d inhibits beta-conglycinin induced activation of rat basophilic leukemia-2H3 cells. *Int Immunopharmacol.* **13(3):** 257–263.

30. Rios JL. (2011) Chemical constituents and pharmacological properties of Poria cocos. *Planta Med.* **77(7):** 681–691.

31. Sun Y. (2014) Biological activities and potential health benefits of polysaccharides from Poria cocos and their derivatives. *Int J Biol Macromol.* **68:** 131–134.

32. Lee JH, Lee YJ, Shin JK, *et al.* (2009) Effects of triterpenoids from Poria cocos Wolf on the serotonin type 3A receptor-mediated ion current in Xenopus oocytes. *Eur J Pharmacol.* **615(1–3):** 27–32.

33. Wang C, Yang S, Gao L, *et al.* (2018) Carboxymethyl pachyman (CMP) reduces intestinal mucositis and regulates the intestinal microflora in 5-fluorouracil-treated CT26 tumour-bearing mice. *Food Funct.* **9(5):** 2695–2704.

34. Yu X, Sun S, Guo Y, *et al.* (2018) Citri reticulatae pericarpium (Chenpi): Botany, ethnopharmacology, phytochemistry, and pharmacology of a frequently used traditional Chinese medicine. *J Ethnopharmacol.* **220:** 265–282.

35. Zhang X, Ji Z, Zhao C. (2012) Effects of Chenpi extract on grastric emptying and small bowel peristalsis in mice in vivo and smooth muscle of ileum of rabbits in vitro (in Chinese). *J Henan Univ (Med Sci).* **31(1):** 12–14.

36. Guo J, Chen J, Lie Z. (2012) Effects of different extracts of Pericarpium citri reticulatae on cold-stagnant qi stagnation model rats. *Chin Tradit Pat Med.* **34(6):** 1158–1160.

37. 宋玉鹏, 陈海芳, 胡源祥, *et al.* (2017) 陈皮及其主要活性成分对脾虚模型大鼠血清胃泌素、血浆乙酰胆碱、P物质、胃动素和血管活性肠肽的影响. *中药药理与临床.* **33(3):** 79–83.

38. Li Q, Liang S, Chu H. (2012) Screening of effective part of gastrointestinal motility in pericarpium citri reticulatae. *Chin Tradit Pat Med.* **34(5):** 941–943.

39. Jain D, Katti N. (2015) Combination treatment of lycopene and hesperidin protect experimentally induced ulcer in laboratory rats. *J Intercult Ethnopharmacol.* **4(2):** 143–146.

40. Selmi S, Rtibi K, Grami D, *et al.* (2017) Protective effects of orange (Citrus sinensis L.) peel aqueous extract and hesperidin on oxidative stress and peptic ulcer induced by alcohol in rat. *Lipids Health Dis.* **16(1):** 152.

41. Chun JM, Kim HS, Lee AY, *et al.* (2016) Anti-inflammatory and antiosteo-arthritis effects of Saposhnikovia divaricata ethanol extract: *In vitro* and *in vivo* studies. *Evid Based Complement Alternat Med.* **2016:** 1984238.

42. Khan S, Shin EM, Choi RJ, *et al.* (2011) Suppression of LPS-induced inflammatory and NF-kappaB responses by anomalin in RAW 264.7 macrophages. *J Cell Biochem.* **112(8):** 2179–2188.

43. Jia Q, Sun W, Zhang L, *et al.* (2019) Screening the anti-allergic components in Saposhnikoviae radix using high-expression Mas-related G protein-coupled receptor X2 cell membrane chromatography online coupled with liquid chromatography and mass spectrometry. *J Sep Sci.* **42(14):** 2351–2359.

44. Okuyama E, Hasegawa T, Matsushita T, *et al.* (2001) Analgesic components of saposhnikovia root (Saposhnikovia divaricata). *Chem Pharm Bull (Tokyo).* **49(2):** 154–160.

45. Hwang YH, Ma JY. (2018) Preventive effects of an UPLC-DAD-MS/MS fingerprinted hydroalcoholic extract of Citrus aurantium in a mouse model of ulcerative colitis. *Planta Med.* **84(15):** 1101–1109.

46. Yang ZH, Yu HJ, Pan A, *et al.* (2008) Cellular mechanisms underlying the laxative effect of flavonol naringenin on rat constipation model. *PLoS One.* **3(10):** e3348.

47. Yin J, Liang Y, Wang D, *et al.* (2018) Naringenin induces laxative effects by upregulating the expression levels of c-Kit and SCF, as well as those of aquaporin 3 in mice with loperamide-induced constipation. *Int J Mol Med.* **41(2):** 649–658.

48. Luo H, Wu H, Yu X, *et al.* (2019) A review of the phytochemistry and pharmacological activities of Magnoliae officinalis cortex. *J Ethnopharmacol.* **236:** 412–442.

49. Tian H, Huang D, Li T, *et al.* (2015) The protective effects of total phenols in Magnolia officinalix rehd. et wils on gastrointestinal tract dysmotility is mainly based on its influence on interstitial cells of cajal. *Int J Clin Exp Med.* **8(11):** 20279–20286.

50. Kim HJ, Han T, Kim YT, *et al.* (2017) Magnolia officinalis bark extract induces depolarization of pacemaker potentials through M2 and M3 muscarinic receptors in cultured murine small intestine interstitial cells of Cajal. *Cell Physiol Biochem.* **43(5):** 1790–1802.

51. Zhang WW, Li Y, Wang XQ, *et al.* (2005) Effects of magnolol and honokiol derived from traditional Chinese herbal remedies on gastro-intestinal movement. *World J Gastroenterol.* **11(28):** 4414–4418.

52. Jeong SI, Kim YS, Lee MY, *et al.* (2009) Regulation of contractile activity by magnolol in the rat isolated gastrointestinal tracts. *Pharmacol Res.* **59(3):** 183–188.

53. Zhang M, Zang KH, Luo JL, *et al.* (2013) Magnolol inhibits colonic motility through down-regulation of voltage-sensitive L-type Ca2+ channels of colonic smooth muscle cells in rats. *Phytomedicine.* **20(14):** 1272–1279.

54. Lin YR, Chen HH, Lin YC, *et al.* (2009) Antinociceptive actions of honokiol and magnolol on glutamatergic and inflammatory pain. *J Biomed Sci.* **16:** 94.

55. Khalid S, Ullah MZ, Khan AU, *et al.* (2018) Antihyperalgesic properties of honokiol in inflammatory pain models by targeting of NF-kappaB and Nrf2 signaling. *Front Pharmacol.* **9:** 140.

56. Peng W, Liu YJ, Wu N, *et al.* (2015) Areca catechu L. (Arecaceae): A review of its traditional uses, botany, phytochemistry, pharmacology and toxicology. *J Ethnopharmacol.* **164:** 340–356.

57. 李晨, 胡兵, 吕涛, 魏睦新. (2011) 槟榔对豚鼠胃平滑肌的作用及机制探讨. *中医学报.* **26:** 1477–1479.

58. 李明, 彭解英, 吴颖芳, *et al.* (2011) 槟榔碱诱导上皮细胞凋亡. *国际病理科学与临床杂志.* **31:** 282–285.

59. 杨颖丽, 程昉, 王慧玲, 司克媛. (2002) 槟榔对动物胃肠运动的影响. *西北师范大学学报(自然科学版).* **38:** 61–63.

60. 袁列江, 李忠海, 郑锦星. (2009) 槟榔提取物对大白鼠血脂调节作用的研究. *Food Science Technology.* **34:** 188–192.

61. 郭喜军. (2008) 槟榔对大鼠胃运动及神经递质的影响. *中国中西医结合消化杂志.* **17:** 300–303.

62. Ni YD, Wang JH, Wang RJ. (2004) Comparative study of the effect of Areca nut and arecoline on gastrointestinal motility. *Pharmacology and Clinics of Chinese Materia Medica.* **20:** 11–12.

63. 李晨, 范尧夫, 吕涛, *et al.* (2013) 槟榔有效组分的提取分离及其对大鼠胃平滑肌收缩作用影响的研究. *中医学报.* **28:** 683–685.

64. Xie DP, Li W, Qu SY, *et al.* (2002) Effect of areca on contraction of colonic muscle strips in rats. *World J Gastroenterol.* **8(2):** 350–352.

65. 邹百仓, 魏兰福, 魏睦新. (2003) 槟榔对功能性消化不良模型大鼠胃运动的影响. *中国中西医结合消化杂志.* **11:** 6–8.

66. Bhandare AM, Kshirsagar AD, Vyawahare NS, *et al.* (2010) Potential analgesic, anti-inflammatory and antioxidant activities of hydroalcoholic extract of Areca catechu L. nut. *Food Chem Toxicol.* **48(12):** 3412–3417.

67. Yimam M, Brownell L, Hodges M, Jia Q. (2012) Analgesic effects of a standardized bioflavonoid composition from Scutellaria baicalensis and Acacia catechu. *J Diet Suppl.* **9(3):** 155–165.

68. Lee JH, Chang SH, Park YS, *et al.* (2004) In-vitro and in-vivo anti-allergic actions of Arecae semen. *J Pharm Pharmacol.* **56(7):** 927–933.

69. Wang CC, Lin YR, Liao MH, Jan TR. (2013) Oral supplementation with areca-derived polyphenols attenuates food allergic responses in ovalbumin-sensitized mice. *BMC Complement Altern Med.* **13:** 154.

70. Hu XG, Xu D, Zhao Y, *et al.* (2009) The alleviating pain effect of aqueous extract from Tong-xie-yao-fang on experimental visceral hypersensitivity and its mechanism. *Biol Pharm Bull.* **32(6):** 1075–1079.

71. Yin Y, Zhong L, Wang JW, *et al.* (2015) Tong Xie Yao Fang relieves irritable bowel syndrome in rats via mechanisms involving regulation of 5-hydroxytryptamine and substance P. *World J Gastroenterol.* **21(15):** 4536–4546.

72. Ma X, Wang X, Kang N, *et al.* (2017) The effect of Tong-xie-yao-fang on intestinal mucosal mast cells in postinfectious irritable bowel syndrome rats. *Evid Based Complement Alternat Med.* **2017:** 9086034.

73. Li J, Cui H, Cai Y, *et al.* (2018) Tong-xie-yao-fang regulates 5-HT level in diarrhea predominant irritable bowel syndrome through gut microbiota modulation. *Front Pharmacol.* **9:** 1110.

74. Chang X, Wang S, Bao YR, *et al.* (2016) Multicomponent, multitarget integrated adjustment — metabolomics study of Qizhiweitong particles curing gastrointestinal motility disorders in mice induced by atropine. *J Ethnopharmacol.* **189:** 14–21.

# 7

# Clinical Evidence for Acupuncture and Other Chinese Medicine Therapies

## OVERVIEW

Acupuncture-related therapies and other Chinese medicine (CM) therapies can be used to treat irritable bowel syndrome (IBS). This chapter evaluates efficacy and safety data on acupuncture-related therapies from 22 randomised controlled trials (RCTs) and two non-randomised controlled clinical trials and presents characteristics data on one non-controlled clinical trial. The chapter also describes results for one RCT using a CM therapy type other than acupuncture. Overall, the evidence for acupuncture is limited and clinicians should use their clinical judgement when considering the use of the described therapies for IBS.

## Introduction

Acupuncture includes a family of techniques that stimulate acupuncture points to correct imbalances in energy and restore health to the body. Methods of stimulating acupuncture points include:

- Acupuncture: Insertion of an acupuncture needle into acupuncture points;
- Acupressure: Application of pressure to acupuncture points;
- Moxibustion: Burning of a herb (usually *ai ye*, 艾叶, *Artemesia vulgaris* L.) close to or on the skin to induce a warming sensation; and
- Transcutaneous electrical acupoint stimulation (TEAS): Application of transdermal electrical current to acupuncture points via conducting pads.

While many of these therapies have ancient roots, several have emerged as new techniques in the last century. This includes electroacupuncture, a therapy involving the attachment of a device that can produce an electrical current to acupuncture needles at acupuncture points.

In addition to Chinese herbal medicine (CHM) and acupuncture therapies, Chinese medicine (CM) includes a range of other therapies to treat disease and maintain health. One study investigating *Baduanjin* 八段锦 is discussed in this chapter.

## Previous Systematic Reviews

From English-language databases, five systematic reviews of randomised controlled trials (RCTs) using acupuncture-related therapies for irritable bowel syndrome (IBS) were identified.[1–5] The reviews evaluated the efficacy and safety of acupuncture-related therapies for IBS but used differing review methods. Three reviews evaluated acupuncture,[1,2,3] and two evaluated moxibustion.[4,5]

Of the three systematic reviews evaluating acupuncture, two were specific to evaluating the therapy for IBS,[1,2] and the other reviewed acupuncture for gastrointestinal disease broadly but included IBS studies.[3]

One IBS-specific review was a Cochrane systematic review of RCTs of acupuncture by Manheimer and colleagues in 2012.[1] The review included 17 RCTs and found no difference between acupuncture and sham acupuncture for IBS symptom severity or health-related quality of life in five RCTs totalling 411 people. Data for these studies was rated "low" risk of bias. Results found acupuncture was superior to the antispasmodic drugs pinaverium bromide and trimebutine maleate for two RCTs. The risk of bias for the non-sham control studies was rated "high" due to the lack of blinding and/or inadequate blinding or allocation concealment.[1]

Chao and Zhang systematically reviewed RCTs of acupuncture for IBS; the review included six RCTs and concluded acupuncture to be superior to controls. Control data was limited to four studies using sham acupuncture, one using pinaverium bromide, and one using usual care. Five of the six included studies were rated "high" quality.[2]

The final acupuncture systematic review, in 2007, included studies from a variety of gastrointestinal diseases, including IBS.[3] The review included two IBS RCTs of 102 people, with one RCT using non-penetrating sham acupuncture as the comparator and the other RCT penetrating sham acupuncture. Neither RCT showed any significant difference between acupuncture and the shams in the improvement of IBS. The review rated the quality of the IBS-included studies as "robust".[3]

Two systematic reviews explored moxibustion for IBS.[4,5] One review included 20 RCTs of 1,625 people of any IBS type.[4] From the included studies (n = 7 RCTs), the review concluded moxibustion reduced IBS symptoms compared to convention pharmacological treatment.[4] The review also found moxibustion plus acupuncture combined therapy to be more effective than pharmacological therapy (n = 4 RCTs). Overall, the risk of bias was rated "high" for the included studies.[4]

The other moxibustion review by Tang and colleagues in 2016 included seven RCTs of 568 persons with IBS with predominant diarrhoea (IBS-D) and found moxibustion to be more effective than pharmacological therapy for global IBS symptoms abdominal pain, abdominal distension, abnormal stool, and defection frequency. The methodological quality of the included studies was reported to be "low".[5]

## Identification of Clinical Studies

A search of English and Chinese databases identified 17,896 citations. Following title and abstract screening, the full texts of 3,838 publications were further screened, with 26 publications meeting acupuncture-related or other therapy study inclusion criteria. Of these publications, 24 reported on RCTs, two reported on non-randomised controlled clinical trials (CCTs), and one reported on a non-controlled study.

From the 24 acupuncture RCT publications, one RCT (A23) was reported in three publications. Data from the multiple publications was merged prior to analysis. Thus, the final study inclusion numbers were 22 acupuncture RCTs, one controlled trial, and one non-controlled study (see Fig. 7.1).

The included studies utilised various acupuncture-related therapies, including manual acupuncture, electroacupuncture, moxibustion and TEAS.

One RCT study (O1) investigated *Baduanjin* 八段锦, classified as an "other CM therapy", is included in Fig. 7.1, and discussed in this chapter.

# Acupuncture

For this section, the information is presented in separate subsections based on the IBS subtype, namely IBS with predominant diarrhoea (IBS-D) and IBS with predominant constipation (IBS-C).

## Irritable Bowel Syndrome with Predominant Diarrhoea

Twelve RCTs (A1–A12) and one non-controlled study (A13) investigated acupuncture for IBS-D.

## Randomised Controlled Studies

Two RCTs had multiple acupuncture intervention arms, with A2 having three acupuncture intervention arms and A4 having an acupuncture arm and an acupuncture (with moxibustion) arm. For these two RCTs, all their arms are described in this section. Two RCTs had three intervention arms, with only one of these arms involving acupuncture and the other two arms involving a CHM and combination therapy; these arms are described in Chap. 5 ("Clinical Evidence for Chinese Herbal Medicine", A5) and Chap. 8 ("Clinical Evidence for Combination Therapies", A12).

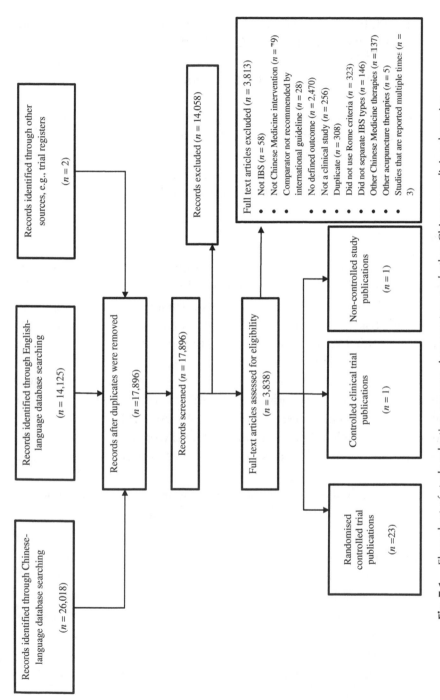

**Fig. 7.1.** Flow chart of study selection process: Acupuncture and other Chinese medicine therapies.

Nine RCTs (A1, A3, A4, A6, A7, A9–A12) investigated acupuncture alone as the intervention, one RCT (A5) investigated electroacupuncture therapy alone, two RCTs (A2, A8) investigated acupuncture plus electroacupuncture, and one RCT (A4) investigated acupuncture plus moxibustion.

Overall, the most frequently reported acupoints for IBS-D type RCTs were ST25 *Tianshu* 天枢 (10 studies), LR3 *Taichong* 太冲 (8 studies), ST36 *Zusanli* 足三里 (8 studies), ST37 *Shangjuxu* 上巨虚 (6 studies), GV20 *Baihui* 百汇 (6 studies), SP6 *Sanyinjiao* 三阴交 (6 studies), and EX-HN3 *Yintang* 印堂 (5 studies).

## Risk of Bias

All 12 RCTs were described as randomised; 11 studies reported adequate details of sequence generation (Table 7.1), while one (A7) did not provide adequate details of randomisation and was judged as "unclear" risk of bias for this domain. For allocation concealment, only one study (A2) clearly stated an appropriate method of concealment. The remaining studies did not provide sufficient information. The blinding of participants and personnel is difficult in acupuncture studies; all studies were judged as "high" risk of bias due to a lack of blinding of personnel. Four studies (A1, A3, A4, A11) did not provide reasons for participant dropout numbers and were judged as "unclear" risk for this domain. Two studies did not report on all planned

Table 7.1.  Risk of Bias of Randomised Controlled Trials: Acupuncture

| Risk of Bias Domain | Low Risk n (%) | Unclear Risk n (%) | High Risk n (%) |
|---|---|---|---|
| Sequence generation | 11 (91.7) | 1 (8.3) | 0 (0) |
| Allocation concealment | 1 (8.3) | 11 (91.7) | 0 (0) |
| Blinding of participants | 0 (0) | 0 (0) | 12 (100) |
| Blinding of personnel* | 0 (0) | 0 (0) | 12 (100) |
| Blinding of outcome assessors | 0 (0) | 0 (0) | 12 (100) |
| Incomplete outcome data | 8 (66.7) | 4 (33.3) | 0 (0) |
| Selective outcome reporting | 0 (0) | 10 (83.3) | 2 (16.7) |

*Blinding of personnel (acupuncturists) is challenging in manual therapy studies.

outcomes and was judged "high" risk of bias for selective outcome reporting. No protocols could be located for the remaining studies, so they were judged as "unclear" risk of bias for selective outcome reporting. Overall, the assessment of the methodological quality of the included studies was limited by inadequate study details.

## Acupuncture vs. Pharmacotherapy

In total, there were 622 participants in the nine RCTs (A1, A3, A4, A6, A7, A9–A12) investigating acupuncture efficacy alone for IBS-D. Eight of the RCTs (A1, A3, A4, A6, A9–12) utilised the Rome III criteria for participant inclusion, and one RCT (A7) utilised Rome II. All the RCTs were conducted in China, with four (A1, A3, A10, A11) conducted in outpatient departments, two (A9, A12) with a mixture of inpatients and outpatients, and one (A6) with participants from the community who were screened in a hospital.

Seven RCTs (A1, A3, A4, A6, A9, A11, A12) had greater numbers of female participants (n = 220) compared to males (n = 173). The lowest mean age in the RCT acupuncture groups was 38.81 years (A1) and the highest was 46.08 years (A12). For the control groups, the lowest mean age was 37.29 years (A3) and the highest was 48 years (A10). The duration of pre-existing IBS in the treatment groups ranged from a mean of 2.09 (A12) to 13.6 years (A9) and in the control groups from 1.98 (A12) to 13.30 years (A9). One study did not report the duration of IBS for participants (A7).

Six RCTs (A1, A3, A6, A9, A11, A12) reported the use of CM syndrome differentiation for diagnosis, with all of these referring to stagnancy or depression of the Liver and deficiency of the Spleen. One of the RCTs (A12) referred to a syndrome of Liver *qi* stagnation overacting on the Spleen.

The duration of the RCTs ranged from between four weeks (A1, A3, A4, A11, A12) and eight weeks (A7, A9), with a treatment period of four weeks being the most common. Only one RCT (A3) reported a follow-up period after the end of the treatment period at three months.

Seven of the RCTs (A3, A4, A6, A7, A9–A11) described a needle retention time of 30 minutes for each treatment. Two RCTs (A1, A12) did not report the needle retention time. The most commonly reported treatment frequency was three times per week (A6, A7, A10) or every second day (A1, A9, A12).

The most frequent control comparator was pinaverium bromide, which was used alone in 7 RCTs (A1, A4, A6, A7, A9–A11) and combined with probiotics in one RCT (A3). One study (A12) used a probiotic alone as the comparator.

## Outcomes

No acupuncture-alone RCTs reported on adequate relief. For IBS symptom measurement outcomes, the IBS Severity Scoring System (IBS-SSS) score,[6] treatment effective rate (TER) based on SSS, stool form and pain based on the TER were reported. For quality of life, the IBS-Quality Of Life (IBS-QOL)[7] was the only outcome measure reported by included RCTs. Analysis of acupuncture alone for each of these outcomes is presented in this section.

### Irritable bowel syndrome severity scoring symptom

Two RCTs (A6, A10; 124 participants) comparing acupuncture to pinaverium bromide reported on IBS-SSS scores and found that acupuncture-alone therapy was superior to pinaverium bromide (MD: −33.01[−65.23, −0.80] $I^2 = 76\%$). One of the studies (A10) also presented data based on the TER for the IBS-SSS and found treatment effects slightly better with acupuncture compared to pinaverium bromide (RR:1.26 [0.99, 1.61]).

### Quality of life

Four studies (A1, A3, A4, A12; 319 participants) reported IBS-QOL data; however, none of these studies reported the total score data using a correct scoring method. One study (A12) used an indeterminable outcome scaling method, and two RCTs (A3, A4) reported IBS-QOL scores outside of the accepted range (0–100). One study

(A3) reported follow-up data at three months, but again the data was above the allowable scale range.

Three RCTs (A1, A3, A12) reported IBS-QOL subdomain data. One of these (A3) used an unclear scaling method, so the data was excluded. One study (A12) mixed two types of IBS-QOL scales, so the reported data could not be analysed. The other study (A1) found acupuncture to be superior to pinaverium bromide for the domains Dysphoria (MD: 7.12 [2.39, 11.85]), Interference with Activity (MD: 9.00 [1.34, 16.66]), Body Image (MD: 6.25 [1.02, 11.48]), Health Worry (MD: 5.83 [1.80, 9.86]), Food Avoidance (MD: 8.45 [2.13, 14.77]), and Social Reaction (MD: 8.22 [1.03, 15.41]), but not for the Sexual (MD: −0.17 [−5.93, 5.59]) or Relationships domains (MD: 1.66 [−6.48, 9.80]).

## Pain/bloating/discomfort

Four RCTs (A4, A7, A9, A11) reported data for pain/bloating/discomfort (269 participants). Two (A7, A11) of these studies' data contained errors and was unable to be verified and so was excluded, while one study (A4) did not report data in a form matching the inclusion criteria. The remaining study provided TER pain and bloating data but found no difference between acupuncture treatment and pinaverium bromide for pain (RR: 1.00 [0.82, 1.22]) or bloating (RR: 1.17 [0.95, 1.43]) (A9).

## Stool form

Data for stool form was reported by three RCTs (A4, A9, A11; 215 participants). Two RCTs (A4, A11) did not use a scoring method matching the outcome inclusion criteria. One RCT (A9) reported the stool form according to the TER based on *Guiding principles of clinical research of Traditional Chinese Medicine*[8], showing that the effect from acupuncture was similar to that of pinaverium bromide: RR 1.17 [0.95, 1.43].

## Electroacupuncture vs. Pharmacotherapy

One RCT (A5; 320 participants) conducted in China had outpatients and inpatients utilising four weeks of electroacupuncture for IBS-D diagnosed using the Rome III criteria. No CM syndrome was reported for participant inclusion or treatment. The mean duration of the condition was 4.8 years for both the control and intervention groups and the mean age of participants was 40 years for both groups.

The RCT (A5) compared four weeks of electroacupuncture twice per day to a combination of conventional therapies: compound diphenoxylate hydrochloride tablets, montmorillonite powder, and amitriptyline. These acupoints received electroacupuncture: bilateral BL18 *Ganshu* 肝俞 and BL20 *Pishu* 脾俞 (left side only), ST36 *Zusanli* 足三里 and LR3 *Taichong* 太冲, four points around the umbilicus, each 2 *cun* away from the umbilicus. Follow-up data was reported at Week 60.

The RCT reported data for the Bristol stool form for IBS symptoms and SF-36 data for quality of life. There was no difference at the end of the treatment between the electroacupuncture and control groups for stool form (MD: 0.00 [−0.15, 0.15]); however, at the end of the follow-up, the stool form was more improved in the electroacupuncture group (MD: −0.44 [−0.64, −0.24]).

The RCT showed that at the end of the treatment, electroacupuncture, when compared to a combination of diphenoxylate hydrochloride, montmorillonite powder, and amitriptyline, was similar for all SF-36 domains: Physical Functioning (PF) (MD:0.15 [−5.91, 6.21]), Role–Physical (RP) (MD:0.15 [−5.91, 6.21]), Bodily Pain (BP) (MD −0.48 [−5.48, 4.52]), General Health (GH) (MD: −0.16 [−5.23, 4.91]), Vitality (VT) (MD: −0.07 [−5.24, 5.10]), Social Functioning (SF) (MD: −0.45 [−5.19, 4.29]), Role–Emotional (RE) (MD: 0.04 [−3.02, 3.10]), and Mental Health (MH) (MD: 0.02 [−8.52, 8.56]).

At a follow-up at 60 weeks, however, the results favoured the electroacupuncture group for all SF-36 domains: PF (MD: 11.67 [8.86, 14.48]), RP (MD: 11.67 [8.86, 14.48]), BP (MD 9.12 [2.30, 15.94]), GH (MD: 9.25 [1.97, 16.53]), VT (MD: 8.48 [1.12, 15.84]), SF (MD: 7.36 [1.72, 13.00]), RE (MD: 8.94 [2.81, 15.07]), and MH (MD: 7.82 [3.97, 11.67]).

## Acupuncture + Electroacupuncture vs. Pharmacotherapy

Two IBS-D studies (A2, A8) conducted in China investigated acupuncture and electroacupuncture for four weeks with a total of 236 IBS-D outpatients. Both studies reported the use of CM syndrome for participant inclusion, including people with Liver *qi* stagnation with Spleen deficiency and people with Large intestine dysfunction. The latter study further randomised participants into three specific intervention arms A2; the *He* group received treatments on LI11 *Quchi* 曲池 and ST37 *Shangjuxu* 上巨虚 bilaterally, the *He-Shu* group received treatments on ST25 *Tianshu* 天枢 and BL25 *Dachangshu* 大肠俞 bilaterally, and the *He-Shu-Mu* group received treatments to LI11 *Quchi* 曲池, ST37 *Shangjuxu* 上巨虚, ST25 *Tianshu* 天枢, and BL25 *Dachangshu* 大肠俞 on one side of the body each session. One study (A8) compared electroacupuncture to the control, spasmolytic pinaverium bromide, and the other study (A2) compared acupuncture and electroacupuncture treatment arms to the antidiarrheal loperamide hydrochloride. Both studies reported follow-up periods, with one study (A2) at four weeks and the other (A8) at three months.

### Stool form and frequency

For stool frequency, one study (A2) reported change data only without standard deviation (SD) data, with results showing a greater reduction for each of the electroacupuncture arms (the *He* group with a decreased mean to six stools per week, *Shu-mu* group with a decreased mean to 4.6 stools per week and *He-Shu-Mu* group with a decreased mean to 4.8 stools per week), as compared to the loperamide hydrochloride's mean decrease to 4.1 stools per week. Data for stool frequency did not match the specified inclusion criteria for this outcome and was not included for analysis (A8).

For stool form, one study (A2) reported data using the Bristol scale but again presented mean data without SD. The mean score of 5.4 at the end of the treatment was the same for the He group, *Shu-mu* group and control (loperamide) group, but the *He-Shu-Mu* group showed a lower mean score (5.0). The other RCT (A8) did not report the data according to the outcome inclusion criteria.

## Quality of life

Data for the SF-36 was reported by one study (A2) with results favouring, but without significant difference, the loperamide group compared to the electroacupuncture plus acupuncture arm for the Physical Functioning, Role–Physical Function and General Health domains. For the Bodily Pain, Vitality, Social Functioning, Role-Emotional Function, and Mental Health domains, the results favoured electroacupuncture plus acupuncture, but again, there was no significant difference.

Study A8 reported on the IBS-QOL; however, the data used incorrect scaling with data outside of the outcome measures range. The domain score data for the IBS-QOL used the correct scaling and showed an improved quality of life for the acupuncture plus electroacupuncture group as compared to the pinaverium bromide group for Dysphoria (MD: 10.18 [5.29, 15.07]), Interference with Activity (MD: 11.13 [5.89, 16.37]), Body Image (MD: 5.00 [0.37, 9.63]), Health Worry (MD: 10.72 [5.06, 16.38]), Food Avoidance (MD: 8.78 [2.41, 15.15]), Social Reaction (MD: 6.61 [2.22, 11.00]), and Relationships (MD: 4.28 [0.24, 8.32]). No difference between the groups was found for the Sexual domain (MD: 5.72 [−0.21, 11.65]).

## Zung self-rating anxiety scale and Zung self-rating depression scale

One study (A8) reported data for the Zung Self-rating Anxiety Scale (SAS) and Zung Self-rating Depression Scale (SDS) scores. Results from the RCT favoured acupuncture and electroacupuncture compared to pinaverium bromide (MD: −3.91 [−6.25, −1.57]). Similarly, SDS results also favoured acupuncture and electroacupuncture (MD: −4.22 [−7.37, −1.07]).

## Recurrence rate

The recurrence rate (RR) was reported in one study (A8). From the results, the RR for IBS at a follow-up at 3 months was 34% (12/35) in the electroacupuncture plus acupuncture group and 51% (18/33) in the pinaverium bromide group; however, the difference was not significant (RR: 0.63 [0.36, 1.09]).

## *Acupuncture + Moxibustion vs. Pharmacotherapy*

One RCT (A4) conducted in China investigated four weeks of acupuncture plus moxibustion in outpatients diagnosed with IBS-D according to the Rome III criteria. The RCT compared two intervention arms to pinaverium bromide in 90 people. The acupuncture-alone intervention arm has been described in the previous section. The acupuncture and moxibustion arm treated 30 participants — 14 males and 16 females — for four weeks. The RCT did not report on the CM syndrome. The participants had a mean duration of IBS of 5.8 years and a mean age of 40 years in the acupuncture plus moxibustion arm, and 5.4 years (mean duration) and 38 years (mean age) in the pinaverium bromide arm.

Indirect moxibustion with ginger slices was administered to ST25 *Tianshu* 天枢 and CV4 *Guanyuan* 关元 for 60 minutes once per day. Acupuncture treatment was applied to GV20 *Baihui* 百汇 and CV12 *Zhongwan* 中脘, and bilaterally to ST25 *Tianshu* 天枢, while ST36 *Zusanli* 足三里, SP9 *Yinlingquan* 阴陵泉, ST39 *Xiajuxu* 下巨虚, and LR3 *Taichong* 太冲 were needled for 30 minutes once per day during the treatment period.

The RCT reported symptom outcome data for pain, stool frequency, and stool form; however, none of this data matched the inclusion criteria methods for calculating these outcomes. For quality of life, the RCT only reported the IBS-QOL total score; however, it used an incorrect scale scoring method with results beyond the pre-specified scale limits, so it was not possible to conduct the analysis.

Adverse events (AEs) data was not reported, and there was no long-term follow-up.

## Non-randomised Controlled Studies

There were no non-randomised controlled studies of acupuncture for IBS-D.

## Non-controlled Studies

There was one included non-controlled acupuncture study (A13). The study (A13) was conducted in Germany and assessed acupuncture to points LR13 *Zhangmen*章门, CV12 *Zhongwan* 中脘, ST25 *Tianshu* 天枢, CV4 *Guanyuan* 关元, LR14 *Qimen* 期门, LI4 *Hegu*合谷, LR3 *Taichong* 太冲, LI11 *Quchi* 曲池, SP9 *Yinlingquan* 阴陵泉, and ST36 *Zusanli* 足三里 in 21 persons with IBS-D. All persons had the CM syndrome of Liver *qi* stagnation with Spleen deficiency, with acupuncture administered for 30 minutes per session, two to three times per week, until 16 sessions were delivered. The study did not report on AEs.

## Frequently Reported Acupuncture Points in Meta-analyses Showing Favourable Effect

Meta-analyses showed the benefit of acupuncture or electroacupuncture over comparators for the improvement of overall symptom severity (see the section "IBS-D Acupuncture vs. Pharmacotherapy, Severity Scoring System"). The acupuncture points of studies included in these meta-analyses were reviewed to identify those that may have contributed to the favourable effects seen. In the two RCTs (A6, A10) included in the meta-analysis for IBS-SSS, both studies used GV20 *Baihui* 百会, ST25 *Tianshu* 天枢, ST36 *Zusanli* 足三里, ST37 *Shangjuxu* 上巨虚, LR3 *Taichong* 太冲, SP6 *Sanyinjiao* 三阴交, and EX-HN3 *Yintang* 印堂.

Among the studies (A1, A8) that contributed to improvements in quality-of-life outcomes, the most frequently used acupuncture points were ST25 *Tianshu* 天枢, ST36 *Zusanli* 足三里, and LR3 *Taichong* 太冲.

One study that showed an improvement in SAS and SDS scores used GV20 *Baihui* 百会, ST25 *Tianshu* 天枢, ST36 *Zusanli* 足三里, ST37 *Shangjuxu* 上巨虚, LR3 *Taichong* 太冲, SP6 *Sanyinjiao* 三阴交, and EX-HN3 *Yintang* 印堂, with electroacupuncture on both ST25 *Tianshu* 天枢 after *de qi* 得气 (A8).

## Assessment using Grading of Recommendations Assessment, Development and Evaluations

An assessment of the quality of the evidence from RCTs was made using Grading of Recommendations Assessment, Development and Evaluations (GRADE). Interventions, comparators and outcomes to be included were selected based on a consensus process, as described in Chap. 4. Acupuncture and electroacupuncture were considered to be important interventions for IBS treatments, and experts considered that comparison with pharmacotherapy, especially pinaverium bromide, for IBS-D would provide valuable information to inform clinical practice.

### *Acupuncture vs. Pinaverium Bromide for Irritable Bowel Syndrome with Predominant Diarrhoea*

Evidence for acupuncture versus pinaverium bromide was of "low" to "very low" quality (Table 7.2). Very low-quality evidence showed that acupuncture was statistically different from pinaverium bromide in reducing the IBS-SSS scores. Low-quality evidence showed that acupuncture significantly improved the quality of life for IBS participants, compared to pinaverium bromide. Low-quality evidence showed that acupuncture was not statistically different from pinaverium bromide for the total effective rate based on pain, bloating and stool form.

Two RCTs (A1, A10; 137 participants) reported no AEs in the acupuncture group. In the pinaverium bromide group, one case of increased diarrhoea was reported.

### *Electroacupuncture vs. Pharmacotherapy for Irritable Bowel Syndrome with Predominant Diarrhoea*

Evidence for electroacupuncture vs. pharmacotherapy was of "moderate" quality (Table 7.3). Evidence from one study showed that acupuncture was statistically different from pharmacotherapy for the Bristol Stool Form Scale score or three months of follow-up but not at the end of eight weeks of treatment.

The RCT did not report on AEs.

**Table 7.2. Acupuncture vs. Pinaverium Bromide for Irritable Bowel Syndrome with Predominant Diarrhoea**

| Outcome; Mean Treatment Duration | Estimated Absolute Effect | | Relative Effect (95% CI) No. RCTs (Participants) | Certainty of Evidence GRADE |
|---|---|---|---|---|
| | Acupuncture | Pinaverium Bromide | | |
| IBS-SSS 6w | **−33.01** MD: 33.01 lower (95% CI: 65.23 lower to 0.8 lower) | 0 | MD −33.01 [−65.23, −0.8] 2 (120) | ⊕○○○ VERY LOW[a,b,c] |
| TER – pain 8w | **87** per 100 Difference: 0 fewer per 1,000 patients (95% CI: 0 difference per 100 patients) | **87** per 100 | RR 1.00 [0.82, 1.22] 1 (60) | ⊕⊕○○ LOW[a,d] |
| TER – bloating 8w | **94** per 100 Difference: 14 more per 100 patients (95% CI: 4 fewer to 34 more per 100 patients) | **80** per 100 | RR 1.17 [0.95, 1.43] 1 (60) | ⊕⊕○○ LOW[a,d] |
| TER – stool form 8w | **94** per 100 Difference: 14 more per 1,000 patients (95% CI: 4 fewer to 34 more per 100 patients) | **80** per 100 | RR 1.17 [0.95, 1.43] 1 (60) | ⊕⊕○○ LOW[a,d] |
| IBS-QOL total score 4w | **90.05** MD: 7.28 higher (95% CI: 2.63 higher to 11.93 higher) | 82.77 | MD 7.28 [2.63, 11.93] 1 (60) | ⊕⊕○○ LOW[a,d] |

Abbreviations: CI, confidence interval; GRADE, Grading of Recommendations Assessment, Development and Evaluation; IBS-QOL, Irritable Bowel Syndrome-Quality of Life; IBS-SSS, IBS-Severity Scoring System; MD, mean difference; RCT, randomised controlled trial; RR: risk ratio; TER, total effective rate; w, weeks.

[a]High risk of bias due to lack of blinding.
[b]Considerable statistical heterogeneity.
[c]Wide CI and small sample size.
[d]Small sample size.

Study references:
IBS-SSS: A6, A10.
TER – pain, TER – bloating, TER – stool form: A9.
IBS-QOL total score: A1.

**Table 7.3.  Electroacupuncture vs. Pharmacotherapy for Irritable Bowel Syndrome with Predominant Diarrhoea**

| Outcome; Treatment Duration | Estimated Absolute Effect | | Relative Effect (95% CI) No. RCTs (Participants) | Certainty of Evidence GRADE |
|---|---|---|---|---|
| | Electroacupuncture | Pharmacotherapy | | |
| Bristol Stool Form Scale 4w | **2.33** MD: 0 (95% CI: 0.15 lower to 0.15 higher) | **2.33** | MD 0 (−0.15, 0.15) 1 (317) | ⊕⊕⊕◯ MODERATE[a] |
| Bristol Stool Form Scale follow-up 4w | **2.36** MD: 0.44 lower (95% CI: 0.64 lower to 0.24 lower) | **2.8** | MD −0.44 (−0.64, −0.24) 1 (317) | ⊕⊕⊕◯ MODERATE[a] |

Abbreviations: CI: confidence interval; GRADE, Grading of Recommendations Assessment, Development and Evaluation; MD, mean difference; RCT, randomised controlled trial; w, weeks.

[a]Unclear allocation concealment. High risk of bias due to lack of blinding of participants and personnel.

Study reference:
Bristol Stool Form Scale: A5.


# Safety of Acupuncture

Six studies (A1–A3, A5, A8, A10) reported on the safety of acupuncture. Among these, two RCTs reported that no AEs occurred during the study in both groups (A1, A3). One study that evaluated acupuncture alone for IBS-D reported no AEs in the intervention group (A10); in the pharmacotherapy group (A10), one case of increased diarrhoea was reported.

One IBS-D study (A5) that evaluated electroacupuncture reported two cases of abdominal pain in the pharmacotherapy group; no AEs were reported in the acupuncture group.

When acupuncture and electroacupuncture were evaluated together for IBS-D (A2), AEs in the intervention group included 1 case of abdominal pain, 1 case of cold limbs, 3 cases of fainting, 4 cases of insomnia, and 1 case of weakness. In the control group receiving loperamide, 1 case of hot flushes was reported.

## Irritable Bowel Syndrome with Predominant Constipation

Five RCTs (A14–A18) investigated acupuncture for IBS-C. No non-randomised controlled studies of acupuncture or non-controlled studies were identified in this review.

## Randomised Controlled Trials of Irritable Bowel Syndrome with Predominant Constipation

A total of five RCTs (A14–A18) evaluated acupuncture and related therapies for IBS-C. Two RCTs (A14, A15) evaluated acupuncture alone for IBS-C, two RCTs (A16, A17) evaluated electroacupuncture for IBS-C, and one RCT (A18) combined acupuncture and electroacupuncture for IBS-C. The most frequently reported acupoints were ST25 *Tianshu* 天枢 and ST36 *Zusanli* 足三里, which were both utilised in 4 out of 5 studies.

Three studies (A14, A15, A18) used random number tables for group allocation, posing "low" risk of bias. Insufficient information was available about how group allocation was assigned in two studies (A16, A17); they were judged as "unclear" risk of bias for sequence generation. All of the studies provided insufficient information on how group allocation was concealed and judged as "unclear" risk of bias for allocation concealment. The lack of blinding of participants, personnel and outcome assessors was considered to pose a "high" risk of bias in all studies. No missing data was reported in three studies (A15, A17, A18), one study (A16) did not report whether there was any missing data, and one study (A14) had missing data but did not report on the reasons for dropouts. No trial protocols or registrations were identified for the studies, posing an "unclear" risk of bias for selective reporting.

### *Acupuncture vs. Pharmacotherapy*

Two RCTs (A14, A15) conducted in China evaluated acupuncture in 161 people with Rome III diagnosed IBS-C. One study (A15) investigated an outpatient population, and the other RCT (A14) did not report where the participants were sourced. Sixty-nine male and 92 female participants, with the mean age of participants being 37.6 years in A15 and 62.1 years in A14. Both studies had a treatment period of four weeks and reported a follow-up period — (A15) 1 month post-intervention, and (A14) 1 month and 3 months post-intervention .

Neither study reported the same outcome measures, with one study (A15) reporting includable outcomes data for each of the IBS-QOL domains and Bristol Stool Form Scale. This RCT (A15) also reported outcome data for pain and bloating, as well as stool frequency, but these outcomes were not based on validated scales or guidelines, and so the study was excluded from the analysis. For IBS-related symptom outcome measures, one RCT only reported IBS-SSS data based on the TER. This RCT (A14) also reported quality-of-life data using the SF-36.

A14 reported includable data for the IBS-SSS, SF-36 and recurrence. For the TER based on the IBS-SSS, there was no difference between the two groups at the end of the treatment (RR: 1.02 [0.90, 1.15]). For the SF-36 at the end of the treatment, the PF (MD: 4.38 [0.94, 7.82]), BP (MD: 11.19 [6.92, 15.46]), GH (MD:6.89 [3.58, 10.20]), VT (MD: 10.69 [6.27, 15.11]), SF (MD: 12.90 [7.60, 18.20]), RE (MD: 7.13 [2.61, 11.65]), and MH (MD: 9.71 [4.26, 15.16]) domains all had better scores in the acupuncture group; however, results from the RP domain showed no difference compared to the mosapride citrate and lactulose group (MD: 3.59 [−1.11, 8.29]). At a one-month follow-up, all the domains were better in the acupuncture group, but at the second follow-up (three months), two domains — RP and SF — no longer showed a difference between the two groups.

A15 showed that acupuncture was superior to testa triticum tricum purif (wheat cellulose particles) for the IBS-QOL domains of Dysphoria (MD: 18.05 [10.67, 25.43]), Interference with Activity (MD: 12.00 [6.28, 17.72]), Body Image (MD: 8.25 [1.86, 14.64]), Health Worry (MD: 16.87 [8.56, 25.18]), Food Avoidance (MD: 19.38 [12.63, 26.13]), Social Reaction (MD: 7.96 [0.48, 15.44]) and Relationships (MD: 6.90 [1.24, 12.56]). The only domain not favouring acupuncture was the Sexual domain, where both groups showed similar effects (MD: 5.77 [−0.91, 12.45]).

For the stool form, there was a difference favouring lower scores in the acupuncture group (MD: 0.61 [0.37, 0.85]). At the follow-up, the results had reversed, and the lower score favoured the testa triticum tricum purif group (MD: −0.60 [−0.84, −0.36]).

## Electroacupuncture

Two RCTs (A16, A17) conducted in China assessed electroacupuncture for IBS-C in 82 outpatients. One RCT used electroacupuncture as integrative medicine, adding one hour of bilateral burst-mode electroacupuncture at 0.5–2 mA to ST36 *Zusanli* 足三里, and the intervention arm additionally received the same control therapies for two weeks. The control group comparator was a combination of live bacteria *clostridium butyricum enterococci* and 10 g of the laxative polyethylene glycol (macrogol 4000 powder) once per day (A17). Study A16 investigated alternating on (2 seconds) and off (3 seconds) electroacupuncture at a frequency of 40 Hz with a wave width of 500 us and output of 10 mA for 30 minutes twice per day, compared to a combination of laxative polyethylene glycol (macrogol 4000 powder), live combined bacillus subtilis, and enterococcus faecium capsules for four weeks.

Both studies reported data for the stool form based on the Bristol score. When electroacupuncture was used as integrative medicine, there was greater improvement in the Bristol score compared to pharmacotherapy alone (MD: 0.78 [0.14, 1.42]) (A17), but not when electroacupuncture was used alone (MD: 0.3 [−0.30, 0.90]) (A16).

One study (A16) reported on the SF-36 domains, SAS and SDS. For the SF-36, results showed that electroacupuncture provided superior SF-36 scores for the GH (MD: 2.90 [0.08, 5.72]), VT (MD: 6.40 [3.39, 9.41]), SF (MD: 4.50 [1.71, 7.29]), and MH (MD: 9.00 [6.39, 11.61]) domains. There was no difference between groups for the PF

(MD: 1.20 [−2.12, 4.52]), RP (MD: 0.70 [−3.99, 2.59]), BP (MD: 2.40 [−0.65, 5.45]) or RE (MD: 1.50 [−1.17, 4.17]) domains. For the SAS, the results favoured electroacupuncture compared to the control group (MD: −3.26 [−3.73, −2.79]), as did the results for the SDS (MD: −1.27 [−1.76, −0.78]).

## *Acupuncture + Electroacupuncture vs. Pharmacotherapy*

One RCT (A18) conducted in China investigated acupuncture and electroacupuncture in 60 outpatients with IBS-C. The treatment period lasted four weeks, with a follow-up at two months. The control group comparator was 15 mL of laxative lactulose administered thrice per day, with acupuncture and electroacupuncture applied once per day for 30 minutes, five times per week at a frequency of 2 Hz/100 Hz in the intervention group. The acupoints stimulated were ST25 *Tianshu* 天枢, ST36 *Zusanli* 足三里, ST37 *Shangjuxu* 上巨虚, LR3 *Taichong* 太冲, SP6 *Sanyinjiao* 三阴交, and EX-HN3 *Yintang* 印堂, and electroacupuncture was performed on ST25 *Tianshu* 天枢 after *de qi* 得气.

The study reported data for the IBS-QOL outcome measure, but the scores were outside of the accepted range (0–100) and were not analysed.

## Frequently Reported Acupuncture Points in Meta-analyses Showing Favourable Effect

Meta-analyses showed the benefit of electroacupuncture over comparators for the outcomes of the Bristol score and quality-of-life questionnaire domains. The acupuncture points of the studies included in these meta-analyses were reviewed to identify those that may have contributed to the favourable effects seen. The most frequently used acupoints were ST25 *Tianshu* 天枢 and ST36 *Zusanli* 足三里.

## Assessment using Grading of Recommendations Assessment, Development and Evaluations

An assessment of the quality of the evidence from RCTs was made using GRADE. Interventions, comparators and outcomes to be included were selected based on a consensus process, as described in Chap. 4. Acupuncture and electroacupuncture were considered to be important interventions for IBS treatments, and experts considered that a comparison with pharmacotherapy for IBS-C would provide valuable information to inform clinical practice.

### Acupuncture vs. Pharmacotherapy for Irritable Bowel Syndrome with Predominant Constipation

Low certainty evidence showed that acupuncture was statistically different from pharmacotherapy for the Bristol Stool Form Scale score (Table 7.4). No statistical difference was found between acupuncture and pharmacotherapy for the TER based on the IBS-SSS and recurrence rate (Table 7.4).

In the one RCT that reported on AEs, no AEs were reported in the acupuncture or pharmacotherapy groups.

### Electroacupuncture vs. Pharmacotherapy for Irritable Bowel Syndrome with Predominant Constipation

Low-certainty evidence showed that electroacupuncture was statistically different to pharmacotherapy for the SAS and SDS scores but not for the Bristol Stool Scale Form scores (Table 7.5).

The RCT did not report on AEs.

## Safety of Acupuncture

Two studies (A14, A17) reported on the safety of acupuncture. One study (A14) reported that no AEs occurred during the study in both groups. One study (A17) had no AEs in the pharmacotherapy group and two cases of broken skin in the electroacupuncture group.

**Table 7.4. Acupuncture vs. Pharmacotherapy for Irritable Bowel Syndrome with Predominant Constipation**

| Outcome; Treatment Duration | Estimated Absolute Effects | | Relative Effect (95% CI) No. RCTs (Participants) | Certainty of Evidence GRADE |
|---|---|---|---|---|
| | Acupuncture | Pharmacotherapy | | |
| Bristol Stool Form Scale<br>4 weeks | **0.71**<br>MD: 0.61 higher<br>(95% CI: 0.37 higher to 0.85 higher) | **0.1** | MD 0.61<br>(0.37, 0.85)<br>1 (41) | ⊕⊕◯◯<br>LOW[a,b] |
| TER – IBS SSS<br>4 weeks | **90**<br>per 100<br>Difference: 2 more per 100 patients<br>(95% CI: 9 fewer to 13 more per 100 patients) | **88**<br>per 100 | RR 1.02<br>(0.90, 1.15)<br>1 (120) | ⊕⊕◯◯<br>LOW[a,b] |
| Recurrence rate at 1 month after end of treatment<br>Treatment duration: 4 weeks | **17**<br>per 100<br>Difference: 15 fewer per 100 patients<br>(95% CI: 23 fewer to 1 more per 1,000 patients) | **32**<br>per 100 | RR 0.53<br>(0.27, 1.01)<br>1 (120) | ⊕⊕◯◯<br>LOW[a,b] |
| Recurrence rate at 3 months after end of treatment<br>Treatment duration: 4 weeks | **25**<br>per 100<br>Difference: 17 fewer per 100 patients<br>(95% CI: 27 fewer to 1 more per 100 patients) | **42**<br>per 100 | RR 0.60<br>(0.35, 1.02)<br>1 (120) | ⊕⊕◯◯<br>LOW[a,b] |

Abbreviations: CI: confidence interval; GRADE, Grading of Recommendations Assessment, Development and Evaluation; IBS-SSS, Irritable Bowel Syndrome-Severity Scoring System; MD, mean difference; RCT, randomised controlled trial; RR: risk ratio; TER, total effective rate.

[a]Unclear allocation concealment. High risk of bias due to lack of blinding of participants and personnel.
[b]Small sample size.

Study references:
Bristol Stool Form Scale: A15.
TER based on IBS Severity Scoring System: A14.
Recurrence rate: A14.

Table 7.5. Electroacupuncture vs. Pharmacotherapy for Irritable Bowel Syndrome with Predominant Constipation

| Outcome; Treatment Duration | Estimated Absolute Effects | | Relative Effect (95% CI) No. RCTs (Participants) | Certainty of Evidence GRADE |
|---|---|---|---|---|
| | Electroacupuncture | Pharmacotherapy | | |
| Zung Self-rating Anxiety Scale (SAS) Treatment duration: 4 weeks | **34.6** MD: 3.26 lower (95% CI: 3.26 lower to 2.79 lower) | **37.86** | MD −3.26 (−3.73, −2.79) 1 (40) | ⊕⊕○○ LOW[a,b] |
| Zung Self-rating Depression Scale (SDS) Treatment duration: 4 weeks | **37.78** MD: 1.27 lower (95% CI: 1.76 lower to 0.78 lower) | **39.05** | MD −1.27 (−1.76, −0.78) 1 (40) | ⊕⊕○○ LOW[a,b] |
| Bristol Stool Scale Form Treatment duration: 4 weeks | **2.65** MD: 0.3 higher (95% CI: 0.3 lower to 0.9 higher) | **2.95** | MD 0.3 (−0.3, 0.9) 1 (40) | ⊕⊕○○ LOW[a,b] |

Abbreviations: CI: confidence interval; GRADE, Grading of Recommendations Assessment, Development and Evaluation; MD, mean difference; RCT, randomised controlled trial; RR: risk ratio.

[a]Unclear randomisation and allocation concealment. High risk of bias due to lack of blinding of participants and personnel.
[b]Small sample size.

Study references:
SAS, SDS, Bristol Stool Form score: A16.

# Moxibustion

Four studies (A19–A22), all RCTs, investigated the efficacy of moxibustion alone for IBS-D in 297 persons. All studies were conducted in China and utilised indirect moxibustion for four weeks. Two studies (A19, A21) recruited participants from hospital outpatients departments, one study (A22) from inpatients and outpatients departments, and one study (A20) from a hospital but did not detail whether the participants were inpatients or outpatients.

One study (A19) utilised a sham moxa as the control, administering the sham to the same acupoints as the intervention group. The other three studies (A20–A22) compared moxibustion to conventional treatment.

Two studies (A21, A22) mentioned using syndrome differentiation at their inclusion. One study (A22) grouped participants into one of three CM syndromes: Liver *qi* stagnation with Spleen deficiency, Spleen and Kidney *yang* deficiency, or Spleen and Stomach weakness. The remaining study (A21) enrolled participants with IBS-D who had the CM syndrome of Spleen *qi* deficiency.

The only common acupuncture point reported between the studies was ST25 *Tianshu* 天枢, reported to be administered moxibustion in two of the studies (A19, A20).

Two studies (A19, A21) reported administering the moxibustion twice per week, one study (A20) once per day, and the remaining study (A22) did not mention the frequency of administration. Two studies (A20, A22) reported having a follow-up period, both at three months.

Random number tables were used for group allocation in two studies (A19, A20), posing "low" risk of bias. The other two studies (A21, A22) did not specify the method of randomisation and were judged as "unclear" risk of bias for sequence generation. One study (A19) used sealed opaque sequentially numbered envelopes and was considered a "low" risk of bias for allocation concealment, while insufficient information was available about how group allocation was concealed in three studies (A20, A21, A22), and these were judged as "unclear" risk for allocation concealment. The lack of blinding of participants, personnel and outcome assessors was considered to pose as a "high" risk of bias in all studies. One study (A19) had high dropout rates in both groups and provided reasons; it was unclear whether this was likely to influence the results. No missing data was reported in the remaining studies. No trial protocols or registrations were identified for the included studies, posing an "unclear" risk of bias for selective reporting.

## Randomised Controlled Trials of Moxibustion

### *Moxibustion vs. Sham Moxibustion for Irritable Bowel Syndrome with Predominant Diarrhoea*

One study (A19; 80 people) investigated moxibustion for IBS-D compared to sham moxibustion. The study applied indirect moxibustion on top of aconite cakes twice per day for four weeks to ST25 *Tianshu* 天枢, CV6 *Qihai* 气海, and CV12 *Zhongwan* 中脘. Sham moxibustion was administered to the same acupoints by placing a round cardboard piece between the aconite cake and the skin. The study reported outcomes for the Birmingham IBS Symptom Scale and IBS-QOL. For the Birmingham Scale, it found moxibustion to be superior to sham moxibustion (MD: −12.46 [−15.57, −9.35]). It was also superior in improving IBS-QOL scores (MD: −25.35 [−30.95, −19.75]).

Using functional magnetic resonance imaging (fMRI), the study also observed brain-imaging changes before and after the moxibustion during rectal balloon distension. It concluded that the moxibustion decreased rectal sensitivity in persons with IBS-D.

### *Moxibustion vs. Conventional Therapy for Irritable Bowel Syndrome with Predominant Diarrhoea*

Three studies compared indirect moxibustion to conventional therapy in 217 persons. Two studies (A21, A22) utilised pinaverium bromide as the control, and the other study (A20) utilised the antidiarrheal loperamide. One study (A21; 40 persons) with Spleen *qi* deficiency used pulverised CM herbs *bai zhu* 白术, *shan yao* 山药, *fu ling* 茯苓, *ding xiang* 丁香, and *wu bei zi* 五倍子 combined with moxa on acupuncture point CV8 *Shenque* 神阙. The other two RCTs did not report the addition of any CHM to the moxa for moxibustion.

One study (A22) administered moxibustion to acupoints according to the CM syndrome of the participants at inclusion. In this study, all three CM syndrome groups received moxibustion to CV4 *Guanyuan* 关元, with the addition of LR14 *Qimen* 期门 for persons in group 1 (Liver *qi* stagnation with Spleen deficiency), BL23 *Shenshu* 肾俞 in group 2 (Spleen and Kidney *yang* deficiency), and group 3

CV12 *Zhongwan* 中脘 (Spleen and Stomach weakness). The remaining studies (A20, A21) applied indirect moxibustion bilaterally to BL25 *Dachangshu* 大肠俞 and ST25 *Tianshu* 天枢.

None of the three studies reported data for the same outcome measures, so they were unable to be combined in the meta-analysis. One study (A22) reported outcome data for the IBS-SSS score and the IBS-SSS based on TER. The study found that compared to conventional therapy, moxibustion significantly improved IBS-SSS scores (MD: −23.1 [−43.53, −2.67]).

One study (A20) reported data for the IBS-QOL but only for the total score, without providing what scoring method it used. The study rated a higher IBS-QOL score as improved quality of life, and the data indicated that moxibustion was superior in improving IBS-QOL scores at the end of the treatment (MD: 6.96 [2.08, 11.84]) and at the end of three months' follow up (MD: 8.82 [3.50, 14.14]). The remaining study (A21) reported the stool form and symptom data based on guidelines; however, it did not present the data in a form suitable for meta-analysis, although it did conclude that when combined, the symptoms reduced significantly at the conclusion of the treatment phase (p < 0.01).

### Safety of Moxibustion

No included studies reported on AEs.

# Transcutaneous Electrical Acupoint Stimulation

One RCT (A23) evaluated TEAS for IBS-D and one non-randomised controlled study (A24) evaluated TEAS for IBS-D.

## Randomised Controlled Trials of Transcutaneous Electrical Acupoint Stimulation

One RCT (A23; 110 outpatients) conducted in China investigated the efficacy of TEAS for IBS-D, with the CM syndrome Liver *qi* stagnation attacking the Spleen. The study applied TEAS bilaterally at an intensity level of 5 for 10 minutes, twice per day, to LR3 *Taichong* 太冲, SP9 *Yinlingquan* 阴陵泉, and ST25 *Tianshu* 天枢. It compared four weeks of TEAS treatment to a placebo TEAS, with the placebo consisting of a simulated intensity applied to the same acupoints as the intervention group. The study reported a follow-up period at eight weeks post-treatment.

Computer-generated randomisation was used for group allocation, posing a "low" risk of bias. Opaque envelopes were used to conceal group allocation, and the study was judged as "low" risk for allocation concealment. A TEAS machine was used, so blinding was achieved for participants, personnel and outcome assessors, resulting in a "low" risk of bias. The study reported one dropout without reasons, and was judged an "unclear" risk for incomplete outcome data. No trial protocol or registration was identified and pre-specified outcomes were not reported in the results section, posing a "high" risk of bias.

Eligible outcome data reporting included data for the IBS-SSS effective rate, IBS-SSS overall score, IBS-DSQ effective rate, stool frequency, and recurrence at a follow-up. For the IBS-SSS, the study found that TEAS was superior to the placebo TEAS (RR 1.6 [1.2, 2.14]) and also for the SSS score (MD: −63.31 [−93.0, −33.63]). For daily stool frequency, the results showed that TEAS was superior to the placebo TEAS (MD: −0.48 [−0.90, −0.06]). For the IBS-DSQ effective rate, the study found that TEAS was superior to the placebo TEAS (RR 1.48 [1.17, 1.87]). For recurrence at a follow-up, the results showed eight recurrences from 33 people completing the follow-up phase in the intervention group and five from 10 people completing the follow-up in the control group, with no significant difference between the groups (RR 0.48 [0.20, 1.15]).

Data was collected on AEs, with the study reporting zero AEs in both groups during the study.

## Non-randomised Controlled Clinical Trials of Transcutaneous Electrical Acupoint Stimulation

One integrative medicine non-randomised CCT (A24) conducted in China investigated the efficacy of TEAS combined with the probiotic

Bifid Triple Viable (containing bacillus acidophilus, bifidobacterium bifidum and faecal streptococci) for IBS-D. The study compared the interventions to the Bifid Triple Viable and the antipsychotic and anti-depressant drug Deanxit® (flupentixol and melitracen) in 100 people for four weeks but did not mention their source. The study also did not mention the use of CM syndrome and applied TENS bilaterally to ST36 *Zusanli* 足三里 and PC6 *Neiguan* 内关 for 40-minute sessions three times per week. The Bifid Triple Viable was administered three times (420 mg each time) per day in both groups, and Deanxit® was administered twice per day in the control group.

The study reported the inclusion eligible outcomes SAS and SDS without reporting on AEs.

## Safety of Transcutaneous Electrical Acupoint Stimulation

One RCT study (A23) reported no AEs, and one CCT (A24) did not report on AEs.

## *Baduanjin* 八段锦

*Baduanjin* 八段锦 is a form of qigong. It includes a routine of eight exercises that coordinate movement and breath. One RCT (O1) conducted in China investigated the efficacy of *Baduanjin* 八段锦 for IBS-C, compared to tegaserod in 60 people from the local community for 12 weeks. The study did not mention the use of CM syndrome. Participants practised 45 minutes of *Baduanjin* 八段锦 twice a day for five days per week. Tegaserod was administered twice (6 mg each time) per day in both groups.

The study did not report on eligible outcomes and did not report on AEs.

## Summary of Acupuncture and Related Therapies: Clinical Evidence

Acupuncture and related therapies for the management of IBS-D and IBS-C have been evaluated in RCTs, non-randomised CCTs, and non-controlled studies. Manual acupuncture and electroacupuncture were the two main types of therapies used in clinical studies. These therapies are frequently used in clinical practice, in and outside of China.

Treatment goals and acupuncture points are different for different types of IBS, so this chapter presented results according to IBS-D and IBS-C clinical studies.

For IBS-D studies, the treatment duration ranged from 4 to 8 weeks, with the median treatment duration of four weeks in 13 RCTs. In the nine clinical studies that reported information on needle retention, eight studies had a needle retention time of 30 minutes. The most commonly reported treatment frequency was thrice per week or every second day. In clinical studies that described the CM syndrome of included IBS-D participants, 87.5% (7 of 8 studies) were related to Liver *qi* stagnation with Spleen deficiency. The Liver and Spleen were the main organs identified to be involved in IBS for these participants. This aligns with the syndromes described in clinical textbooks and guidelines (see Chap. 2).

The comparators used in the IBS-D clinical studies included pharmacotherapy and probiotics; of the pharmacotherapy used, pinaverium bromide was the most frequently used in the included clinical studies (8 of 12 studies, 75%). For IBS-D symptoms, acupuncture was more effective than pinaverium bromide for the IBS-SSS score and TER based on the IBS-SSS. No significant difference was found between acupuncture and pinaverium bromide for pain, bloating or discomfort, or TER based on stool form; this data was based on results from single studies. For quality-of-life outcomes, the included studies did not report on the total score data using a correct scoring method, so the data could not be used in meta-analyses. Using the correct tool and scoring method is essential in future clinical studies. Only a third of the clinical studies (4 of 12) had a follow-up period; future studies may consider investigating the long-term effect of acupuncture for IBS-D. Only one included study in the IBS-D type reported on the SAS and SDS.

The assessment of clinically important questions using the GRADE framework highlighted that the strength and quality of evidence ("certainty") ranged from "very low" to "low" when acupuncture was compared with pinaverium bromide in reducing IBS-SSS scores. Low-quality evidence showed no benefit of acupuncture over pinaverium bromide for pain, bloating and stool form, or quality of life for IBS participants. Moderate evidence from one RCT showed no benefit of electroacupuncture over a combination of pharmacotherapy.

For IBS-C studies, the treatment duration ranged from 2 to 4 weeks, with the median treatment duration of four weeks in five RCTs. In the five clinical studies that reported information on needle retention, four studies had a needle retention time of 30 minutes, and the other study retained the needles for an hour. The most commonly reported treatment frequency was five days a week. None of the included studies described CM syndrome for IBS-C.

The Bristol score favoured lower scores in the acupuncture groups at the end of the treatment, but the results reversed, favouring pharmacotherapy at the end of a one-month follow-up. No benefit was seen in acupuncture over pharmacotherapy for the TER based on the IBS-SSS. Quality-of-life outcome measures showed the benefit of acupuncture over pharmacotherapy in some domains, but not for all. The RR of IBS-C at 1 month and 3 months after treatment was lower in the acupuncture group.

The assessment of the studies using the GRADE framework showed low-quality evidence favouring acupuncture over pharmacotherapy for the Bristol Stool Form Scale score and low-quality evidence favouring electroacupuncture over pharmacotherapy for SAS and SDS scores. Low-quality evidence showed no statistical difference between acupuncture and pharmacotherapy for the TER based on the IBS-SSS and RR and Bristol Stool Form Scale scores.

Few clinical studies were available for the assessment of moxibustion and TEAS therapies. There were no moxibustion studies for IBS-C; all included studies were on IBS-D. Moxibustion was found to be beneficial in improving Birmingham IBS symptom questionnaire scores and IBS-QOL scores. When TEAS was compared to the sham TEAS, results showed an improvement in the TEAS group for IBS-SSS, daily stool frequency, IBS-DSQ effective rate, and recurrence rate.

In terms of safety, acupuncture therapies are generally well-tolerated. In the included acupuncture studies, no AEs were reported in the acupuncture group. One electroacupuncture study reported similar numbers of AEs in the treatment group and pharmacotherapy group. AEs were not well reported in the moxibustion and TEAs studies, indicating future studies may include this outcome to contribute to the knowledge of the safety profiles of these therapies.

One RCT assessed the effect of *Baduanjin* 八段锦 plus tegaserod; however, no eligible outcomes were included in the study and, therefore, it lacked clinical evidence.

# References

1. Manheimer E, Cheng K, Wieland LS, *et al.* (2012) Acupuncture for treatment of irritable bowel syndrome. *Cochrane Database Syst Rev.* **5:** CD005111.

2. Chao GQ, Zhang S. (2014) Effectiveness of acupuncture to treat irritable bowel syndrome: A meta-analysis. *World J Gastroenterology.* **20(7):** 1871–1877.

3. Schneider A, Streitberger K, Joos S. (2007) Acupuncture treatment in gastrointestinal diseases: A systematic review. *World J Gastroenterol.* **13(25):** 3417–3424.

4. Park JW, Lee BH, Lee H. (2013) Moxibustion in the management of irritable bowel syndrome: Systematic review and meta-analysis (provisional abstract). *BMC Complement Altern Med.* **13(2):** 247.

5. Tang B, Zhang J, Yang Z, *et al.* (2016) Moxibustion for diarrhea-predominant irritable bowel syndrome: A systematic review and meta-analysis of randomized controlled trials. *Evid Based Complement Alternat Med.* **2016:** 5105108.

6. Francis CY, Morris J, Whorwell PJ. (1997) The Irritable Bowel Severity Scoring System: A simple method of monitoring irritable bowel syndrome and its progress. *Aliment Pharmacol Ther.* **11(2):** 395–402.

7. Patrick DL, Drossman DA, Frederick IO, *et al.* (1998) Quality of life in persons with irritable bowel syndrome: Development and validation of a new measure. *Dig Dis Sci.* **43(2):** 400–411.

8. 郑筱萸. (2002) *中药新药临床研究指导原则*. 中国医药科技出版社, 中国北京.

# References for Included Acupuncture Therapies Clinical Studies

| Study No. | Reference |
|---|---|
| A1 | Sun JH, Wu XL, Xia C, *et al.* (2011) Clinical evaluation of Soothing Gan and invigorating Pi acupuncture treatment on diarrhea-predominant irritable bowel syndrome. *Chin J Integr Med.* **17(10):** 780–785. |
| A2 | Zheng H, Li Y, Zhang W, *et al.* (2016) Electroacupuncture for patients with diarrhea-predominant irritable bowel syndrome or functional diarrhea: A randomized controlled trial. *Medicine.* **95(24):** e3884. |
| A3 | 占道伟. (2013) 疏肝健脾法针刺对腹泻型肠易激综合征患者血清 5-HT、NPY和 CGRP 水平变化的影响. 南京中医药大学硕士学位论文, 中国南京. |
| A4 | 孔素平, 王文琴, 肖宁, 谭奇纹. (2014) 针刺配合隔姜灸治疗腹泻型肠易激综合征临床研究. *上海针灸杂志.* **33(10):** 895–898. |
| A5 | 张超贤. (2016) 针刺联合参苓健脾胃颗粒治疗肠易激综合征腹泻型的近远期疗效观察. *中华中医药学刊.* **34(4):** 854–859. |
| A6 | 徐大可. (2016) 调神健脾针法治疗腹泻型肠易激综合征患者的疗效观察及对血浆胃动素的影响. 南京中医药大学硕士学位论文, 中国南京. |
| A7 | 李彬, 杨丽娟, 冯毅. (2007) 针刺治疗腹泻型肠易激综合征的疗效观察. *北京中医药大学学报：中医临床版.* **14(6):** 19–21. |
| A8 | 李浩. (2011) 疏肝健脾法针刺治疗腹泻型肠易激综合征临床疗效观察. 南京中医药大学硕士学位论文, 中国南京. |
| A9 | 李雪青, 穆世英, 陆听, 陆霞. (2015) 灵龟八法为主针刺治疗腹泻型肠易激综合征疗效观察. *上海针灸杂志.* **34(1):** 22–24. |
| A10 | 李静, 陆瑾, 孙建华, *et al.* (2017) 调神健脾"配穴针刺改善腹泻型肠易激综合征症状和睡眠质量:随机对照试验. *中国针灸.* **37(1):** 9–13. |
| A11 | 裴丽霞, 孙建华, 夏晨, *et al.* (2012) 针灸治疗腹泻型肠易激综合征肝郁脾虚证临床研究. *南京中医药大学学报.* **28(1):** 27–29. |
| A12 | 刘启泉. (2010) 隔山逍遥方配合针刺疗法对肠易激综合征患者生活质量影响的临床观察. *浙江中医药大学学报.* **34(4):** 510–511. |
| A13 | 陆永辉, 唐旭东. (2011)《灵枢》针刺深度法治疗腹泻型肠易激综合征. *中国针灸.* **31(11):** 975–977. |
| A14 | 李湘力, 蔡敬宙, 林泳, *et al.* (2015) 腹针治疗老年便秘型肠易激综合征的疗效及对生活质量的影响. *中国老年学杂志.* **35(19):** 5552–5554. |

*(Continued)*

**(*Continued*)**

| Study No. | Reference |
|---|---|
| A15 | 韩光研. (2011) 疏肝调神通腑法针刺治疗便秘型肠易激综合征的疗效观察. 南京中医药大学硕士学位论文, 中国南京. |
| A16 | 彭随风, 杨家耀, 石拓, *et al.* (2013) 电针治疗便秘型肠易激综合征患者的临床观察. *中国中西医结合消化杂志*. **21(8):** 426–428. |
| A17 | 潘晨, 杨杰, 张永宏. (2012) 足三里电刺激辅助治疗便秘型肠易激综合征的疗效观察. *临床荟萃*. **27(17):** 1545–1547. |
| A18 | 裴丽霞, 朱莉, 孙建华, *et al.* (2015) 调神健脾配穴针刺治疗便秘型肠易激综合征:随机对照研究. *中国针灸*. **35(11):** 1095–1098. |
| A19 | Zhu Y, Wu Z, Ma X, *et al.* (2014) Brain regions involved in moxibustion-induced analgesia in irritable bowel syndrome with diarrhea: A functional magnetic resonance imaging study. *BMC Complement Altern Med.* **14:** 500. |
| A20 | 张狄, 吴华军, 李鹏, *et al.* (2016) 温和灸大肠俞募穴治疗腹泻型肠易激综合征临床观察. *浙江中西医结合杂志*. **26(12):** 1096–1098. |
| A21 | Chen S, Du D, Ma Y, *et al.* (2011) Clinical study on herbal cone-partitioned moxibustion for irritable bowel syndrome due to Spleen *qi* deficiency. *J Acupunct Tuina Sci.* **9(5):** 265–268. |
| A22 | 虞露长. (2016) 基于新型易灸器灸法治疗腹泻型肠易激综合征的临床疗效观察. *按摩与康复医学*. **7(7):** 9–11. |
| A23 | 陈明显, 叶开升, 金曼, 蔡淦. (2013) 经皮穴位电刺激法治疗腹泻型肠易激综合征的随机对照临床研究. *中华中医药学刊*. **31(5):** 1053–1055. |
| A24 | 李志婷, 张国顺, 张秀静. (2016) 经皮穴位电刺激治疗腹泻型肠易激综合征的临床研究. *中国煤炭工业医学杂志*. **19(11):** 1636–1638. |
| O1 | 冯毅翀, 卞伯高, 潘华山, *et al.* (2010) 八段锦运动对老年便秘型肠易激综合征的疗效观察. *体育科研*. **31(2):** 89–90, 98. |

# 8

# Clinical Evidence for Combination Therapies

## OVERVIEW

Chinese medicine clinical practice often uses two or more types of therapies, such as Chinese herbal medicine plus acupuncture. This chapter includes clinical studies that use a combination of treatment therapies for irritable bowel syndrome (IBS). Seven randomised controlled studies are included, and the most common combination of therapies is Chinese herbal medicine with acupuncture. Results show some benefits in IBS symptom improvement, quality of life, and mental well-being.

## Introduction

Combination Chinese medicine (CM) therapies are defined as two or more CM interventions from different categories administered together, for example, Chinese herbal medicine (CHM) plus acupuncture. This approach is common in clinical practice. Previous systematic reviews of combination therapies were not identified in the database searches.

## Identification of Clinical Studies

A search of electronic databases identified 40,145 potentially relevant citations. After the removal of duplicates, the titles and abstracts of citations were read, and more than 14,000 irrelevant citations were excluded (Fig. 8.1). The full texts of the remaining articles were

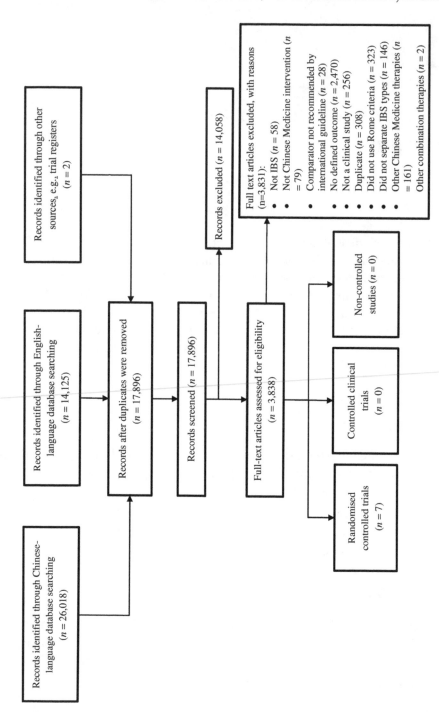

**Fig. 8.1.** Flow chart of study selection process: Combination therapies.

reviewed, and two studies that used interventions not commonly practised outside of China were excluded. In total, seven clinical studies that evaluated combinations of CM therapies were included. Studies are indicated by "C" and then a number, and the references for the studies can be found at the end of the chapter.

# Randomised Controlled Trials of Combination Therapies

All seven studies were identified as randomised controlled trials (RCTs) of combination therapies (C1–C7, Fig. 8.1). All included studies were RCTs investigating the effect of combination therapies on irritable bowel syndrome (IBS) with predominant diarrhoea (IBS-D). Therapies included:

- CHM plus acupuncture (3 studies; C1–C3);
- CHM plus moxibustion (1 study, C4);
- CHM plus ear-acupressure (1 study, C5);
- CHM plus transcutaneous electrical acupuncture stimulation (TEAS) (1 study, C6);
- CHM enema plus acupuncture plus moxibustion (1 study, C7).

One study (C6) using CHM plus TEAS was compared to the placebo CHM and sham TEAS, while the remaining studies used pharmacotherapy as comparators. There were four studies with three arms or four arms; in this chapter, the arm, including combination therapy, is included, while the other arms using CHM are presented in Chap. 5 (C2, C3, C5, C6) and acupuncture therapies in Chap. 7 (C2, C3).

## Clinical Evidence for Combination Therapies from Randomised Controlled Trials for Irritable Bowel Syndrome with Diarrhoea

Seven studies with a total of 1,618 participants diagnosed according to the Rome III diagnostic criteria were included; all studies were done in China. In the treatment group, the mean age was 41.9 years and the mean duration of disease was 41.32 months. In the control group, the mean age was 41.3 years and the mean duration of disease was 40.76 months. The treatment duration ranged from 4 to 8 weeks. Four studies (C2, C4, C5, C7) described syndrome differentiation for participants; these include Liver *qi* stagnation with Spleen deficiency, Spleen *qi* deficiency, Spleen *qi* deficiency with damp stagnation, Liver stagnation overacting on Spleen, and Spleen and Stomach deficiency.

Two studies had follow-up periods of one year (C7) and 60 weeks (C3), respectively.

In the included studies, the most common combination of therapies was CHM with acupuncture. Two studies (C4, C5) used modified *Shen ling bai zhu san* 参苓白术散. The most commonly used herbs were *bai zhu* 白术 (6 studies), *chen pi* 陈皮 (4 studies), *fu ling* 茯苓 (4 studies), *bai shao* 白芍 (4 studies), and *bai bian dou* 白扁豆 (4 studies) (Table 8.1). In studies that evaluated acupuncture therapies, the most frequently reported points were LR3 *Taichong* 太冲 (5 studies), ST25 *Tianshu* 天枢 (4 studies), and ST36 *Zusanli* 足三里 (4 studies) (Table 8.1).

## Risk of Bias

The included studies all mentioned "randomisation"; six studies (C2–C7) used either computer software or a random number table for sequence generation and were assessed as "low" risk of bias. One study (C6) used sealed opaque envelopes for allocation concealment and was judged as a "low" risk of bias; the other studies did not describe the method of allocation concealment and were assessed as "unclear" risks. One study (C6) used placebo medication and a placebo TEAS machine and so was judged as a "low" risk for the blinding of participants, personnel and assessors. The remaining studies were judged as "high" risk for blinding due to the nature of the interventions and comparators. Four studies (C1, C2, C4, C5) had no dropouts, and one study (C3) reported the reasons for dropouts, and the dropout numbers were balanced between the groups. Therefore,

**Table 8.1. Frequently Reported Herbs and Acupuncture Points in Randomised Controlled Trials**

| Most Common Herb | | | Most Common Acupuncture Point | |
|---|---|---|---|---|
| Herb Name | Scientific Name | Frequency of Use | Point Name | Frequency of Use |
| Bai zhu 白术 | *Atractylodes macrocephala* Koidz. | 6 | LR3 *Taichong* 太冲 | 5 |
| Chen pi 陈皮 | *Citrus reticulata* Blanco | 4 | ST25 *Tianshu* 天枢 | 4 |
| Fu ling 茯苓 | *Poria cocos* (Schw.) Wolf | 4 | ST36 *Zusanli* 足三里 | 4 |
| Bai shao 白芍 | *Paeonia lactiflora* Pall. | 4 | BL20 *Pishu* 脾俞 | 2 |
| Bai bian dou 白扁豆 | *Dolichos lablab* L. | 4 | SP9 *Yinlingquan* 阴陵泉 | 2 |
|  |  |  | ST37 *Shangjuxu* 上巨虚 | 2 |
|  |  |  | SP6 *Sanyinjiao* 三阴交 | 2 |

these five studies were assessed as "low" risk of bias for incomplete outcome data. Two studies (C6, C7) had dropouts but did not report on the reasons or which arm the dropouts were in and were thus judged as "high" risk for this domain. Two studies did not report on all planned outcomes and were assessed as "high" risk of bias for selective reporting. No protocols were identified for the included studies, so it was not possible to judge whether all the planned outcomes were reported, so all studies were assessed as "unclear" risk of bias for selective reporting (Table 8.2).

## Chinese Herbal Medicine + Acupuncture vs. Pharmacotherapy

Three RCTs (C1, C2, C3) compared the effect of CHM plus acupuncture to pharmacotherapy alone.

**Table 8.2.  Risk of Bias of Randomised Controlled Trials: Combination Therapies**

| Risk of Bias Domain | Low Risk n (%) | Unclear Risk n (%) | High Risk n (%) |
|---|---|---|---|
| Sequence generation | 6 (85.7) | 1 (14.3) | 0 (0) |
| Allocation concealment | 1 (14.3) | 6 (85.7) | 0 (0) |
| Blinding of participants | 1 (14.3) | 0 (0) | 6 (85.7) |
| Blinding of personnel | 1 (14.3) | 0 (0) | 6 (85.7) |
| Blinding of outcome assessors | 1 (14.3) | 0 (0) | 6 (85.7) |
| Incomplete outcome data | 5 (71.4) | 2 (28.6) | 0 (0) |
| Selective outcome reporting | 1 (14.3) | 6 (85.7) | 0 (0) |

One study (C1; 216 participants) assessed the effect of a combination of CHM and electroacupuncture, compared to pinaverium bromide for IBS-D; the study reported on the Zung Self-rating Anxiety Scale (SAS) scores. After four weeks of treatment, results showed that CHM, in combination with electroacupuncture, significantly reduced SAS scores compared to pinaverium bromide (MD: −12.49 [13.57, −11.41]).

One study (C3; 320 participants) compared the effect of combination therapies (CHM and acupuncture) to antidepressants for IBS-D for the Short-Form Health Survey (SF-36) and Bristol Stool Form Scale. After four weeks of treatment, results showed that the combination of CHM and acupuncture therapies was superior in improving stool form according to the Bristol Stool Form Scale (lower was better) (MD: −1.08 [−1.16, −1.00]). In terms of the SF-36, the overall score was not reported; results for each section of the SF-36 showed that people in the combination CM therapies group had higher scores than those in the antidepressant group, indicating better health quality.

In 162 participants, the authors assessed the effect of CHM plus acupuncture on probiotics after four weeks of treatment; the study (C2) reported on the IBS-Quality of Life scale. The study included information from two different scales, so the results are not presented here.

## Chinese Herbal Medicine + Transcutaneous Electrical Acupuncture Stimulations vs. Placebo CHM + Sham Transcutaneous Electrical Acupuncture Stimulations

One RCT (C6; 162 participants) compared four weeks of a combination of CHM and TEAS to a placebo CHM and sham TEAS for IBS-D. The results showed that the combination therapy was superior to the placebo in the improvement of the IBS-SSS score (RR: 1.90 [1.47, 2.46]).

## Chinese Herbal Medicine + Moxibustion vs. Pharmacotherapy

One RCT (C4) assessed *Shen ling bai zhu san* 参苓白术散 plus moxibustion compared with the anti-diarrhoea agent loperamide in stool form and frequency change score in 60 IBS-D participants.[1] After four weeks of treatment, the results showed that the combination therapy was superior in reducing the stool form and frequency scores (MD: −0.60 [−0.74, −0.46]).

## Chinese Herbal Medicine + Ear-acupressure vs. Pharmacotherapy

One RCT (C5; 40 participants) assessed *Shen ling bai zhu san* 参苓白术散 plus ear-acupressure compared with trimebutine plus probiotics in the stool frequency score. Thirty days of treatment showed that the combination therapy was superior in reducing the stool form and frequency scores based on the *Consensus Opinion of Traditional Chinese Medicine Diagnosis and Treatment Strategy for Irritable Bowel Syndrome*[2] (MD: −2 [−2.87, −1.13]).

## Chinese Herbal Medicine Enema + Acupuncture + Moxibustion vs. Pharmacotherapy

One RCT (C7; 100 participants) compared CHM enema plus acupuncture plus moxibustion to pinaverium bromide. The study reported on the IBS-SSS effective rate; results showed that although there was a trend for improvement in the IBS-SSS effective rate, there was no significant difference between the groups (RR: 1.10 [0.94, 1.27]).

# Controlled Clinical Trials of Combination Therapies

No non-randomised controlled clinical trials of combination therapies for IBS were identified.

# Non-Controlled Studies of Combination Therapies

No non-controlled studies of combination therapies for IBS were identified.

### Safety of Combination Therapies

Four studies (C2, C3, C4, C5) reported on adverse events (AEs) in 620 participants. Two studies (C2, C5) reported that there were no AEs. Two studies (C3, C4) with 380 participants reported AEs from both the combination therapies group and the pharmacotherapy group. AEs in the combination therapies group included a skin burn (1 case, C4). AEs in the pharmacotherapy group included two cases (C3, C4) of constipation, one case of abdominal cramp, and two cases of abdominal pain.

# Summary of Combination Therapies Evidence

This chapter has evaluated the combination of two or more CM therapies used to manage IBS symptoms. All studies included were RCTs investigating the effect of combination therapies on IBS-D. Among included studies, CHM plus acupuncture was the most commonly used combination. Aside from one study that evaluated CHM as an enema, CHM was administered orally and was the most commonly used therapy (6 of 7 studies, 85.7%).

*Shen ling bai zhu san* 参苓白术散 was used in 2 out of 7 included studies. The most frequently used herbs were *bai zhu* 白术, *chen pi* 陈皮, *fu ling* 茯苓, *bai shao* 白芍, and *bai bian dou* 白扁豆. The key aim of the CHM treatment was to tonify the Spleen and Stomach. In studies that evaluated acupuncture therapies, the most frequently reported points were ST25 *Tianshu* 天枢, LR3 *Taichong* 太冲, and ST36 *Zusanli* 足三里. Studies used different combinations of herbs and acupuncture points, and no clear conclusion about the best combination can be drawn from the current research.

Diversity was seen in the CM combination therapies, comparators and outcomes, which were used for IBS, and so it was not possible to perform meta-analyses. Results from single studies showed that the combination of CHM and acupuncture improved the IBS-QOL score and SF-36 score, as well as the SAS score and the Bristol Stool Form Scale. In terms of IBS severity and stool form and frequency, results from single studies also showed the benefits of CM combination therapies.

Overall, CM combination therapies appear to be safe for the management of IBS symptoms. Results from current research do not provide strong enough evidence to make specific recommendations for clinical practice. Further research is needed to evaluate CM combination therapies for IBS. Based on the evidence on individual CM therapies (see Chaps. 5 and 7) and combination therapies, practitioners should consider their use on an individual basis.

# References

1.  郑筱萸. (2002) *中药新药临床研究指导原则*. 中国医药科技出版社, 中国北京.
2.  中华中医药学会脾胃病分会. (2010) 肠易激综合征中医诊疗共识意见. *中华中医药杂志*. **25(7):** 1062–1065.

# References for Included Combination Therapies: Clinical Studies

| Study No. | Reference |
|---|---|
| C1 | 韩宝娟, 冯丽英. (2013) 药针联合治疗对焦虑状态的腹泻型肠易激综合征患者细胞因子的影响. *临床合理用药杂志*. **6(5B):** 121–122. |
| C2 | 刘启泉. (2010) 隔山逍遥方配合针刺疗法对肠易激综合征患者生活质量影响的临床观察. *浙江中医药大学学报*. **34(4):** 510–513. |
| C3 | 张超贤, 郭李柯, 秦咏梅. (2016) 针刺联合参苓健脾胃颗粒治疗肠易激综合征腹泻型的近远期疗效观察. *中华中医药学刊*. **34(4):** 854–859. |
| C4 | 谢文堂, 李茂清, 周三林, *et al.* (2015) 参苓白术散与艾灸对肠易激综合征患者血清脑肠肽的影响. *中国中医药信息杂志*. **22(3):** 36–38. |
| C5 | 李玲. (2015) 参苓白术散配合耳穴按压治疗腹泻型肠易激综合征（脾虚湿阻证）的临床研究. 湖南中医药大学. |
| C6 | 李熠萌, 林江, 蔡淦, 陈明显. (2014) 肠吉泰联合经皮穴位电刺激法治疗腹泻型肠易激综合征的随机, 双盲, 安慰剂对照研究. *中国中西医结合消化杂志*. **22(1):** 1–4. |
| C7 | 匡小霞, 吴小慧. (2015) 针药结合治疗腹泻型肠易激综合征 50 例. *湖南中医杂志*. **31(12):** 88–90. |

# 9

# Summary and Conclusions

## OVERVIEW

This chapter summarises the main findings of the previous chapters, including those from classical literature, clinical trial evidence, and experimental evidence. Chinese medicine therapies, including Chinese herbal medicine and acupuncture, are discussed regarding the clinical management of irritable bowel syndrome. Limitations of the available evidence are reported and future directions identified for clinical and experimental research.

## Introduction

Irritable bowel syndrome (IBS) is a type of functional bowel disorder causing symptoms of abdominal pain and altered bowel habits. Depending on the sufferer's predominant clinical bowel habits, IBS is classified into subtypes IBS-C (constipation predominant), IBS-D (diarrhoea predominant), IBS-M (a mix of constipation and diarrhoea), and IBS-U (where the person's condition does not fit into any of the previous three subtypes).[1-3]

Currently, there is no cure for IBS. Behavioural therapy (psychological and dietary mainly) focus on the management of IBS. Drugs are predominantly used to ameliorate specific symptoms. Integrated care has the best results in IBS management in clinical practice. Diet and lifestyle modifications are also recommended for IBS sufferers, as restricting some types of foods can assist in managing IBS symptoms.[4-6] Regular exercise has also been shown to reduce IBS symptoms.[7]

This monograph includes a "whole-evidence" analysis of Chinese medicine (CM) for the management of IBS subtypes. A review of clinical guidelines and textbooks has identified the main syndromes for IBS and recommended CM treatments, including oral Chinese herbal medicine (CHM) and acupuncture (Chap. 2). A review of classical literature identified the traditional use of CHM (Chap. 3). The full methodologies of identifying, extracting, evaluating and analysing modern literature clinical evidence are presented in Chap. 4. Findings from meta-analyses of clinical studies revealed some benefits of CHM, acupuncture and combination therapies for IBS symptom relief and quality of life (Chaps. 5, 7 and 8). Current available evidence from experimental studies has also been reviewed to explain the possible action mechanisms of the commonly used herbs in IBS (Chap. 6).

## Chinese Medicine Syndrome Differentiation

Different syndromes are categorised for IBS-D and IBS-C; current clinical guidelines and textbooks categorise CM syndromes according to the presenting signs and symptoms.[8-10] For each syndrome, formulae with modifications according to different symptoms are suggested as a guide for clinical practice (Chap. 2).

The CM syndromes described in Chap. 2 for IBS-D include Liver stagnation and Spleen deficiency, Spleen and Stomach deficiency or Spleen deficiency with dampness, Spleen and Kidney *yang* deficiency, dampness-heat in the Spleen and Stomach, and complex cold-heat syndrome. Modern literature suggested the CM syndromes of Spleen–Stomach deficiency, Liver *qi* stagnation, Spleen *yang* deficiency, and Spleen deficiency and dampness are also cited in classical literature (Chap. 3). Classical literature citations described the pathogenesis of IBS-D with symptoms such as extreme abdominal pain with diarrhoea. Irregularity in diet can cause weakness in the Spleen and Stomach, causing difficulties in the Stomach and Spleen functions of receiving, transforming and transporting food, resulting in food accumulation, in turn causing abdominal pain with diarrhoea, with a reduction in pain after diarrhoea. Classical texts also described how anger could lead to Liver stagnation, which damages the Spleen *qi*, resulting in vomiting, bloating, diarrhoea, abdominal pain, and difficulty with diet. Another passage described how a deficiency in the Spleen *yang* could cause symptoms such as bloating and fullness in the chest and abdomen, an inability to digest food, abdominal pain and borborygmus, constant diarrhoea, and anxiety.

In IBS-D clinical studies of CHM, 82 studies used CM syndrome differentiation. A few studies used syndrome differentiation as inclusion criteria or criteria for selecting the formula to be used. The most common syndromes were consistent with those mentioned in the clinical practice guidelines (Chap. 2). In IBS-D studies that described CM syndromes, the common syndromes included Liver *qi* stagnation and Spleen deficiency, Spleen and/or Kidney *yang* deficiency, and Spleen deficiency with damp retention.

In randomised controlled trials (RCTs) using acupuncture and related therapies for IBS-D, the most mentioned syndrome was Liver *qi* stagnation with Spleen deficiency. In the non-controlled acupuncture study for IBS-D, Liver *qi* stagnation and Spleen deficiency were reported.

In the seven combination CM therapy RCTs for IBS-D, four studies described syndrome differentiation for participants; these include Liver *qi* stagnation with Spleen deficiency, Spleen *qi* deficiency, Spleen *qi* deficiency with damp stagnation, Liver stagnation overacting on Spleen, and Spleen and Stomach deficiency.

As for IBS-C, the CM syndromes described in Chap. 2 include Liver *qi* stagnation, heat accumulating in the Stomach and the Large Intestine, Spleen and Kidney *yang* deficiency, and Lung and Spleen deficiency. In classical text citations describing abdominal pain with constipation, the most frequently mentioned aetiology was the stagnation of dampness, food or a pathogen, and the most frequently mentioned pathogenesis was stagnation in *qi* movement.

Clinical studies on CHM for IBS-C (4 out of 14 RCTs) reported on different syndromes, including *qi* stagnation and intestinal dryness, *qi* stagnation (or with *yin* deficiency with internal heat), Liver *qi* stagnation and Spleen deficiency, and Spleen deficiency and *qi* stagnation.

Acupuncture clinical studies for IBS-C did not report on CM syndrome differentiation. One study assessing other CM therapies (*Baduanjin* 八段锦) for IBS-C also did not mention syndrome differentiation.

## Chinese Herbal Medicine

This section summarises the evidence from Chaps. 2, 3 and 5. CHM treatment is an integral part of CM IBS treatment. A summary of key clinical textbooks' and clinical guidelines' treatment recommendations for IBS is presented in Chap. 2, with traditional formulae and manufactured products based on CM syndrome differentiation. The herbal treatments can be used via oral administration, topical application or as an enema.

In the classical literature, more than 80% of the included citations described CHM treatment; this suggests CHM treatments were the main method for treating IBS-like disease in ancient times. More IBS-D-like citations (n = 512) than IBS-C-like citations (n = 80) were identified. Clinical studies of CHM for the IBS-D and IBS-C subtypes were identified and evaluated, but no IBS-M or IBS-U clinical studies were found. Randomised controlled trials (RCTs) were the main study type, in which CHM was compared to conventional medicines, or a combination of CHM and conventional medicines was compared to conventional medicines alone. CHM interventions were orally administrated or used as an enema.

Overall, in people with IBS, CHM showed promising effects in improving the IBS Severity Scoring System (IBS-SSS) score, stool frequency, stool form, quality of life, and mental well-being. CHM showed a good safety profile for use in people with IBS.

Experts in IBS and CM were consulted to identify important clinical questions. Grading of Recommendations Assessment, Development and Evaluation (GRADE) assessments were used to assess the quality of the evidence (Chap. 5, Tables 5.19, 5.20, 5.21 and 5.27).

The following section summarises the evidence from Chaps. 2, 3 and 5 for IBS-D and IBS-C separately.

## Irritable Bowel Syndrome with Predominant Diarrhoea

The earliest IBS-D treatment-related citation is found in the *Tai Ping Sheng Hui Fang* 太平圣惠方 (c. 992, by Wang Huai Yin, Song and Jin dynasties). All but one citation described an oral form of CHM for IBS-D, while one formula cited a topical herb use describing the use of *suan* 蒜 (garlic). The most frequently cited formulae were *Ba wei wan* 八味丸 and *Si shen wan* 四神丸.

In total, 112 clinical studies evaluated CHM for IBS-D. In the included IBS-D clinical studies, various outcome measures had sufficient data suitable for pooling. These included overall condition severity-related outcomes such as adequate relief, IBS-SSS score, stool form and frequency, abdominal pain, discomfort and bloating, IBS recurrence rate, and adverse events (AEs). Further, health-related quality-of-life questionnaires were also assessed, including those that measure physical and mental health states, including the IBS-Quality Of Life scales, 36-Item Short-Form Survey (SF-36), Zung Self-rating Anxiety Scale (SAS), Zung Self-rating Depression Scale (SDS), and Hospital Anxiety and Depression Scale (HADS). IBS-specific quality-of-life questionnaires such as the IBS-36 and the Gastrointestinal Quality of Life Index, which are specific to people with gastrointestinal diseases, and the Gastrointestinal Symptom Rating Scale, were not reported. Data was provided for the end of the treatment period, ranging from two weeks to two months in the included IBS-D studies. Of the conventional drugs, pinaverium bromide was the most frequently used in IBS-D clinical trials.

For each available pre-specified outcome, results from RCTs and controlled clinical trials (CCTs) using CHM were analysed and presented in Chap. 5.

Compared to a placebo, oral CHM improved the total effective rate (TER) of the IBS-SSS, adequate relief (AR), IBS-SSS score, Bristol Stool Form Scale score, and stool frequency. CHM also improved SF-36 subscale scores and scores for the Hamilton Anxiety Rating

Scale and Hamilton Depression Rating Scale. Heterogeneity was low for the TER of the IBS-SSS. Heterogeneity was high for studies with adequate relief and IBS-SSS scores, and subgroup analysis was not possible; the source of heterogeneity may be the different CHM interventions in terms of treatment duration, ingredients, dosage, and medication compliance. For other outcomes, only one study was included. The sample size was small in the meta-analysis, and the meta-analysis results were graded with a "very low to moderate" certainty.

Meta-analyses results showed the benefits with oral CHM compared to pharmacotherapy in improving the TER of the IBS-SSS, total IBS-SSS score, SF-36 domains, and subscales of IBS quality of life in Dysphoria and Interference with Activity at the end of the treatment. Compared to pharmacotherapy, oral CHM showed the benefit of improving abdominal pain, including bloating or discomfort and improving stool frequency and form. Despite the encouraging results, due to the limited number of studies with small sample sizes and the low quality of the included studies, the results are of "very low to low" certainty.

When oral CHM and conventional therapies such as probiotics and pharmacotherapy were used together, meta-analyses results showed the added benefits of CHM for the TER of the IBS-SSS, SF-36 domains (Vitality and Mental Health), SAS, SDS, Hamilton Anxiety Rating Scale, and improved stool frequency and form. The number of studies was limited for the meta-analyses.

In terms of the safety of CHM, the total AEs in the CHM groups, with either CHM alone or integrative CHM, were fewer than in the control groups.

## Chinese Herbal Medicine Formulae in Key Clinical Guidelines and Textbooks, Classical Literature and Clinical Studies

Overall, the CHMs used for IBS-D were different between classical literature, contemporary clinical practice guidelines, and clinical trials, with some consistencies (Table 9.1).

**Table 9.1.  Summary of Chinese Herbal Medicine Traditional Formulae for Irritable Bowel Syndrome with Predominant Diarrhoea**

| Formula Name | Clinical Guidelines (Chap. 2) | Classical Literature (No. Citations) (Chap. 3) | Clinical Studies (No. Studies) (Chap. 5) | | | Combination Therapies (Chap. 8) |
|---|---|---|---|---|---|---|
| | | | RCTs (No. Studies) | CCTs (No. Studies) | NCSs (No. Studies) | |
| *Tong xie yao fang* 痛泻要方 | Yes | 18 | 17 | 0 | 0 | 1 |
| *Shen ling bai zhu san* 参苓白术散 | Yes | 1 | 9 | 0 | 0 | 2 |
| *Fu zi li zhong tang* 附子理中汤 | Yes | 10 | 2 | 0 | 0 | 0 |
| *Si shen wan* 四神丸 | Yes | 10 | 2 | 0 | 0 | 0 |
| *Ge gen huang qin huang lian tang* 葛根黄芩黄连汤 | Yes | 0 | 0 | 0 | 0 | 0 |
| *Wu mei wan* 乌梅丸 | Yes | 0 | 0 | 0 | 0 | 0 |
| *Si ni san* (including modified) 四逆散（加减） | No | 1 | 6 | 0 | 0 | 0 |
| *Ban xia xie xin tang* 半夏泻心汤 | No | 3 | 2 | 0 | 0 | 0 |
| *Wen shen jian pi fang* 温肾健脾方 | No | 0 | 2 | 0 | 0 | 0 |
| *Jia wei huang qi jian zhong tang* (including modified) 加味黄芪建中汤（加减） | No | 2 | 2 | 0 | 0 | 0 |
| *Li zhong tang /Li zhong wan* (including modified) 理中汤/理中丸（加减） | No | 13 | 2 | 0 | 0 | 0 |

Abbreviations: CCT, controlled clinical trial; NCS, non-controlled studies; RCT, randomised controlled trial.

Comparing classical text citations with modern clinical guidelines for CHM treatment of IBS shows that the frequently cited classical formulae for IBS-D are still recommended. Used classically and identified in clinical studies, *Tong xie yao fang* 痛泻要方 is recommended in modern guidelines for the treatment of IBS-D with Liver *qi* stagnation and Spleen deficiency syndrome.[9] *Si shen wan* 四神丸 and *Fu zi li zhong tang* 附子理中汤 are recommended for the Spleen and Kidney *yang* deficiency syndrome.[9] Two traditional formulae, *Ge gen huang qin huang lian tang* 葛根黄芩黄连汤 and *Wu mei wan* 乌梅丸, are recommended in guidelines but not found in classical literature or clinical studies (Table 9.1). *Li zhong tang* or *Li zhong wan* 理中汤/理中丸 was cited in classical literature texts and tested in clinical studies but is not recommended by the guidelines.

In the IBS-D clinical studies, the most commonly used formula was *Tong xie yao fang* 痛泻要方, which appeared in 17 RCTs. It was recommended in clinical guidelines for IBS-D with the CM syndrome of Liver stagnation and Spleen deficiency. It was also the most cited in classical literature. In classical literature, *Tong xie yao fang* 痛泻要方 was recommended for the treatment of "abdominal pain" and "diarrhoea". Compared to conventional medicines, *Tong xie yao fang* 痛泻要方 improved the TER based on the IBS-SSS.

Table 9.2 summarises the manufactured CHM products that have been found in contemporary and classical literature and tested in clinical studies. For IBS-D, the manufactured product *Tong xie ning ke li* 痛泻宁颗粒 is recommended in clinical textbooks and guidelines (see Chap. 2). However, though it has been tested in clinical studies, it is not found in classical literature. Three other manufactured products — *Chang ji tai* 肠吉泰, *Chang an I hao fang* 肠安I号方, *Chang ji ling* (including modified) 肠激灵 (加减) — were also tested in clinical studies, but there are likewise no recommendations in guidelines or classical texts. *Chang ji tai* 肠吉泰 was a popular product used in five included RCTs; its formula is based on *Tong xie yao fang* 痛泻要方. Although found to be more effective than a placebo and conventional treatments, the analysis in this review found limited evidence to support its use in clinical practice due to the small number of studies available.

Three formulae that were recommended in textbooks are neither found in classical literature nor tested in clinical studies: *Shen ling bai zhu ke li* 参苓白术颗粒, *Bu pi yi chang wan* 补脾益肠丸, *Gu ben yi chang pian* 固本益肠片, and *Feng liao chang wei kang ke li* 枫蓼

**Table 9.2. Summary of Chinese Herbal Medicine Manufactured Products for Irritable Bowel Syndrome with Predominant Diarrhoea**

| Formula Name | Clinical Guidelines (Chap. 2) | Classical Literature (No. Citations) (Chap. 3) | Clinical Studies (No. Studies) (Chap. 5) | | | Combination Therapies (Chap. 8) |
|---|---|---|---|---|---|---|
| | | | RCTs (No. Studies) | CCTs (No. Studies) | NCSs (No. Studies) | |
| *Tong xie ning ke li* 痛泻宁颗粒 | Yes | 0 | 2 | 0 | 0 | 0 |
| *Shen ling bai zhu ke li* 参苓白术颗粒 | Yes | 0 | 0 | 0 | 0 | 0 |
| *Bu pi yi chang wan* 补脾益肠丸 | Yes | 0 | 0 | 0 | 0 | 0 |
| *Gu ben yi chang pian* 固本益肠片 | Yes | 0 | 0 | 0 | 0 | 0 |
| *Feng liao chang wei kang ke li* 枫蓼肠胃康颗粒 | Yes | 0 | 0 | 0 | 0 | 0 |
| *Chang ji tai* 肠吉泰 | No | 0 | 5 | 0 | 0 | 1 |
| *Chang an I hao fang* 肠安I号方 | No | 0 | 2 | 0 | 0 | 0 |
| *Chang ji ling* (including modified) 肠激灵 （加减） | No | 0 | 2 | 0 | 0 | 0 |

Abbreviations: CCT, controlled clinical trial; NCS, non-controlled studies; RCT, randomised controlled trial.

肠胃康颗粒. While not included in identified clinical studies, there may be evidence to support the use of these products that were not included in this review.

## Irritable Bowel Syndrome with Predominant Constipation

The earliest IBS-C treatment-related citation is found in the *Jin Gui Yao Lue Fang Lun* 金匮要略方论 (c. 206, by Zhang Zhong Jin, Dong Han dynasty). One case report described topical CHM for IBS-C using *sheng jiang* 生姜, *cong tou* 葱头, *lai fu zi* 莱菔子, *xiang fu* 香附 and salt.

The remainder of the citations reported on the oral use of CHM. The most frequently cited formulae were *Hou pu san wu tang* 厚朴三五汤 and *Da cheng qi tang* 大乘气汤. Both formulae were used for excess heat syndrome.

A total of 17 clinical studies evaluating CHM for IBS-C have been analysed in this monograph. When oral CHM was compared to conventional medicine, meta-analyses showed the benefits of oral CHM in improving all SF-36 domains and the three domains of Social Functioning, Role Functioning and Mental Health when CHM was used in combination with conventional medicine. When CHM was added to conventional therapy, added benefits were seen in the reduction of the SDS and improved stool frequency. One RCT using an enema for IBS-C showed a favourable effect using CHM for the Bristol scale.

In terms of the safety of CHM, the total AEs in the CHM groups, either CHM alone or integrative CHM, were fewer than in the comparison groups.

## Chinese Herbal Medicine Formulae in Key Clinical Guidelines and Textbooks, Classical Literature and Clinical Studies

Overall, the CHMs used for IBS-C were different between classical literature, contemporary clinical practice guidelines, and clinical trials, with some consistencies (Table 9.2).

Recommendations for IBS-C formulae in contemporary texts and guidelines were not cited in classical texts nor evaluated in the included clinical studies. These formulae included *Liu mo tang* 六磨汤, *Ma zi ren wan* 麻子仁丸, *Ji chuan jian* 济川煎, and *Huang qi tang* 黄芪汤. Their actions include regulating *qi*, moving *qi* to remove stagnation, and relaxing the bowels to relieve constipation.[11]

The formulae used in the included clinical studies varied across all studies, and it was difficult to identify a core formula. One formula, *Tong bian tang* 通便汤, was identified for use in clinical studies; however, it was not recommended in clinical guidelines or cited in classical texts.

Many other formulae have been evaluated in clinical trials, including those listed in Table 9.3, that are not recommended in the clinical guidelines given in Chap. 2.

For IBS-C, one formula, *Si mo tang kou fu ye* 四磨汤口服液, recommended in clinical textbooks and guidelines in Chap. 2, was tested

**Table 9.3.  Summary of Chinese Herbal Medicine Traditional Formulae for Irritable Bowel Syndrome with Predominant Constipation**

| Formula Name | Clinical Guidelines (Chap. 2) | Classical Literature (No. Citations) (Chap. 3) | Clinical Studies (No. Studies) (Chap. 5) | | | Combination Therapies (Chap. 8) |
|---|---|---|---|---|---|---|
| | | | RCTs (No. Studies) | CCTs (No. Studies) | NCSs (No. Studies) | |
| *Liu mo tang* 六磨汤 | Yes | 0 | 0 | 0 | 0 | 0 |
| *Ma zi ren wan* 麻子仁丸 | Yes | 0 | 0 | 0 | 0 | 0 |
| *Ji chuan jian* 济川煎 | Yes | 0 | 0 | 0 | 0 | 0 |
| *Huang qi tang* 黄芪汤 | Yes | 0 | 0 | 0 | 0 | 0 |
| *Tong bian tang* 通便汤 | No | 0 | 0 | 0 | 1 | 0 |

Abbreviations: CCT, controlled clinical trial; NCS, non-controlled studies; RCT, randomised controlled trial.

**Table 9.4. Summary of Chinese Herbal Medicine Manufactured Products for Irritable Bowel Syndrome with Predominant Constipation**

| Formula Name | Clinical Guidelines (Chap. 2) | Classical Literature (No. Citations) (Chap. 3) | Clinical Studies (No. Studies) (Chap. 5) | | | Included in Combination Therapies (Chap. 8) |
| --- | --- | --- | --- | --- | --- | --- |
| | | | RCTs (No. Studies) | CCTs (No. Studies) | NCSs (No. Studies) | |
| *Qi rong run chang kou fu ye* 芪蓉润肠口服液 | Yes | 0 | 0 | 0 | 0 | 0 |
| *Si mo tang kou fu ye* 四磨汤口服液 | Yes | 0 | 0 | 1 | 0 | 0 |
| *Ma ren wan* 麻仁丸 | Yes | 0 | 0 | 0 | 0 | 0 |
| *Ma ren run chang wan* 麻仁润肠丸 | Yes | 0 | 0 | 0 | 0 | 0 |
| *Bian mi tong* 便秘通 | Yes | 0 | 0 | 0 | 0 | 0 |
| *Wu ling* capsule 乌灵胶囊 | No | 0 | 1 | 0 | 0 | 0 |

Abbreviations: CCT, controlled clinical trial; NCS, non-controlled studies; RCT, randomised controlled trial.

in clinical studies but was not found in classical literature. Another formula, *Wu ling* capsule 乌灵胶囊, has been tested in clinical studies but is not recommended in the guidelines given in Chap. 2 or found in classical texts. Limited evidence has been found in this review to support the *Wu ling* capsule for clinical use. A summary of CHM-manufactured products for IBS-C is presented in Table 9.4.

## Acupuncture and Related Therapies

This section summarises the evidence from Chaps. 2, 3 and 7. The clinical guidelines and CM textbooks (Chap. 2) recommend manual acupuncture based on IBS subtype and CM syndrome differentiation. Acupuncture and moxibustion were the only therapies recommended in textbooks and guidelines and described in classical texts. Further, acupuncture therapies for IBS have been tested in clinical studies alone or combined with other CM therapies. Moxibustion was tested alone and in combination with other CM therapies. The evidence for acupuncture for IBS is limited and is currently insufficient to make recommendations for clinical practice.

Transcutaneous electrical acupoint stimulation was tested in three clinical studies; however, textbooks or guidelines do not recommend it. It is also not found in classical texts because it is a therapy that uses modern technology.

Ear acupuncture is recommended for the relief of constipation in the guidelines. However, only one-ear acupressure combined with other CM therapies for IBS-D was identified in this review, reflecting that acupuncture and moxibustion are the more commonly used and tested therapies.

## Acupuncture Therapies in Key Clinical Guidelines and Textbooks, Classical Literature and Clinical Studies

Further to identifying different therapies of use from different sources, acupuncture points were also analysed for history and their frequency of use. The points recommended in clinical guidelines and textbooks for each intervention are described in Table 9.5 for IBS-D and Table 9.6 for IBS-C.

For IBS-D, the most frequently used acupuncture point in clinical studies are ST25 *Tianshu* 天枢 (19 studies), ST36 *Zusanli* 足三里 (16 studies), and LR3 *Taichong* 太冲 (16 studies). They are acupuncture points from the Stomach and Liver meridians; these points benefit the Stomach, Spleen and Liver, which are the main organs affected by IBS-D. ST25 *Tianshu* 天枢 and ST36 *Zusanli* 足三里 are also commonly cited in classical texts as identified to be related to IBS-D. ST25 *Tianshu* 天枢 regulates the intestines, regulates the Spleen and Stomach, and resolves dampness and damp-heat.[12] The earliest classical citation related to acupuncture for IBS-D described

**Table 9.5.** **Summary of Acupuncture and Related Therapies for Irritable Bowel Syndrome with Predominant Diarrhoea**

| Intervention | Clinical Guidelines and Textbooks (Chap. 2) | Classical Literature (Chap. 3) (No. Citations) | Clinical Studies (Chap. 7) | | | Combination Therapies (Chap. 8) (No. Studies) |
|---|---|---|---|---|---|---|
| | | | RCTs (No. Studies) | CCTs (No. Studies) | NCSs* (No. Studies) | |
| Acupuncture | Yes | 39 | 12 | 0 | 1 | 4 |
| Massage | Yes | 0 | 0 | 0 | 0 | 0 |
| Electromagnetic heat treatment | Yes | NA | 0 | 0 | 0 | 0 |
| Transcutaneous electrical acupoint stimulation | No | NA | 1 | 1 | 0 | 1 |
| Ear-acupuncture/ acupressure | Yes | 0 | 0 | 0 | 0 | 1 |
| Moxibustion | Yes | 62 | 4 | 0 | 0 | 1 |
| **Acupuncture Point** | | | | | | |
| ST36 *Zusanli* 足三里 | Yes | 2 | 10 | 1 | 1 | 4 |
| ST25 *Tianshu* 天枢 | Yes | 5 | 14 | 0 | 1 | 4 |
| SP6 *Sanyinjiao* 三阴交 | Yes | 3 | 6 | 0 | 0 | 2 |
| BL20 *Pishu* 脾俞 | Yes | 3 | 2 | 0 | 0 | 2 |
| LR13 *Zhangmen* 章门 | Yes | 0 | 0 | 0 | 1 | 0 |
| GV4 *Mingmen* 命门 | Yes | 0 | 0 | 0 | 0 | 0 |
| CV4 *Guanyuan* 关元 | Yes | 2 | 1 | 0 | 1 | 0 |
| SP4 *Gongsun* 公孙 | Yes | 3 | 0 | 0 | 0 | 0 |
| BL23 *Shenshu* 肾俞 | Yes | 1 | 1 | 0 | 0 | 1 |
| BL18 *Ganshu* 肝俞 | Yes | 0 | 2 | 0 | 0 | 1 |

Table 9.5. (*Continued*)

| Intervention | Clinical Guidelines and Textbooks (Chap. 2) | Classical Literature (Chap. 3) (No. Citations) | Clinical Studies (Chap. 7) | | | Combination Therapies (Chap. 8) (No. Studies) |
|---|---|---|---|---|---|---|
| | | | RCTs (No. Studies) | CCTs (No. Studies) | NCSs* (No. Studies) | |
| LR2 *Xingjian* 行间 | Yes | 0 | 0 | 0 | 0 | 0 |
| GV20 *Baihui* 百汇 | Yes | 0 | 6 | 0 | 0 | 0 |
| LR3 *Taichong* 太冲 | Yes | 1 | 10 | 0 | 1 | 5 |
| ST37 *Shangjuxu* 上巨虚 | No | 10 | 6 | 0 | 0 | 2 |
| EX-HN3 *Yintang* 印堂 | No | 0 | 5 | 0 | 0 | 1 |
| BL25 *Dachangshu* 大肠俞 | No | 10 | 4 | 0 | 0 | 1 |
| SP14 *Fujie* 腹结 | No | 7 | 0 | 0 | 0 | 0 |
| **Moxibustion** | | | | | | |
| CV8 *Shenque* 神阙 | Yes | 11 | 1 | 0 | 0 | 0 |
| **Ear Acupuncture Point** | | | | | | |
| CO4 Stomach 胃 | Yes | 0 | 0 | 0 | 0 | 1 |
| CO7 Large intestine 大肠 | Yes | 0 | 0 | 0 | 0 | 1 |
| CO6 Small intestine 小肠 | Yes | 0 | 0 | 0 | 0 | 0 |
| HX2 Rectum直肠 | Yes | 0 | 0 | 0 | 0 | 0 |
| AH6 Sympathetic 交感 | Yes | 0 | 0 | 0 | 0 | 0 |
| AT4 Subcortex 皮质下 | Yes | 0 | 0 | 0 | 0 | 1 |
| CO17 Triple Energizer三焦 | Yes | 0 | 0 | 0 | 0 | 0 |

*Some studies used more than one intervention, e.g., acupuncture plus moxibustion. They are counted separately in this table.

Abbreviations: CCT, controlled clinical trial; NA, not applicable; NCS, non-controlled studies; RCT, randomised controlled trial.

**Table 9.6.** Summary of Acupuncture and Related Therapies for Irritable Bowel Syndrome with Predominant Constipation

| Intervention | Clinical Guidelines and Textbooks (Chap. 2) | Classical Literature (Chap. 3) (No. Citations) | Clinical Studies (Chap. 7) | | | Combination Therapies (Chap. 8) (No. Studies) |
|---|---|---|---|---|---|---|
| | | | RCTs (No. Studies) | CCTs (No. Studies) | NCSs* (No. Studies) | |
| Acupuncture | Yes | 45 | 5 | 0 | 0 | 0 |
| Massage | Yes | 0 | 0 | 0 | 0 | 0 |
| Electromagnetic heat treatment | Yes | NA | 0 | 0 | 0 | 0 |
| Transcutaneous electrical acupuncture stimulation | No | NA | 0 | 0 | 0 | 0 |
| Ear-acupuncture/ acupressure | Yes | 0 | 0 | 0 | 0 | 0 |
| Moxibustion | Yes | 29 | 0 | 0 | 0 | 0 |
| **Acupuncture Point** | | | | | | |
| ST36 *Zusanli* 足三里 | No | 5 | 4 | 0 | 0 | 0 |
| BL25 *Dachangshu* 大肠俞 | Yes | 0 | 0 | 0 | 0 | 0 |
| ST25 *Tianshu* 天枢 | Yes | 0 | 4 | 0 | 0 | 0 |
| TE6 *Zhigou* 支沟 | Yes | 0 | 0 | 0 | 0 | 0 |
| ST40 *Fenglong* 丰隆 | Yes | 0 | 0 | 0 | 0 | 0 |
| LI4 *Hegu* 合谷 | Yes | 0 | 0 | 0 | 0 | 0 |
| LI11 *Quchi* 曲池 | Yes | 0 | 0 | 0 | 0 | 0 |
| CV12 *Zhongwan* 中脘 | Yes | 0 | 0 | 0 | 0 | 0 |
| LR2 *Xingjian* 行间 | Yes | 0 | 0 | 0 | 0 | 0 |
| SP6 *Sanyinjiao* 三阴交 | No | 0 | 2 | 0 | 0 | 0 |

**Table 9.6.** (*Continued*)

| Intervention | Clinical Guidelines and Textbooks (Chap. 2) | Classical Literature (Chap. 3) (No. Citations) | Clinical Studies (Chap. 7) | | | Combination Therapies (Chap. 8) (No. Studies) |
|---|---|---|---|---|---|---|
| | | | RCTs (No. Studies) | CCTs (No. Studies) | NCSs* (No. Studies) | |
| BL20 *Pishu* 脾俞 | Yes | 0 | 0 | 0 | 0 | 0 |
| BL21 *Weishu* 胃俞 | Yes | 0 | 0 | 0 | 0 | 0 |
| CV6 *Qihai* 气海 | Yes | 0 | 0 | 0 | 0 | 0 |
| GV20 *Baihui* 百汇 | No | 0 | 2 | 0 | 0 | 0 |
| LR3 *Taichong* 太冲 | No | 0 | 2 | 0 | 0 | 0 |
| ST37 *Shangjuxu* 上巨虚 | No | 0 | 2 | 0 | 0 | 0 |
| EX-HN3 *Yintang* 印堂 | No | 0 | 2 | 0 | 0 | 0 |
| **Moxibustion** | | | | | | |
| ST36 *Zusanli* 足三里 | No | 5 | 0 | 0 | 0 | 0 |
| BL25 *Dachangshu* 大肠俞 | Yes | 8 | 0 | 0 | 0 | 0 |
| KI16 *Huangshu* 肓俞 | No | 4 | 0 | 0 | 0 | 0 |
| BL28 *Pangguangshu* 膀胱俞 | No | 4 | 0 | 0 | 0 | 0 |

*Some studies used more than one intervention, e.g., acupuncture plus moxibustion. They are counted separately in this table.

Abbreviations: CCT, controlled clinical trial; NA, not applicable; NCS, non-controlled studies; RCT, randomised controlled trial.

the use of ST36 *Zusanli* 足三里 for symptoms of abdominal pain, diarrhoea, bloating and borborygmus in the book *Zhen Jiu Jia Yi Jing* 针灸甲乙经 (c. 282, by Huang Pu Yi). ST36 *Zusanli* 足三里 harmonises the Stomach, tonifies the Spleen and *qi*, and relieves pain. LR3

*Taichong* 太冲 spreads the Liver *qi* and regulates the lower *jiao* 焦, addressing Liver *qi* stagnation.

In addition to ST25 *Tianshu* 天枢, ST36 *Zusanli* 足三里, and LR3 *Taichong* 太冲, other frequently used acupuncture points in clinical studies include ST37 *Shangjuxu* 上巨虚 (8 studies), which regulates the Spleen and Stomach, clears damp-heat and alleviates diarrhoea and dysenteric disorders.[12] ST37 *Shangjuxu* 上巨虚 was the most cited acupuncture point in classical texts identified to be related to IBS-D. This acupuncture point was not recommended in textbooks or guidelines.

GV20 *Baihui* 百会 (7 studies) and EX-HN3 *Yintang* 印堂 (5 studies) are also commonly used acupuncture points in clinical studies; they help calm the spirits. These acupuncture points are used in clinical studies that had favourable results in the SAS and SDS scores, suggesting that it is possible to support psychological states in people with IBS-D using acupuncture.

In classical texts, CV8 *Shenque* 神阙 is the most frequently cited acupuncture point for moxibustion. However, only one RCT was identified in this review.

The number of clinical studies for IBS-C identified for this review was small. The most frequently used acupuncture point in clinical studies for IBS-C were ST25 *Tianshu* 天枢 (4 studies) and ST36 *Zusanli* 足三里 (4 studies). These points are from the Stomach and the Spleen meridians. They regulate the Spleen and the Stomach and harmonise the Stomach. Interestingly, ST25 *Tianshu* 天枢 is recommended in textbooks and guidelines and cited in classical text, while ST36 *Zusanli* 足三里 is cited in classical texts but not recommended by textbooks or guidelines for IBS-C.

In classical texts, the most frequently cited IBS-C treatment acupoints are from the Bladder, Stomach and Kidney Channels, KI16 *Huangshu* 肓俞, and BL28 *Pangguangshu* 膀胱俞. In clinical guidelines, BL28 is also recommended for IBS-C.

For IBS-C, moxibustion is recommended in textbooks and guidelines where cold is present. However, no clinical studies assessed the effects of moxibustion for IBS-C. Acupuncture points used for moxibustion included BL25 *Dachangshu* 大肠俞, ST36 *Zusanli* 足三里, KI16 *Huangshu* 肓俞, and BL28 *Pangguangshu* 膀胱俞.

In clinical studies, no subtypes of IBS-mixed (IBS-M) or IBS-unclassified (IBS-U) were identified. In classical texts, acupuncture points could treat symptoms of both "possible" IBS-D and "possible" IBS-C. This suggests that classically, these acupuncture points were likely understood to be able to either stimulate or reduce intestinal peristalsis, and they may be a potential treatment option for people with IBS-M. One of the acupoints identified with this dual-action is BL25 *Dachangshu* 大肠俞, with a classical text stating that it can be used for the symptoms of "bloating, pain around umbilical, borborygmus, diarrhoea, dysentery and stool difficulty" (*Gu Jin Yi Tong Da Quan* 古今医统大全). BL25 *Dachangshu* 大肠俞 was also used in the clinical studies of IBS-D, but not in the included studies of IBS-C. In classical texts, two other acupoints that could treat both IBS-D-like and IBS-C-like conditions were BL28 *Pangguangshu* 膀胱俞 and BL60 *Kunlun* 昆仑.

## Other Chinese Medicine Therapies

This section summarises the evidence from Chaps. 2, 3 and 7. Guidelines recommend managing emotions and using diet therapy for the management of IBS.[10,11,13,14] In classical texts, diet therapy for IBS-D included eating wheat noodles and soup with ginger, black bean and pepper (Chap. 3). While diet therapy is mentioned by the guidelines as a preventive therapy for IBS, it is not described as a treatment therapy.[10] Diet therapy was not assessed in the clinical studies.

Modern guidelines did not mention *Qigong* 气功 as a treatment for IBS. In classical texts, *Qigong* 气功 was used for the relief of constipation and abdominal pain. One study using *Baduanjin* 八段锦 (a form of *Qigong* 气功) for IBS-C was identified; however, the study did not report on eligible outcomes, so the effect of *Baduanjin* for IBS-C could not be assessed.

**Table 9.7.** Summary of Other Chinese Medicine Therapies for Irritable Bowel Syndrome

| Intervention | Clinical Guidelines and Textbooks (Chap. 2) | Classical Literature (Chap. 3) (No. Citations) | Clinical Studies (Chap. 7) | | | Combination Therapies (Chap. 8) |
| --- | --- | --- | --- | --- | --- | --- |
| | | | RCTs (No. Studies) | CCTs (No. Studies) | NCSs (No. Studies) | |
| Diet therapy | Yes | 7 | 0 | 0 | 0 | 0 |
| *Qigong* 气功 (*Baduanjin* 八段锦) | No | 6 | 0 | 0 | 1 | 0 |

Abbreviations: CCT, controlled clinical trial; NCS, non-controlled studies; RCT, randomised controlled trial.

Little clinical trial evidence was found for IBS management using other CM therapies, and the information was presented in Chap. 7 (Table 9.7). No studies used other CM therapies for IBS-D.

Due to the small number of studies and the lack of eligible outcomes for assessment, it was not possible to draw a conclusion on the effectiveness or safety of these therapies for IBS.

# Limitations of Evidence

For this review, considerable effort was made to collect and analyse data from a variety of sources, including classical texts, modern textbooks and guidelines, clinical studies, and experimental studies. However, it is still possible to have omissions from the datasets. An overview of the current CM clinical practice for IBS, presented in Chap. 2, has been taken from authoritative clinical practice guidelines and CM textbooks. This is, however, not a comprehensive list, and some syndromes and treatments that are not widely used are not included in Chap. 2. Therefore, clinical practice recommendations could change in the future.

In Chap. 3, a comprehensive summary of the treatment for IBS in classical texts has been presented. We used the *Encyclopaedia of Chinese Medicine* (*Zhong Hua Yi Dian* (ZHYD)). It is the largest searchable resource, but it does not contain all the historical CM texts, and some books may not have been included. To identify IBS-related citations in classical texts, three groups of search terms representing the most prominent features of IBS were used: *fu tong* 腹痛, *xie xie* 泄泻, and *bian mi* 便秘. In total, 21 search terms were used to find IBS citations in classical texts, but more citations might be identified if more search terms were used. More citations describing IBS-D were identified compared to those describing IBS-C; it is unknown whether IBS-C citations were inadvertently omitted from the search.

In Chaps. 5, 7 and 8, clinical trial evidence from a comprehensive search of the Chinese and English scientific databases has been presented. However, errors or misclassifications may have occurred during the screening process. Where appropriate, meta-analysis was conducted to provide aggregate data from multiple studies. Of studies included in meta-analyses, demographic features, disease severity, diagnostic criteria, and outcome measurements varied. Further, meta-analysis largely focused on the overall effect of CHM or acupuncture on different outcomes. CHM treatment details, such as formula ingredients, herb dosage and treatment duration, varied from study to study; acupuncture treatment details including acupuncture point selection, needle retention time, and treatment frequency also varied from study to study. Therefore, substantial statistical heterogeneity was observed in pooled results; sometimes, this was reduced by subgroup analysis, but in some instances, the heterogeneity still could not be explained via a subgroup analysis. To account for the heterogeneity, a random effects model was used to provide conservative estimations of effect sizes.

Further, some methodological shortfalls of the included clinical studies were observed; these included a lack of information on random sequence allocation, a lack of blinding of participants and personnel, and small sample sizes. As a result, these methodological shortfalls led to the downgrading of the evidence quality for the included published clinical evidence.

For CHM clinical studies, different measurements of the Bristol Stool Form Scale score led to studies not being able to be grouped for meta-analysis, resulting in a small sample size and poor values for the measurement.

Moreover, AEs were insufficiently reported in the included studies.

The representativeness of the included studies also needs to be taken into consideration when interpreting the results, as over 98% of the clinical studies were conducted in China and hospitals.

Scarce clinical evidence was available for the synthesis of other CM therapies, such as CM diet therapy, *baduanjin* 八段锦, *taichi* 太极, and *tuina* 推拿.

No included clinical studies assessed the effects of CM therapies for IBS-M and IBS-U, so the clinical evidence on these subtypes of IBS is very limited.

The limitations discussed above should be taken into consideration when interpreting the results in this monograph.

## Implications for Practice

IBS is a disease with subtypes and presents with many CM syndromes. A summary of information from the clinical guidelines and CM textbooks (Chap. 2) provides important guidance for syndrome differentiation and the selection of appropriate CM treatments for people with IBS. The main organs involved are the Liver, Spleen, Stomach and Large Intestines.

To develop a treatment plan most beneficial and suitable for the individual and IBS subtype, clinicians need to take into consideration the presenting symptoms and signs of patients and treat the root cause of the disease. Diet plays a large part in the causes and triggers of IBS symptoms; to avoid intestinal dysfunction, people are advised to have meals at regular intervals, avoid overconsumption of fatty, cold and fried foods, and exclude foods from any diet that could be potentially irritating.

### Irritable Bowel Syndrome with Predominant Diarrhoea

For IBS-D, Liver *qi* stagnation and Spleen and Stomach deficiencies have been described across contemporary, classical and clinical trial evidence and should be considered the main syndrome.

The formula recommended by contemporary texts and guidelines for IBS-D, described in classical literature, and is the most studied in included clinical studies is *Tong xie yao fang* 痛泻要方. This formula removes Liver *qi* stagnation and strengthens the Spleen; experimental evidence also supports its use in IBS-D rats. Other formulae have also been evaluated by clinical studies and are recommended in textbooks, guidelines and classical texts. These include *Fu zi li zhong tang* 附子理中汤 and *Si shen wan* 四神丸; these formulae warm and tonify Spleen and Kidney.

Meta-analysis showed improvements in several IBS-D outcome categories with oral CHM. Where meta-analyses indicated a superior effect with CHM alone or as integrative medicine, analysis was undertaken to identify the herbs that may have contributed to the effect. Some of the most frequently used herbs used in studies included in meta-analysis favouring CHM were: *bai zhu* 白术, *bai shao* 白芍, *chen pi* 陈皮, *fu ling* 茯苓, *fang feng* 防风, and *gan cao* 甘草. Many of these herbs have demonstrated actions of anti-gastrointestinal inflammation, anti-gut hypersensitivity, and improvement in intestinal motility (see Chap. 6).

In meta-analyses showing benefits of acupuncture in the IBS-SSS, improvements in quality of life and improved SAS and SDS scores, some of the frequently used acupuncture points were: ST25 *Tianshu* 天枢, ST36 *Zusanli* 足三里, ST37 *Shangjuxu* 上巨虚, LR3 *Taichong* 太冲, and GV20 *Baihui* 百汇. Study numbers and study sample sizes were small, so this needs to be taken into consideration.

According to classical texts, irregular diet, emotional upsets, and deficiencies of the Spleen, Stomach and Kidneys can all lead to abdominal pain and diarrhoea. A diet recommendation for IBS-D details the use of foods that are warm in nature and support the Spleen and the Stomach, such as ginger, *sheng jiang* 生姜, black bean, *dou chi* 豆豉, and pepper, *hu jiao* 胡椒.

## Irritable Bowel Syndrome with Predominant Constipation

For IBS-C, *qi* stagnation is the main syndrome that is described across contemporary, classical and clinical trial evidence.

Formulae that were recommended by contemporary textbooks and guidelines for IBS-C included *Liu mo tang* 六磨汤, *Ma zi ren wan* 麻子仁丸, *Ji chuan jian* 济川煎, and *Huang qi tang* 黄芪汤. Their actions include regulating and moving *qi* to remove stagnation and relaxing the bowels.

In meta-analyses favouring CHM either alone or as integrative medicine for IBS-C that improved stool habit and quality of life, frequently used herbs were: *bin lang/da fu pi* 槟榔/大腹皮 and *zhi shi/zhi qiao* 枳实/枳壳. These herbs have demonstrated actions of improving gastrointestinal motility and anti-gut hyperalgesic effect (see Chap. 6).

The most commonly studied acupuncture points with a favourable effect for IBS-C were ST25 *Tianshu* 天枢 and ST36 *Zusanli* 足三里. Further, KI18 *Shiguan* 石关 and BL28 *Pangguangshu* 膀胱俞 were recorded for treating IBS-C in ancient texts.

*Qigong* therapy for symptom treatment of IBS-C was recorded in classical texts; however, there is no clinical evidence, and recommendations cannot be made.

## Implications for Research

Many clinical studies evaluated the effect and safety of CM therapies for IBS. Encouraging evidence is available for CHM and acupuncture therapies, but the evidence is lacking for other CM therapies. For other CM therapies such as CM diet therapy, *baduanjin* 八段锦, *taichi* 太极, and *tuina* 推拿, only one clinical study was identified in this review. Although CHM and acupuncture-related therapies are more used in the treatment of IBS, other CM therapies may be good supplementary therapy for the maintenance of treatment results and prevention of IBS. Thus, other CM therapies for IBS may be an area for exploration.

IBS-specific quality-of-life questionnaires such as the IBS-36 and Gastrointestinal Quality of Life Index, which is specific to people with gastrointestinal diseases, were not reported. Future trials could incorporate these outcome measures, as they are specifically designed for IBS and gastrointestinal diseases, with questions that are more specific and relatable to the condition, rather than general quality-of-life questionnaires.

Complete spontaneous bowel movement is an important outcome measure for IBS-C; however, this outcome was not reported in the included clinical studies. Future trials could consider including this outcome.

Using the correct tool and scoring method is essential in future clinical studies.

Rigorous methodology is needed when designing future clinical trials of CM therapies for IBS. Methods of sequence generation and allocation concealment should be clearly stated. Future RCTs should have their protocols published and be registered to minimise reporting bias and increase transparency in the reporting of the results.

Few studies included follow-up data, so the long-term effect of CHM on IBS-D and IBS-C is unknown. Future studies could consider investigating the long-term effects of CM therapies for IBS.

The use of CM syndromes for the selection of CHM or acupuncture interventions was not specified in most of the included clinical studies. CM therapies should be performed where possible based on the specific syndrome and specificity of the condition. This would validate the theory of CM and improve outcome translation into clinical practice.

In this monograph, the majority of the RCTs were assessed as "unclear" risk of bias for several domains due to the insufficiency of the information published. Future clinical studies should follow the items required by the Consolidated Standards of Reporting Trials (CONSORT)[15] and its extensions for herbal medicine, traditional CM and acupuncture.[16–19] Accurate and comprehensive reporting of trial protocols, reasons for intervention selection and comparators, and results of validated outcome measures would provide high-level clinical evidence that would be beneficial for patients, practitioners and researchers.

# References

1. Engsbro AL, Simren M, Bytzer P. (2012) Short-term stability of subtypes in the irritable bowel syndrome: Prospective evaluation using the Rome III classification. *Aliment Pharmacol Ther.* **35(3):** 350–359.

2. Quigley EM, Fried M, Gwee KA, *et al.* (2016) World Gastroenterology organisation global guidelines irritable bowel syndrome: A global perspective (update: September 2015). *J Clin Gastroenterol.* **50(9):** 704–713.

3. National Institute for Health and Care Excellence (NICE). (2017) Irritable bowel syndrome in adults: Diagnosis and management (CG61). In: *National Institute for Health and Care Excellence.* United Kingdom.

4. Bohn L, Storsrud S, Tornblom H, *et al.* (2013) Self-reported food-related gastrointestinal symptoms in IBS are common and associated with more severe symptoms and reduced quality of life. *Am J Gastroenterol.* **108(5):** 634–641.

5. Staudacher HM, Whelan K, Irving PM, Lomer MC. (2011) Comparison of symptom response following advice for a diet low in fermentable carbohydrates (FODMAPs) versus standard dietary advice in patients with irritable bowel syndrome. *J Hum Nutr Diet.* **24(5):** 487–495.

6. Whelan K, Martin LD, Staudacher HM, Lomer MCE. (2018) The low FODMAP diet in the management of irritable bowel syndrome: An evidence-based review of FODMAP restriction, reintroduction and personalisation in clinical practice. *J Hum Nutr Diet.* **31(2):** 23–55.

7. Johannesson E, Simren M, Strid H, *et al.* (2011) Physical activity improves symptoms in irritable bowel syndrome: A randomized controlled trial. *Am J Gastroenterol.* **106(5):** 915–922.

8. 中华中医药学会脾胃病分会. (2010) 肠易激综合征中医诊疗共识意见. *中华中医药杂志.* **25(7):** 1062–1065.

9. 中华中医药学会脾胃病分会. (2017) 肠易激综合征中医诊疗专家共识意见. **58**(18).

10. 中国中西医结合学会消化系统疾病专业委员会. (2011) 肠易激综合征中西医结合诊疗共识意见. *中国中西医结合杂志.* **31(5):** 587–590.

11. 中华中医药学会脾胃病分会. (2017) 肠易激综合征中医诊疗专家共识意见. **58(18):** 1615–1620

12. Deadman P, Al-Khafaji M, Baker K. (2000) A manual of acupuncture. *Journal of Chinese Medicine Publications.*

13. 张声生, 沈洪, 王垂杰, 唐旭东. (2016) *中华脾胃病学.* 人民卫生出版社, 中国北京.

14. 陈志强, 杨关林. (2016) *中西医结合内科学*. 中国中医药出版社, 中国北京.

15. Schulz KF, Altman DG, Moher D. (2010) CONSORT 2010 Statement: Updated guidelines for reporting parallel group randomised trials. *Trials*. **11:** 32.

16. Bian Z, Liu B, Moher D, *et al*. (2011) Consolidated standards of reporting trials (CONSORT) for traditional Chinese medicine: Current situation and future development. *Front Med*. **5(2):** 171–177.

17. Gagnier JJ, Boon H, Rochon P, *et al*. (2006) Reporting randomized, controlled trials of herbal interventions: An elaborated CONSORT statement. *Ann Intern Med*. **144(5):** 364–367.

18. 18. MacPherson H, Altman DG, Hammerschlag R, *et al*. (2010) Revised STandards for Reporting Interventions in Clinical Trials of Acupuncture (STRICTA): Extending the CONSORT statement. *J Evid Based Med* **3(3):** 140–155.

19. MacPherson H, White A, Cummings M, Jobst K, Rose K, Niemtzow R. (2002) Standards for reporting interventions in controlled trials of acupuncture: The STRICTA recommendations. STandards for Reporting Interventions in Controlled Trails of Acupuncture. *Acupunct Med* **20(1):** 22–25.

# Glossary

| Terms | Acronym | Definition | Reference |
|---|---|---|---|
| 95% confidence interval | 95% CI | A measure of the uncertainty around the main finding of a statistical analysis. Estimates of unknown quantities, such as the odds ratio comparing an experimental intervention with a control, are usually presented as a point estimate and a 95% confidence interval. This means that if someone were to keep repeating a study in other samples from the same population, 95% of the confidence intervals from those studies would contain the true value of the unknown quantity. Alternatives to 95%, such as 90% and 99% confidence intervals, are sometimes used. Wider intervals indicate lower precision; narrow intervals, greater precision. | http://handbook.cochrane.org/ |
| Acupuncture | — | The insertion of needles into humans or animals for remedial purposes or its methods. | WHO international standard terminologies of traditional medicine in the Western Pacific Region. World Health Organization. (2007) |
| Allied and Complementary Medicine Database | AMED | Alternative medicine bibliographic database. | http://www.ovid.com/site/catalog/databases/12.jsp |
| Antihyperglycaemic agents | — | Drugs that can reduce the blood glucose level to reach a target glucose level. | — |
| Australian New Zealand Clinical Trial Registry | ANZCTR | Australian clinical trial registry. | http://www.anzctr.org.au/ |

*(Continued)*

277

**(Continued)**

| Terms | Acronym | Definition | Reference |
|---|---|---|---|
| Birmingham IBS symptom questionnaire | — | A self-administered 11-item symptom scale based on the Rome II criteria scored on a 6-point Likert scale and responses relevant for the previous four weeks. | Roalfe AK, Roberts LM, Wilson S. (2008) Evaluation of the Birmingham IBS symptom questionnaire. *BMC Gastroenterol.* **8:** 30. |
| Bristol Stool Form Scale | — | A scale that provides visual images and written descriptions for the classification of the form of stools. Stools can be classified into one of seven types, with types 3 and 4 recognised to be normal stools. Types 1 and 2 indicate constipation, with type 1 indicating greater severity. Types 5–7 indicate diarrhoea; the higher the number type, the greater the severity. | Lewis SJ, Heaton KW. (1997) Stool form scale as a useful guide to intestinal transit time. *Scand J Gastroenterol.* **32(9):** 920–924. |
| China National Knowledge Infrastructure | CNKI | Chinese language bibliographic database. | http://www.cnki.net |
| Chinese Biomedical Literature Database | CBM | Chinese language bibliographic database. | http://www.imicams.ac.cn/ |
| Chinese Clinical Trial Registry | ChiCTR | Chinese clinical trial registry. | http://www.chictr.org/ |
| Chinese herbal medicine | CHM | Chinese herbal medicine. | — |
| Chinese medicine | CM | — | — |
| Chongqing VIP Information Company | CQVIP | Chinese language bibliographic database. | http://www.cqvip.com |
| ClinicalTrials.gov | — | Clinical trial registry. | https://clinicaltrials.gov/ |
| Cochrane Central Register of Controlled Trials | CENTRAL | Bibliographic database that provides a highly concentrated source of reports of controlled trials. | http://community.cochrane.org/editorial-and-publishing-policy-resource/cochrane-central-register-controlled-trials-central |
| Combination therapies | — | Two or more Chinese medicines from different therapy groups (e.g., Chinese herbal medicine, acupuncture therapies or other Chinese medicine therapies) administered together. | — |
| Controlled clinical trials | CCT | An experimental study in which people are allocated to different interventions using methods that are not random. | http://handbook.cochrane.org/ |

# Glossary

| Terms | Acronym | Definition | Reference |
|---|---|---|---|
| Convention on International Trade in Endangered Species of Wild Fauna and Flora | CITES | — | https://www.cites.org/eng/disc/text.php |
| Cumulative Index of Nursing and Allied Health Literature | CINAHL | Bibliographic database. | https://www.ebscohost.com/nursing/about |
| Cupping therapy | — | Suction by using a vaccumised cup or jar. | World Health Organization. (2007) WHO international standard terminologies of traditional medicine in the Western Pacific Region. |
| Effect size | — | A generic term for the estimate of effect of treatment for a study. | http://handbook.cochrane.org/ |
| Electroacupuncture | — | Electric stimulation of the needle following insertion. | World Health Organization. (2007) WHO international standard terminologies of traditional medicine in the Western Pacific Region. |
| EU Clinical Trials Register | EU-CTR | European clinical trial registry. | https://www.clinicaltrialsregister.eu |
| Excerpta Medica database | Embase | Bibliographic database. | http://www.elsevier.com/solutions/embase |
| Gastrointestinal Symptom Rating Scale | GSRS | A self-administered rating scale for people with IBS or peptic ulcer disease, it consists of 15 items related to clinical symptoms that are graded on a 4-point Likert verbal scale. | Svedlund J, Sjodin I, Dotevall G. (1988) GSRS — A clinical rating scale for gastrointestinal symptoms in patients with irritable bowel syndrome and peptic ulcer disease. *Dig Dis Sci.* **33(2):** 129–134. |
| Grading of Recommendations, Assessment, Development and Evaluation | GRADE | Approach used to grade quality of evidence and strength of recommendations. | http://www.gradeworkinggroup.org/ |
| Hamilton Anxiety Rating Scale | HAMA | A 14-item instrument describing the symptoms and measures for anxiety. | |
| Hamilton Rating Scale of Depression | HRSD | Questionnaire that rates the severity of depression. | Hamilton M. (1960) A rating scale for depression. *J Neurol Neuosurg Psychiatry.* **23(1):** 56–62. |

*(Continued)*

(Continued)

| Terms | Acronym | Definition | Reference |
|---|---|---|---|
| Heterogeneity | — | Used in a general sense to describe the variation in, or diversity of, participants, interventions, and measurement of outcomes across a set of studies, or the variation in internal validity of those studies. Used specifically as statistical heterogeneity to describe the degree of variation in the effect estimates from a set of studies. Also used to indicate the presence of variability among studies beyond the amount expected due solely to the play of chance. | http://handbook.cochrane.org/ |
| Homogeneity | — | Used in a general sense to mean that the participants, interventions, and measurement of outcomes are similar across a set of studies. Used specifically to describe the effect estimates from a set of studies where they do not vary more than would be expected by chance. | http://handbook.cochrane.org/ |
| Hospital Anxiety and Depression Scale | HADS | A 14-item instrument consisting of two sections. The first section contains seven items related to anxiety and the second section contains seven items related to depression. | Snaith RP. (2003) The Hospital Anxiety and Depression Scale. *Health Qual Life Outcomes.* **1(1):** 29. |
| Irritable Bowel Syndrome | IBS | A type of functional bowel disorder causing symptoms of abdominal pain and altered bowel habits such as diarrhoea or constipation. | National Institute for Health and Care Excellence (NICE). (2017) Irritable bowel syndrome in adults: Diagnosis and management (CG61). In: *National Institute for Health and Care Excellence.* United Kingdom. |
| Irritable Bowel Syndrome with Predominant Constipation | IBS-C | A type of functional bowel disorder causing symptoms of abdominal pain and altered bowel habits with predominant constipation. | National Institute for Health and Care Excellence (NICE). (2017) Irritable bowel syndrome in adults: Diagnosis and management (CG61). In: *National Institute for Health and Care Excellence.* United Kingdom. |

**(*Continued*)**

| Terms | Acronym | Definition | Reference |
|---|---|---|---|
| Irritable Bowel Syndrome with Predominant Diarrhoea | IBS-D | A type of functional bowel disorder causing symptoms of abdominal pain and altered bowel habits with predominant diarrhoea. | National Institute for Health and Care Excellence (NICE). (2017) Irritable bowel syndrome in adults: Diagnosis and management (CG61). In: *National Institute for Health and Care Excellence.* United Kingdom. |
| Irritable Bowel Syndrome with Mixed Bowel Habits | IBS-M | IBS with mixed bowel habits consisting of both constipation and diarrhoea. | National Institute for Health and Care Excellence (NICE). (2017) Irritable bowel syndrome in adults: Diagnosis and management (CG61). In: *National Institute for Health and Care Excellence.* United Kingdom. |
| Irritable Bowel Syndrome-Quality of Life | IBS-QOL | A 34-item self-reported instrument that measures quality of life specifically related to IBS. | Patrick DL, Drossman DA, Frederick IO, *et al.* (1998) Quality of life in persons with irritable bowel syndrome: Development and validation of a new measure. *Dig Dis Sci.* **43(2):** 400–411. |
| Irritable Bowel Syndrome Severity Scoring System | IBS-SSS | A scoring system that consists of the severity of abdominal pain, frequency of abdominal pain, distension, satisfaction of stool frequency and consistency, and interference with life in general. | Francis CY, Morris J, Whorwell PJ. (1997) The irritable bowel severity scoring system: A simple method of monitoring irritable bowel syndrome and its progress. *Aliment Pharmacol Ther.* **11(2):** 395–402. |
| Irritable Bowel Syndrome Unclassified | IBS-U | IBS where the condition does not meet IBS-C, IBS-D or IBS-M. | — |
| $I^2$ | — | A measure of study heterogeneity that indicates the percentage of variance in a meta-analysis. | http://handbook.cochrane.org/ |
| Integrative medicine | — | Chinese herbal medicine combined with pharmacotherapy or other conventional therapy. | — |

(*Continued*)

**(Continued)**

| Terms | Acronym | Definition | Reference |
|---|---|---|---|
| Low-density lipoprotein | LDL | Transports cholesterol from the liver to the tissues and cells of the body. | — |
| Mean difference | MD | In meta-analysis: A method used to combine measures on continuous scales, where the mean, standard deviation and sample size in each group are known. The weight given to the difference in means from each study (e.g., how much influence each study has on the overall results of the meta-analysis) is determined by the precision of its estimate of effect; mathematically, this is equal to the inverse of the variance. This method assumes that all of the trials have measured the outcome on the same scale. | http://handbook.cochrane. org/ |
| Meta-analysis | — | The use of statistical techniques in a systematic review to integrate the results of included studies. Sometimes misused as a synonym for systematic reviews, where the review includes a meta-analysis. | — |
| Non-controlled studies | — | Observations made on individuals, usually receiving the same intervention, before and after an intervention but with no control group. | http://handbook.cochrane. org/ |
| Numerical rating scale | NRS | An 11-point scale (0–10) is the most common; however, other number scales are possible. For pain, an increasing score on the scale is indicative of increasing severity, and a score of zero would indicate that there is no pain. | — |
| Other Chinese medicine therapies | — | Other Chinese medicine therapies include all traditional therapies except Chinese herbal medicine and acupuncture, such as, *tai chi* 太极 *qigong* 气功, *tuina* 推拿,and cupping. | — |
| PubMed | PubMed | Bibliographic database. | http://www.ncbi.nlm.nih. gov/pubmed |
| Randomised controlled trial | RCT | Clinical trial that uses a random method to allocate participants to treatment and control groups. | — |

(*Continued*)

| Terms | Acronym | Definition | Reference |
|---|---|---|---|
| Risk of bias | — | Assessment of clinical trials to indicate if the results may overestimate or underestimate the true effect because of bias in study design or reporting. | http://handbook.cochrane.org/ |
| Risk ratio (relative risk) | RR | The ratio of risks in two groups. In intervention studies, it is the ratio of the risk in the intervention group to the risk in the control group. A risk ratio of one indicates no difference between comparison groups. For undesirable outcomes, a risk ratio that is less than one indicates that the intervention was effective in reducing the risk of that outcome. | http://handbook.cochrane.org/ |
| Short-Form 36 | SF36 | A 36-item instrument that surveys the quality of life generically based on self-reported health status. | RAND Health. (nd) 36-Item Short Form Survey (SF-36) scoring instructions. The RAND Corporation. https://www.rand.org/health/surveys_tools/mos/36-item-short-form/scoring.html. (Cited: 2018) |
| Standardised mean difference | SMD | In meta-analysis: A method used to combine results for continuous scales that measure the same outcome but in different ways (e.g., with different scales). The results of studies are standardised to a uniform scale to allow data to be combined. | http://handbook.cochrane.org/ |
| Summary of findings | — | Presentation of results and rating the quality of evidence based on the GRADE approach. | http://www.gradeworkinggroup.org/ |
| *Tuina* 推拿 | — | Chinese massage: Rubbing, kneading, or percussion of the soft tissues and joints of the body with the hands, usually performed by one person on another, especially to relieve tension or pain. | World Health Organization. (2007) WHO international standard terminologies of traditional medicine in the Western Pacific Region. |
| Visual analogue scale | VAS | A measure that uses a 100 mm horizontal line. For the measure of pain, the higher end of this scale is associated with increasing severity of pain and the lower end is a decrease in reported pain severity. | — |

(*Continued*)

(Continued)

| Terms | Acronym | Definition | Reference |
|---|---|---|---|
| Wangfang database | Wanfang | Chinese language bibliographic database. | www.wanfangdata.com |
| World Health Organization | WHO | WHO is the directing and coordinating authority for health within the United Nations system. It is responsible for providing leadership on global health matters, shaping the health research agenda, setting norms and standards, articulating evidence-based policy options, providing technical support to countries, and monitoring and assessing health trends. | http://www.who.int/about/en/ |
| *Zhong Hua Yi Dian* 中华医典 | ZHYD | The Zhong Hua Yi Dian (ZHYD) "Encyclopaedia of Traditional Chinese Medicine" is a comprehensive series of electronic books on compact disk. The collection was put together by the Hunan electronic and audio-visual publishing house. It is the largest collection of Chinese electronic books and includes the major Chinese ancient works, many of which are from rare manuscripts and are the only existing copies. These books cover the period from ancient times up to the period of the Republic of China (1911–1948). | Hu R, ed. (2000) *Zhong Hua Yi Dian [Encyclopaedia of Traditional Chinese Medicine]*. 4th ed. Hunan Electronic and Audio-Visual Publishing House, Chengsha. |
| Zung Self-rating Anxiety Scale | SAS | A 20- item self-administered instrument measuring anxiety levels. | Zung WW. (1971) A rating instrument for anxiety disorders. *Psychosomatics.* **12(6):** 371–379. |
| Zung Self-rating Depression Scale | SDS | A 20-item, self-administered instrument measuring depression status. | Zung WW, Richards CB, Short MJ. (1965) Self-rating depression scale in an outpatient clinic. Further validation of the SDS. *Arch Gen Psychiatry.* **13(6):** 508–515. |

# Index

# Evidence-based Clinical Chinese Medicine

*(Continued from page ii)*